DRUGS AND SENSORY FUNCTIONS

BIOLOGICAL COUNCIL

THE CO-ORDINATING COMMITTEE FOR SYMPOSIA ON DRUG ACTION

A Symposium on

DRUGS AND SENSORY FUNCTIONS

Editor

ANDREW HERXHEIMER
M.B., B.S.

with 85 Illustrations

LITTLE, BROWN AND COMPANY
BOSTON
1968

Standard Book Number
7000 1321 0

Library of Congress
Catalog Card Number
68-20972

Printed in Great Britain

PREFACE

Scientists concerned with various aspects of the 'special' senses work in many different disciplines and tend to be isolated from one another. Physiologists, experimental psychologists, pharmacologists and toxicologists seemingly inhabit different worlds; even physiologists concerned with vision, hearing, taste and smell rarely meet. Such a traditional division of interests may be convenient because we have got used to it, but it obscures much that could be valuable. For example the physiology of the chemical senses, taste and smell, could be regarded as a part of pharmacology, since it deals with the action of foreign substances on receptors. Perfume chemists have long been studying structure-activity relationships, but pharmacologists have taken little interest in their work. In this Symposium scientists with widely differing interests in drugs and sensory functions were brought together for mutual enlightenment and provocation. The book includes all but three of the papers given at the symposium; those by A. Summerfield, W. K. Noell and R. Fatehchand have had to be omitted.

The Symposium was organized by a Committee consisting of G. B. Arden, F. Bergel, P. B. Bradley, J. Diamond, A. Herxheimer (Secretary), R. Hinchcliffe, G. E. Paget and Hannah Steinberg (Chairman). The following societies participated in the Symposium: The Biochemical Society, The British Association of Otolaryngologists, The British Pharmacological Society, The British Psychological Society, The European Society for the Study of Drug Toxicity, The International Society for Clinical Electroretinography, The Physiological Society, and the Royal Society of Medicine.

The Symposium was held at the Royal College of Physicians in London, and was attended by more than 250 members of the participating societies. The Organizing Committee is grateful to the officers and staff of the Royal College of Physicians for their help. The Wellcome Trust generously gave a grant which made it possible to invite participants from Europe and the United States, and the Ciba Foundation helped greatly by providing hospitality for overseas visitors.

I am very grateful to Miss G. Blunt, Miss Jill Bacon and Mrs. Diana Lawson for their excellent organizational and secretarial help. Dr. G. B. Arden gave valuable help with the editing. It has been a pleasure to work with Mr. J. A. Rivers and J. & A. Churchill Ltd.

A. Herxheimer.

CONTENTS

Session IV: Vision

Chairmen: Sir Stewart Duke-Elder and E. S. Perkins

Session V: Central Effects

Chairman: J. A. B. Gray

AUTHOR INDEX, *List of chairmen (C), speakers and their co-authors, and participants in the discussions.*

The affiliations and addresses are those current at the time of the Symposium.

		Pages
J. A. B. Gray (C)	University College, Gower Street, London W.C.1.	
S. P. Grossman	Department of Psychology, University of Chicago, Illinois 60637, U.S.A.	18, *101*, 137–139, 165, 284
R. Harper	A.R.C. Food Research Institute, Earlham Laboratory, Recreation Road, Norwich NOR 26G.	*39*, 89, 98, 100, 127, 254
J. E. Hazelton	114 Herbert Gardens, London N.W.10.	36
A. Herxheimer	Department of Pharmacology, London Hospital Medical College, London E.1.	38, 89, 98/9, *131*, 255, 269
R. Hinchcliffe (C)	Institute of Laryngology and Otology, Grays Inn Road, London W.C.1.	139, 150
W. M. Hollyhock	Committee on Safety of Drugs, Queen Anne's Mansions, Queen Anne's Gate, London S.W.1.	12, 18
L. Hösli	Physiological Institute, University of Basel, Switzerland.	196
Hisako Ikeda	Department of Neurophysiology, Institute of Ophthalmology, Judd Street, London W.C.1.	*229*
B. J. Key	Department of Experimental Neuropharmacology, Medical School, University of Birmingham, Birmingham 15.	*153*
A. R. King	Neuropharmacology Research Unit, Medical School, University of Birmingham, Birmingham 15.	36, 166
H. W. Kosterlitz	Physiology Department, Marischal College, University of Aberdeen.	90
M. Kramer	Department of Psychiatry, University of Cincinnati, c/o VA Hospital, 3200 Vine Street, Cincinnati, Ohio 45220, U.S.A.	299
D. G. Land	A.R.C. Food Research Institute, Earlham Laboratory, Recreation Road, Norwich NOR 26G.	98, 130
D. Legge	Department of Psychology, University College, Gower Street, London W.C.1.	*245*
Phyllis C. Lemon	Smith, Kline and French Research Institute, Welwyn Garden City, Herts.	*5*

		Pages
S. A. Lewis	University Department of Psychiatry, Royal Edinburgh Hospital, Morningside Park, Edinburgh 10.	*287*
P. G. Lundquist	Department of Otolaryngology, Karolinska Hospital, Stockholm 60.	*142*
J. L. Malcolm	Physiology Department, Marischal College, University of Aberdeen.	255, 260, 270/1
H. McIlwain	Biochemistry Department, Institute of Psychiatry, Denmark Hill, London S.E.5.	12, 97
R. W. Moncrieff	The Gables, Hambrook, Chichester, Sussex.	11, *22* 98
R. A. Nicoll	Laboratory of Neuropharmacology, Division of Special Mental Health Research Programs, National Institute of Mental Health, at St. Elizabeth's Hospital, Washington, D.C. 20032, U.S.A.	*73*
W. K. Noell	Department of Physiology, University of New York, Buffalo, N.Y., U.S.A.	
Hugh Norris	Department of Pharmacology, University College, Gower Street, London W.C.1.	196
P. H. Ornstein	Department of Psychiatry, University of Cincinnati, Ohio 45220, U.S.A.	*299*
G. E. Paget	Smith, Kline and French Research Institute, Welwyn Garden City, Herts.	*5*
M. W Parkes	Pharmacological Laboratory, Roche Products Ltd., Welwyn Garden City, Herts.	37
E. S. Perkins (C)	Institute of Ophthalmology, Judd Street, London W.C.1.	
A. J. Philipszoon	Louis Davidsstraat 5, The Hague, Holland.	150, *175*
J. P. Quilliam	Department of Pharmacology, St. Bartholomew's Hospital Medical College, London E.C.1.	12, 254
A. D. J. Robertson	National Physical Laboratory, Teddington, Middlesex.	326, 328
G. C. Salmoiraghi	Laboratory of Neuropharmacology, Division of Special Mental Health Research Programs, National Institute of Mental Health at St. Elizabeth's Hospital, Washington D.C. 20032, U.S.A.	*73*, 270/1, 283

		Pages
G. Salomon	E.N.T. Department, Copenhagen Country Hospital in Gentofte, Hellerup, Denmark.	164
I. Siegel	Institute of Ophthalmology, Judd Street, London W.C.1.	*210*
J. T. Silverstone	Department of Psychological Medicine, St. Bartholomew's Hospital, London E.C.1.	139
Phyllis J. Spear	Physiology Department, Marischal College, University of Aberdeen.	*260*
Hannah Steinberg	Department of Pharmacology, University College, Gower Street, London W.C.1.	207
A. Summerfield	Department of Psychology, Birkbeck College, Malet Street, London W.C.1.	283
P. Turner	St. Bartholomew's Hospital, London E.C.1.	*91*, 97/8, 254
V. Udall	Wellcome Research Laboratories, Langley Court, Beckenham, Kent.	
O. L. Wade (C)	Department of Therapeutics, Queen's University, Grosvenor Road, Belfast 12.	*3*, 89, 126
R. H. J. Watson	Department of Nutrition, Queen Elizabeth College, Campden Hill Road, London W.8.	138
J. Wersäll	Department of Otolaryngology, Karolinska Hospital, Stockholm 60.	12, *142*
I. C. Whitfield	Neurocommunications Research Unit, Medical School, University of Birmingham, Birmingham 15.	*167*, 206, 271
R. M. Whitman	Department of Psychiatry, University of Cincinnati, Ohio 45220, U.S.A.	*299*
C. W. M. Wilson	Department of Pharmacology, Trinity College, Dublin.	137
J. H. Wolstencroft	Department of Neuropharmacology, Medical School, University of Birmingham, Birmingham 15.	

Session I

Introductory Session

Chairman: O. L. Wade

THE CLINICAL PROBLEM

O. L. WADE

Department of Therapeutics, Queen's University, Belfast

THE physiological basis of sensation lies in the proper functioning of the central nervous system and the organs of special sense. Any drugs which affect the nervous system directly by stimulating or depressing neuronal function, or indirectly by affecting its blood supply or its metabolism, or any drugs which affect the organs of special sense are the concern of this Symposium. We are particularly concerned with psychotropic drugs and drugs which affect the special senses: vision, hearing, smell and taste. Anaesthetics, hypnotics and analgesics have been purposely omitted. Physicians do not use the sensory effects of drugs for therapeutic ends but they are familiar with some of the toxic effects on the sensory system of drugs at present in use. The peripheral neuritis which can occur after continued use of thalidomide is now notorious. Antibiotics can alter taste. Streptomycin and kanamycin damage the vestibular nerve, dihydrostreptomycin the auditory nerve. That atropine can precipitate glaucoma has long been known; it is perhaps surprising that anaesthetists so seldom run into this trouble. Scotomata can be caused by the anti-malarial drug chloroquine, used in rheumatoid arthritis. Triparanol ('MER 29'), a drug used evanescently to lower the blood cholesterol level, can cause cataracts.

Drugs which produce mood changes, cerebral excitation or hallucinations as adverse reactions are of particular interest, and some of them are of course used in therapy. Isoniazid was noted quite unexpectedly to modify mood in patients receiving it as part of their antituberculous therapy: this led to the use of iproniazid, the first of the monoamine oxidase inhibitors. In Belfast we now screen the urine of young adolescents diagnosed as suffering from schizophrenia, because the mental excitement and occasionally the paranoia or hallucinations produced by chronic amphetamine intoxication may be clinically indistinguishable from schizophrenia.

The field of adverse reactions is a rich source of pharmacological knowledge which is only now beginning to be tapped. Study of the ways in which drugs can affect sensory functions is likely to help us understand not only the actions of drugs but also sensory mechanisms. Careful observation and recording of adverse reactions involving sensation is a valuable starting point for investigation; particularly since only human subjects can report and describe sensory effects.

TOXICOLOGICAL ASPECTS

G. E. PAGET and PHYLLIS LEMON

Smith, Kline & French Research Institute, Welwyn Garden City, Herts.

TOXICOLOGICAL evaluation of drugs involves two separate processes. First, the possible adverse effects of the drug on laboratory animals must be detected and their nature must be understood. Only then is it possible to evaluate the significance of these effects for the proposed use of the drug in human beings. The effects of drugs on sensory functions present difficulties in both these phases of the investigation, and they will be discussed separately.

The common method used for the detection of effects on laboratory animals is simple. The drug under examination is administered in the largest possible doses to large groups of animals of at least two, and preferably more species, for long periods. During the period of dosing the animals are observed and clinical, biochemical and other tests are carried out on them. At the end of the period of dosing the animals are killed and their tissues examined histologically. A serious interference with the functioning of a major organ system that is concerned with the day-to-day well-being of the animals can hardly be overlooked. The animals will appear physically unwell, and some may die, often in a characteristic manner. Abnormalities in the tests carried out on the live animals may suggest the site of the damage and the eventual histological preparations will reveal unmistakable damage of the affected tissues, or at least such abnormality of the tissue as will provoke further and more detailed investigation.

The situation is very different with the major sense organs. Clinical observation of laboratory animals may fail completely to provide any evidence of the integrity of these. Small laboratory rodents probably rely little or not at all upon vision for the conduct of their lives. Many investigators believe that the Wistar rat at least is virtually blind, and guinea-pigs are either blind or so stupid that they ignore the messages from their eyes almost completely. While working with guinea-pigs some years ago and trying to decide whether minimal impairment of vision had occurred, our efforts were frustrated by the fact that even healthy and apparently normal guinea-pigs would walk into objects or off the edges of tables and showed no apparent reaction to visual stimuli. Dogs are well known to rely less upon vision than on smell and anyone who has observed a household with a blind dog in it will be aware of how little disability the animal displays in its familiar environment. Hearing is perhaps more easily tested, but the simple tests that are carried out will probably detect only the grossest defects. The other senses are virtually inaccessible to examination. How can one imagine seeking defects in the sense of smell of a rat or in the sense of fine touch in a dog? Despite this, we must assume that these senses are at equal risk with the major senses of sight and hearing.

Sophisticated methods of investigation, particularly of the structure of the eye during life, do exist and are routinely used in man. Perhaps the most powerful tool in the investigation of the transparent media of the eye is the slit lamp. This instrument, however, requires some training in its use and also requires a co-operative subject and a certain minimum size of eye. It is nevertheless becoming increasingly used in toxicological studies and in our laboratories in Philadelphia all the dogs on chronic toxicity tests are examined repeatedly with this instrument by a skilled ophthalmologist. This technique is however available in very few toxicological laboratories.

In principle it is possible to test hearing by establishing conditioned reflexes to an auditory stimulus. Again the elaborate technique and the apparatus required make it unsuitable for routine investigation during chronic toxicity tests. Indeed, one can envisage snags that might vitiate the results even if the technique were regularly and conscientiously used.

The most powerful method at the disposal of the toxicologist for evaluating tissue damage is that of histopathology. Here again the special sense organs present peculiar difficulties. The preparation of sections of the whole eye is perhaps the most difficult job that the histological technician has to perform routinely. Much can be done using appropriate methods and by technical skill, but even so failures will occur quite unpredictably and cause artefacts that may be interpreted as lesions or obscure the existence of actual lesions. In addition the present extensive routine examination of animal eyes makes it clear that spontaneous disease of the eye is as frequent in laboratory animals as spontaneous diseases of other organs.

To our knowledge, no toxicology laboratory would willingly undertake the routine histological examination of the organs of hearing, but there may be exceptions. Here again preparative difficulties and unfamiliar histology present major problems. The same is true of the olfactory mucosa and other sensory organs. The detection of even major changes in the sensorium of experimental animals may therefore be extremely difficult. Minor changes would probably be missed unless attention were drawn to them by major changes or by some other unusual circumstances.

Thus far the difficulty of detecting changes in the major sense organs has been considered. Other difficulties may confound the toxicologist. It is well known that streptomycin severely damages the human auditory mechanism. This effect can be produced in animals, but is only detected easily in cats. For various reasons that are not relevant here cats are not generally used in chronic toxicity tests. Undoubtedly people dealing with streptomycin-like agents will examine their effects in this species, but with chemically and biologically unrelated substances a similar action would probably even now be undetected in animal experiments. A further difficulty has been brought to light by Baker and Alcock (1965). They were working with a substance careful toxicity tests on which had failed to disclose an ocular effect. Such toxicity tests had been carried out on the basis of dosing only 5 days a week. When the substance was re-examined using 7-days-a-week dosing, cataracts appeared in the experimental rats and were detected easily. This substance had had fairly wide usage in man by this time, but no visual ill effects had been noted.

Before passing to the evaluation of effects that are discovered in animals, one can summarize to what extent it is reasonable to expect a competent and conscientious toxicological laboratory to study the special senses. It is, of course, presumed that such studies will be carried out as a part of toxicity tests that are fundamentally sound, since study of any organ system in a poorly designed experiment will have no validity at all. In small animals the only practicable instrumental examination of the special senses is simple ophthalmoscopic examination of the eye. Clinical observation should, therefore, be confined to looking carefully at the eye when the animal is surveyed by the attendant and by the toxicologist carrying out the test. Such examination will certainly disclose advanced changes in the transparent media of the eye. Any attempt to estimate auditory acuity or the activity of any other sense in small animals is not worth the effort, since so many imponderables enter into any possible response to a test situation.

In larger animals more detailed examination of the eye is possible, and instrumental examination is certainly desirable for animals receiving large amounts of drug for long periods. Direct ophthalmoscopy is within the reach of anyone sufficiently qualified to conduct toxicity tests, and recourse to a slit lamp and an attendant expert is probably desirable in cases of doubt. In large animals simple tests of hearing are possible and advisable. However, careful observation by an experienced animal attendant will detect auditory defects as reliably as more formal tests.

When the animals are killed, histological preparations of the eye are essential. The pathological laboratory concerned with the evaluation of the results of toxicity tests must face the difficulty of such preparations and produce a technique that can cope with eyes of rats, dogs, and other species. Many techniques have been recommended for this. In our experience, a technique which works well is hard to transplant, and in laboratories staffed by competent technicians it is probably best to allow the technician to develop his own modification of some published procedure. In our laboratories some promising results have been achieved by embedding whole eyes in 'Araldite' (an epoxy resin, used in the preparation of electron microscopy blocks). Surprisingly large sections can be cut of this material and its hardness and rigidity offer advantages in an organ of such varying consistency as the eye.

The histologist must also become familiar with the appearance of the eye as sectioned in his own laboratory, and with the changes produced by agents known to damage the eye, although some of these changes may be elusive in ordinary sections stained with haematoxylin and eosin. It is not reasonable to recommend routine histological examination of any other special sense organ; the technical difficulties are enormous and the probability of return on the technical outlay is vanishingly small.

Thus, the detection of changes in special sense organs in experimental animals is singularly difficult. These difficulties are however technical and are, in theory at least, surmountable. Fundamental difficulties arise in the evaluation of changes that are successfully detected, but these difficulties beset the evaluation of all toxicity tests in animals before a substance is used in man. This difficulty is illustrated by an astonishing toxic effect on the eye investigated some years ago (Paget, 1962).

The substances in question were thought to be promising antibacterial agents. The colleague who was investigating their anti-bacterial properties, and who was a particularly careful observer, noticed that the guinea-pigs that he was using as 'bacteriological' rather than 'toxicological' animals, showed curious opacities in their eyes shortly after he had administered doses of the compounds. More detailed examination showed that one or two oral doses of the most active of these compounds produced an easily observed opacity of the guinea-pig eye. Histologically this early change within a few hours of the dose of the compound was accompanied by vacuolation and then necrosis of the cells of the lens epithelium. At the same time cellular infiltration of the cornea occurred. Even in the absence of further dosing profound changes occurred in the lens, leading to vacuolation and disruption of the lens fibres with resultant complete opacity. Other remarkable changes also occurred in these eyes.

The guinea-pigs suffering from this drug-induced blindness showed no other major defects, and histologically their other organs were apparently normal. When these substances were given to other species a perplexing picture was obtained. No ocular changes whatsoever could be detected in rats, mice, dogs or cows. Rabbits showed minimal changes in the lens and monkeys also showed slight changes. In both these species the changes were of a type that one would believe to be reversible. Plainly, the question of the likelihood of such changes occurring in man was not to be easily resolved, and indeed was never resolved. Some biochemical study of the mechanism of this toxic effect proved unrewarding (Duncan, 1963). Hence, the possibility of determining whether the system poisoned by this substance in the guinea-pig would also have been poisoned in man, had to be excluded. The hard decision was taken not to try these substances in human beings. Such a decision is always as unsatisfactory scientifically as commercially. Until the biochemical study of such mechanisms is more advanced, however, it will remain necessary to err on the side of safety.

Other problems in evaluation arise when transient ocular disturbances are noted in experimental animals. Fortunately their very

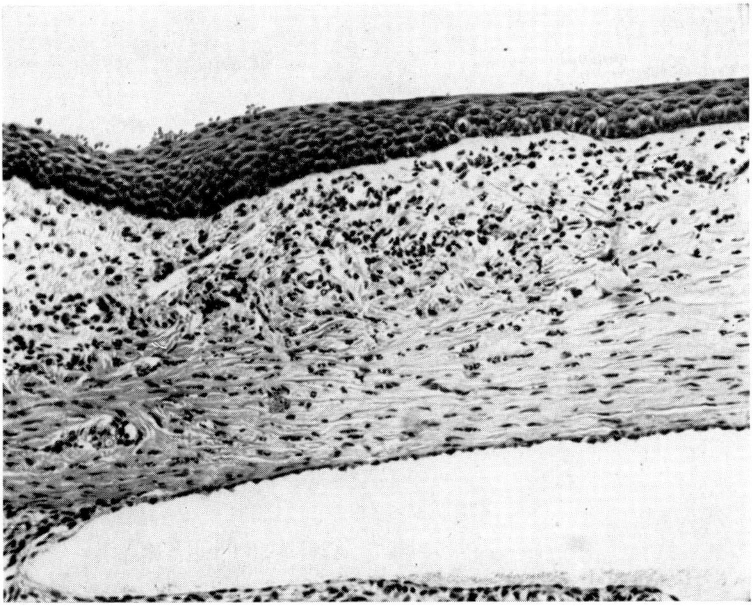

All sections are of guinea-pig eyes.

FIG. 1. Vacuolation of lens epithelium and underlying fibres 8 hours after oral dose of a quinolone. H & E × 570.

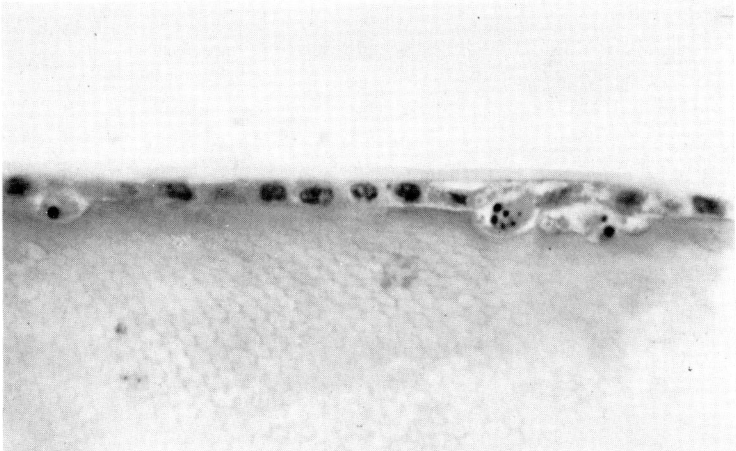

FIG. 2. Necrosis of cells of lens epithelium 16 hours after dose. H & E × 565.

facing page 10

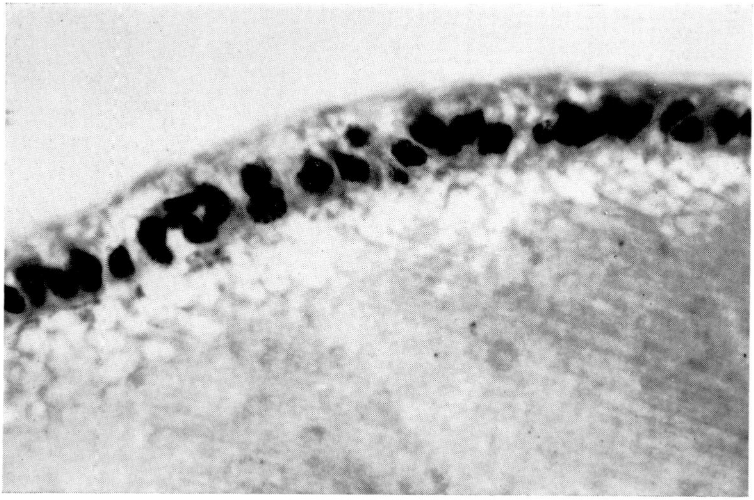

FIG. 3. Cellular infiltration of cornea 24 hours after dose. H & E × 160.

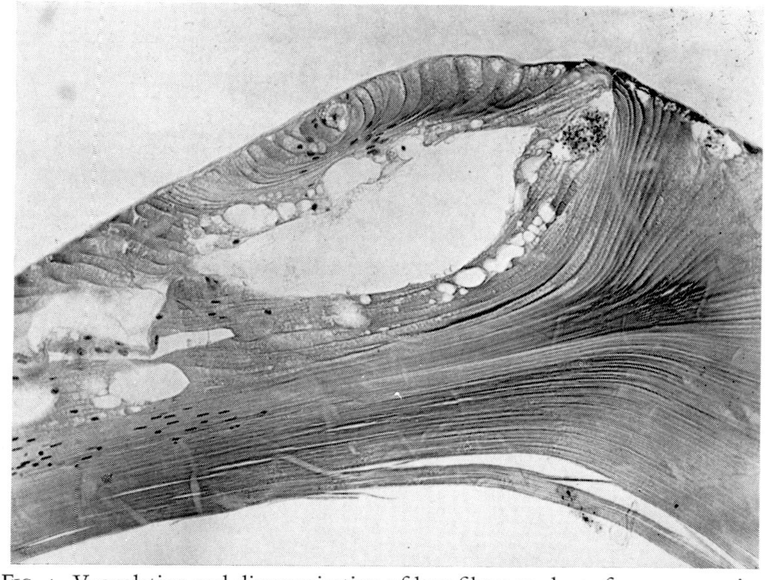

FIG. 4. Vacuolation and disorganization of lens fibres 12 days after commencing oral dosing. H & E × 95.

transience makes them less serious should they be encountered in man; and one could draw comfort from the observation (Weinstock and Stewart, 1961) that morphine and similar opiates have been shown to cause transient opacities in the eyes of mice, although such opacities have not, to my knowledge, been encountered in human medicine.

As often in toxicology one is compelled to recite a list of technical and intellectual difficulties of which no resolution appears in sight. This is, of course, partly the gloomy view of the professional toxicologist surveying the hardness of his lot and bemoaning it. It is not the whole story, as the general safety of most drugs will attest. The special sense organs are but another area to which the toxicologist must extend his skills.

REFERENCES

Baker, S. B. de C. and Alcock, Shirley J. (1965). An apparent change in toxicity of a compound when dosed for seven days a week instead of five. *Proc. Europ. Soc. Study of Drug Toxicity*, **VI,** 213–218.

Duncan, W. A. M. (1963). The importance of metabolism studies in relation to drug toxicity. 2. A general review. *Proc. Europ. Soc. Study of Drug Toxicity*, **II,** 67–77.

Paget, G. E. (1962). Correlation with potential toxicity to man of toxic effects in animals. *Clin. Pharmacol. Therap.*, **3,** 381–384.

Weinstock, M. and Stewart, H. C. (1961). Occurrence in rodents of reversible drug-induced opacities of the lens. *Brit. J. Ophthalmol.*, **45,** 408–414.

DISCUSSION

Moncrieff: Does the more emphatic nature of the reactions of animals to odours not enable their behaviour to show if drug administration has damaged their capacity to smell? If you offer a bottle of musk lactone to a man to smell he would probably say it was very nice, if you offer it to a dog it will smell the bottle and then come nearer and lick the neck of the bottle. If on the other hand you offered an unpleasant odour such as oil-soluble chlorophyll to a human he would say he did not like it; but a dog would slink away from it as though he had been chastised or hurt.

Lemon: We haven't tried testing the sense of smell in dogs. I think one can gain insight into the general sensory reactions of dogs by carefully observing them. This is where it pays to have a really good animal technician.

Blane: The ICI anti-gonadotrophin that was found to be non-toxic when administered to rats on a 5-day week dose schedule but toxic on continuous daily dosing may have been accumulating rather slowly at the dose levels used and taking six or seven days to reach blood levels which resulted in pathological signs in the eye. A respite at the weekend was apparently sufficient to limit accumulation to sub-toxic levels. With regard to the eye, wouldn't it be possible to label your compound with, say, carbon-14 and then just take the eye out and find whether there has been any accumulation of radioactivity in the eye? If the compound does not reach the eye in the first instance then this would rule out the possibility that it can be directly responsible for the damage.

Lemon: I know that at ICI this, or similar techniques, were tried with various compounds. In the case of the particular compound mentioned, which produced cataracts in rats when dosed 7 days a week, the results of tests were not entirely consistent, but it appeared that the compound was cleared from the eyes while it was still detectable in the blood, suggesting that drug accumulation is not a factor. Possibly the effect might be mediated through a deficiency state.

Hollyhock: We have found, in the Committee on Safety of Drugs, that dosing for 5 days out of 7 may mask toxicity. Would you agree that dosing on every day should be routine and not just in special cases?

Lemon: Yes, I think this is absolutely essential. Some years ago now when we were dosing 5 days a week at I.C.I. for routine chronic toxicity tests, it was very noticeable that the animals' weights on the top dose would increase only slightly during the week, but would rise sharply over the weekend, so that the weight curve went up in a series of steps. I can only put this down to the fact that over the weekend the animals recovered from the effects of the drug. I think it is essential to dose 7 days a week, but it is terribly difficult to know whether one should extend the principle further and dose three times a day, seven days a week. Perhaps this will come in time, if the staffing problems can be overcome.

McIlwain: Isn't it rather surprising that rats and guinea pigs seem largely to ignore visual cues? Can it be that this applies only to strains of laboratory-bred animals selected for other reasons, and that selection for visual acuity could be advantageous in animals used for toxicological work within daylight hours?

Lemon: Yes, I think you are probably right about that.

Wersäll: Testing suspected toxicity related to the inner ear or visual system is so complicated that it is hardly realistic to expect all laboratories to adopt the necessary technique for such testing. It would, however, be of great value if a screening test of hearing and vestibular function could be done in all laboratories and where ototoxic effects are suspected the drug could be referred to a special laboratory for testing. International collaboration could probably be arranged for such special testing.

Lemon: Yes. We have really been discussing routine chronic toxicity tests where one hopes to pick up an effect if it occurs. Where one is dealing with a compound which is suspected of causing or of being likely to cause such effects, then other tests have to be designed specifically to look for them. Here a specialist laboratory could be of enormous help. With regard to the inner ear, one can certainly notice cerebellar ataxia quite easily in a dog and I imagine that if the vestibular mechanism was seriously disturbed, one would notice this also.

Quilliam: During studies on corneal damage arising from toxic vapours, I was impressed with the ease with which the cornea of the rabbit could be examined with a loupe or a slit lamp when the animal was restrained in a rabbit box. In your search for toxic actions of drugs upon the uveal tract, have you had any experience of using the rabbit because its eye offers a large organ for examination by either indirect or direct ophthalmoscopy whereas primates are less co-operative with those intending to carry out ophthalmoscopy on them?

Lemon: We have not used rabbits in this way. On this question it seems to me that the important thing is not to find a species of test animal which may be easier to test than some other animal, but to define those species which are susceptible to particular drug effects or to particular compounds. For instance, monkeys are much more sensitive to the general neurotoxic effects of the 8-aminoquinolines than most other laboratory animals. If one relied only on rabbits one might miss something detectable in other species.

Crawford: Has any use been made of the electro-physiological response in some form? A very interesting correlation has recently been reported between such a response and the sense of smell or the response to scented or odoriferous substances in birds. Demonstration of the sense of smell in birds is otherwise rather difficult. I wonder whether a similar technique, admittedly complicated, might be of use in this context, because the threshold response electro-physiologically appears to be not very far above the threshold response in a human in similar circumstances.

Lemon: That is a very interesting suggestion.

NEUROPHYSIOLOGICAL INVESTIGATION

P. B. BRADLEY

Department of Experimental Neuropharmacology, University of Birmingham

NEUROPHYSIOLOGICAL techniques have been extensively used for investigating drug action on the nervous system and a considerable volume of literature exists on the subject. The results of such investigations, particularly those relating to drug effects on the interaction between the organism and its environment, are greatly enhanced if the neurophysiological data can be correlated with behavioural changes. Thus, the development of chronic animal preparations carrying implanted electrodes has enabled changes in electrophysiological potentials to be correlated with changes in behaviour when drugs are given (Bradley and Elkes, 1953). Experiments with such preparations have shown that a dissociation is produced between the electrical activity of the cortex and behaviour when certain drugs are administered, whilst other drugs which modify behaviour by actions on the central nervous system induce appropriate changes in the E.E.G. (Bradley and Elkes, 1957). Such studies, together with the results of experiments on unanaesthetized acute preparations such as the *encéphale isolé* and the *cerveau isolé*, have led to the suggestion that the sites of action of certain drugs, particularly those affecting levels of wakefulness, are closely related to mechanisms in the brain stem reticular formation (Bradley and Elkes, 1957). Studies of the effect of these drugs on arousal thresholds (Bradley and Key, 1958) using arousal produced by electrical stimulation of the brain stem reticular formation and also arousal induced by sensory stimulation, have confirmed the earlier hypothesis and, in addition, have enabled the effects of drugs on the central nervous system to be quantified. However, whereas the effects of drugs which modify levels of wakefulness and consciousness, such as the barbiturates and amphetamine, appear to do so by directly depressing or exciting the brain stem reticular formation activating system, other drugs which are more potent in modifying responses to environmental stimuli, such as chlorpromazine and lysergide (LSD 25; *d*-lysergic acid diethylamide), seem to have little direct action on arousal mechanisms in the brain stem, but produce their effects by actions related to sensory influences on this system (Bradley and Key, 1958).

An extension of these investigations using conditioned and non-conditioned arousal responses has confirmed these findings (Key and Bradley, 1960) and studies of sensory generalization and of habituation to sensory stimuli have shown that chlorpromazine simulates the habituation process, reducing the significance level of all sensory stimuli very rapidly to a level at which no responses occur. Lysergide on the other hand, appears to simulate the process of conditioning, and increases the significance level of stimuli to which animals were previously unresponsive (Key, 1961a, b). The actions of these two drugs thus appear to be very closely linked with the processes of filtering and integration of sensory information in the nervous system. These actions are discussed in more detail by Dr. B. J. Key (p. 153).

The methods described so far enable some localization of drug action in the nervous system to be made but do not pinpoint these actions very precisely, particularly as regards the neuronal mechanisms themselves. The recent development of the technique of micro-iontophoresis by means of multi-barrelled microelectrodes enables drugs to be applied to the surface of single neurones whilst the activity of the neurone is recorded (Curtis, 1965). The pharmacological properties of neurones in the brain stem have been studied with this technique (Bradley and Wolstencroft, 1965) and it has been found that neurones respond to acetylcholine,

5-hydroxytryptamine, and noradrenaline, all of which are possible candidates for the role of synaptic transmitters in the nervous system. Each of these substances can have an excitatory or inhibitory action and in the case of acetylcholine, these two actions have different pharmacological properties (Bradley, Dhawan and Wolstencroft, 1966). In addition many neurones respond to more than one of these substances and mixed effects can be observed. Thus, there is a wide variety of responses of the neurones in this part of the brain. If these responses reflect the pharmacological properties of the neurones, there is considerable diversity in these properties and this may be related to the diversity of functions which they subserve. It had not yet been possible to produce any precise information on the relationship between the pharmacology and function but we have some indication that the neurones in one particular nucleus we have studied, the paramedian reticular nucleus, are more homogeneous in their pharmacological properties than those in other parts of the brain stem (Avanzino, Bradley and Wolstencroft, 1966). These studies are still in their infancy and a great deal more needs to be done. It is perhaps interesting to note that the two drugs whose actions on sensory functions have been studied extensively, lysergide and chlorpromazine, both depress neuronal activity when applied iontophoretically (Bradley and Wolstencroft, 1964). We are now investigating some of the many possible explanations for this depressant action.

REFERENCES

Avanzino, G. L., Bradley, P. B. and Wolstencroft, J. H. (1966). Pharmacological properties of neurones of the paramedian reticular nucleus. *Experientia*, **22**, 410.

Bradley, P. B., Dhawan, B. N. and Wolstencroft, J. H. (1966). Pharmacological properties of cholinoceptive neurones in the medulla and pons of the cat. *J. Physiol.*, **183**, 658–674.

Bradley, P. B. and Elkes, J. (1953). A technique for recording the electrical activity of the brain in the conscious animal. *EEG clin. Neurophysiol.*, **5**, 451–456.

Bradley, P. B. and Elkes, J. (1957). The effects of some drugs on the electrical activity of the brain. *Brain*, **80**, 77–117.

Bradley, P. B. and Key, B. J. (1958). The effect of drugs on arousal responses produced by electrical stimulation of the reticular formation of the brain. *EEG clin. Neurophysiol.*, **10**, 97–110.

Bradley, P. B. and Wolstencroft, J. H. (1964). The action of drugs on single neurones in the brain stem. *In* Neuro-Psychopharmacology, **3**, 237–240 (ed. Bradley, P. B., Flügel, F. and Hoch, P.) Amsterdam: Elsevier.

Bradley, P. B. and Wolstencroft, J. H. (1965). Actions of drugs on single neurones in the brain-stem. *Brit. med. Bull.*, **21**, 15–18.

Curtis, D. R. (1965). Actions of drugs on single neurones in the spinal cord and thalamus. *Brit. med. Bull.*, **21**, 5–9.

Key, B. J. (1961a). Effects of chlorpromazine and lysergic acid diethylamide on the rate of habituation of the arousal response. *Nature*, **190**, 275–277.

Key, B. J. (1961b). The effect of drugs on discrimination and sensory generalisation of auditory stimuli in cats. *Psychopharmacologia*, **2**, 352–363.

Key, B. J. and Bradley, P. B. (1960). The effects of drugs on conditioning and habituation to arousal stimuli in animals. *Psychopharmacologia*, **1**, 450–462.

DISCUSSION

Grossman: Did you imply, Professor Bradley, that neurones which share common pharmacological properties, which, for instance are excited by acetylcholine or inhibited by 5-hydroxytryptamine are likely to be part of a particular functional system?

Bradley: No, I wasn't making that particular point. That is a very attractive hypothesis and one which we should bear in mind. I personally think it will be a bit more complicated than that. We might find a differential distribution of neurones with different pharmacological properties, so that one region of the brain stem might contain a greater proportion of one type of neurone and smaller proportions of others, but that is a hypothesis which we are investigating at present.

Hollyhock: Have you been able to achieve any histological location of neurones with these differential responses? Do they appear in a scattered distribution, or aggregated in discrete groups of separate function?

Bradley: At this stage we have data for only one particular group—our initial studies were done without too careful consideration of the position of the neurones; we were just examining the pharmacological properties of brain-stem neurones. Now we are attempting to determine to what nuclei they belong and we have one group in the paramedian reticular nucleus which appears to be homogeneous in this respect.

Arden: Can I ask you two questions, which may be very naïve: (1) When you are dealing with habituation what evidence have you about the stimuli to the neurone, especially about their constancy? and (2) How sure are you from these recordings that the site of action of the drug is localized to the specific cell which you are investigating?

Bradley: The parameters of the acoustic stimuli are quite well controlled; it is true that they are applied through a loud-speaker and one has the imperfections of the electro-mechanical side but they are reproducible within the limits of this equipment. One can readily observe the effects of changing one of the parameters, if an animal is habituated to one particular stimulus, it responds again when the parameter is changed slightly.

Of course we are not certain that the site of action of the drug is localized to the neurone being recorded, but we hope that the drug is acting on that neurone, especially where it is producing an immediate effect. We cannot completely exclude the possibility of an indirect effect although we have in some instances recorded from two units simultaneously: in some experiments one has been facilitated and one inhibited by acetylcholine. This seems to exclude an indirect effect in these cases.

Session II

Smell and Taste

Chairman: W. Feldberg

MOLECULAR CONFIGURATION AND ODOUR

R. W. MONCRIEFF

Chichester

SOME materials are odorous, others are not. Flowers, fruits, oils and foods are as a rule odorous; water, sugar, salt, wood, stone, brick, metals, paper, fabrics and fibres are basically inodorous. The differences are usually clear-cut and exceptions are readily accounted for, e.g. cedarwood is odorous because it contains a proportion of an odorous oil, but most woods are almost without odour. Is the essential difference between the two groups of substances, odorous and inodorous, due to their molecular configuration or is it unrelated to it? The connection between the two is in fact a good deal less close than is commonly thought.

Pre-requisites for odour

There are only three pre-requisites for a substance to be odorous:

(1) It must be volatile, not necessarily very volatile like ether or alcohol or even like water, but sufficiently to lose molecules continually to the atmosphere, and so that these can be breathed into the nose and can come in contact with the olfactory apparatus. Contact of odorant molecules with the olfactory sensitive region is essential and this can come about only as a result of volatility. For example, the vapour pressure of 'artificial musk' has been reported to be $1 \cdot 3 \times 10^{-6}$ atmospheres at 37°C (Mullins, 1955), whilst that of amyl acetate, a typically volatile strong-smelling substance (pear drops odour) is given as

$1 \cdot 3 \times 10^{-2}$ atmospheres and that of ethyl ether as $1 \cdot 1$ atmospheres under the same conditions. The vapour pressure of odorous materials can vary within wide limits, but it must have a significant value. Substances such as stone, metals, cotton and nylon which are non-volatile are thereby inodorous.

(2) It must be a substance which can be adsorbed on the sensitive surface of the olfactory epithelium. I have demonstrated the sorptive nature of the olfactory stimulus (Moncrieff, 1955, 1956) and this has been unambiguously proved by the design and construction of an instrument for detecting and measuring odours, which faithfully reproduces many of the features of animal olfaction. This instrument depends upon the energy liberated when odorant molecules are adsorbed on to films, which function as a model of the olfactory epithelium (Moncrieff, 1961, 1964). In effect almost all volatile substances are capable of being adsorbed easily, and the only important group that cannot be are the light gases: hydrogen, nitrogen, oxygen, helium, argon and so on. There is a close analogy between liquefaction and adsorption; adsorption can be regarded as the liquefaction on a surface and in a very thin layer, of a gas. Those gases, the light gases, that are difficult to liquefy, are correspondingly difficult to adsorb and they have no smell. But most gases and vapours lend themselves readily to liquefaction and to adsorption, and they are correspondingly odorous.

(3) It must be a substance which is not already present on the olfactory epithelium, so that when it arrives there, carried by the inspired air, it brings about a change. Only change brings sensation. For example, water vapour carried by the inspired air will not stimulate the sense of smell, because water is already present on and in the tissues.

Molecular configuration not critical for stimulation

So, the three pre-requisites for odour are: volatility, a capacity for being adsorbed, and a customary absence from the olfactory region. Apart from such materials as are evidently non-volatile, and apart from the light gases and water, this leaves the field wide open. There may be a few special cases, notably of substances such as the glycols and of high molecular weight (say 220–300) compounds that require further investigation, but generally any substances which are appreciably volatile are likely to be odorous. The stimulus for olfaction is sorptive in character and because adsorption is itself a basic physical process that is going on all the time in every corner of our world, we live amongst a multitude of odorous substances. Molecular configuration is not at all critical for olfactory stimulation; a multitude of substances drawn from almost every class of compounds are odorous, e.g. the halogens, ozone, sulphides, paraffins, alcohols, aldehydes and ketones, acids, benzenoid compounds, phenols, and the macrocyclic compounds. Odorous materials are ubiquitous and to be found in a large variety of molecular shapes and sizes.

The quality of odour

Molecular configuration is relatively unimportant in determining whether a substance is odorous, but it is very important in determining the kind or quality of the odour that is perceived. There are thousands of different smells, no one knows how many; the range is wide, we can picture a deep red rose such as *Ena Harkness* at one end, and the foul-smelling methyl mercaptan which gives its characteristic odour to faeces somewhere near the other end. There is no present knowledge of the extent of the range; new odours are continually being discovered, odours quite different from those we already know; some men might prefer the synthetic indane musk, Phantolide, to a deep red rose; some people think that thiomalic acid is more objectionable than methyl mercaptan. This state of affairs is very different from that which prevails with colour vision or hearing where the frequency range is known and well explored, so that the production of a hitherto unexperienced colour or sound is almost impossible. A new kind of smell might be discovered tomorrow because chemical compounds with novel molecular configurations are being synthesized every day. The capacity of the nose to characterize the multitude of synthetic substances that have been made is amazing; such well-known and characteristic odours as those of benzene, naphthalene and paradichlorbenzene are not to be found in nature, but the nose copes with them well enough and unequivocally, too. There is, built into our olfactory equipment, an analytical device which enables it to sort out thousands of different odours effortlessly, indeed involuntarily and spontaneously.

Analytical equipment for discrimination

The nature of our analytical equipment has come in for a good deal of investigation. Thus Le Gros Clark (1956, 1957) has reported differences between one olfactory receptor and another in the following respects: in the length and attenuation of the olfactory rod, in the size of the terminal swelling, in the number of olfactory hairs attached thereto, and in the sensitivity of the hairs to silver staining, some of them staining more deeply than others; indeed, the same applies to the receptors themselves 'for in certain regions individual receptors may stand out more conspicuously by their much denser silver staining'. The observations were made on fixed and stained sections of the rabbit's olfactory epithelium. Perhaps some of these differences are significantly related to odour discrimination, but which ones and how they play their part so far eludes us.

Specificity of receptors

We are driven back to the broad postulate that there are different kinds of olfactory cells with different specificities of response but we are not yet sure to what their specific qualities are due. Today's view is that all the olfactory receptors are slightly responsive to all smells but very responsive indeed to one smell or to a small group of smells. Experimental support for this view has been provided by Adrian (1953, 1955), Gesteland *et al.* (1963) and others. Adrian's work (1955) showed that the olfactory mitral cells respond specifically and he thought that the receptor cells must also have a specific sensitivity to certain chemicals and that there might perhaps be fifty kinds of specialized receptor cells. Le Gros Clark has suggested that there might be something of the order of 500. At present we can only guess, but there seem to be many different kinds of olfactory receptors.

Complementary shapes of molecules and receptors

Why should some receptor sites be specifically susceptible to certain odorants? The idea that the shape of one must be complementary to that of the other has appealed to many people. Ruzicka (1920) put forward a theory of osmophores and osmoceptors.

Bogert (1936) studied some substituted benzothiazoles; these compounds contained sulphur in their molecule but instead of having unpleasant odours, as might have been expected, they were pleasant. Thus, 2-phenyl benzothiazole

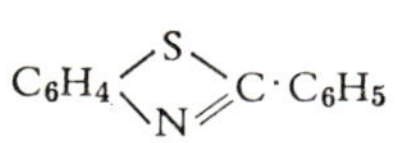

had a pleasant tea-rose odour, and so had some similar benzoselenazoles; this was still more surprising because selenium compounds usually smell even worse than sulphur compounds. Bogert realized that the sulphur or selenium atom in the ring was olfactorily harmless and he concluded that the odour was related to the architectural type of the molecule, and that the structure was more important than the elements concerned. This was a significant step forward. A study of odour in relation to constitution led me to conclude similarly that the general architectural design of the molecule determines its odour and that only in small molecules can any one group exert a determining influence (Moncrieff, 1944a). Later it seemed 'likely that to be odorous a substance must have molecules of prescribed shapes which will fit on certain available molecular sites in the olfactory receptors' (Moncrieff, 1951).

More recently Amoore (1964) has greatly elaborated the theory by postulating that there are seven primary odours: ethereal, camphoraceous, musky, floral, minty, pungent and putrid. For each of the first five a receptor site of specific size and shape is postulated; that for the ethereal odours is a narrow slot, accepting only thin molecules, that for the camphoraceous odours is hemispherical in shape, about 7 Å in diameter, the musky site is a larger elliptical flat-bottomed pan and so on. Pungency and putridness are deemed to depend not on molecular size and shape but on the electronic status, electrophilic or nucleophilic, of the odorant molecules. The most striking evidence in support of the theory was that 21 compounds selected from Beilstein as having been reported to have camphoraceous odours, were found when their molecular models (Catalin) were made, to fit well into the hemispherical postulated site and badly into the other sites. It was well-known from Timmermans' (1938, 1954) earlier observations that a spherical molecular configuration was characteristic of compounds smelling like camphor. But Amoore's work showed that the relation was more consistent and closer than had been known. Amoore's views have received much support from Johnston (1965) and indeed from others, but other workers again have found that their results are incompatible with Amoore's theories and at Corvallis in September 1965 it was stated that much of the theory had been withdrawn. A relationship can often be discerned between molecular shape and odour, but it is sporadic and inconsistent. What is abundantly clear is that any attempt to limit odour quality to seven primary types is very unlikely to succeed.

Molecular structure

Aside from the special cases of odorant and receptor having complementary shapes, the general relation between structure and odour has intrigued many people. Many parallelisms are to be found. Thus if a homologous series such as that of the paraffins or of the aliphatic alcohols is ascended, odour which at first is only weak (e.g. methanol) or even absent (e.g. methane) grows in strength and becomes very strong at about the C_6 to C_8 members and thereafter weakens again and disappears altogether at about C_{15} to C_{20}, partly because of the falling off in volatility as the molecular weight increases. The odours of fruits and fruit essences are largely due to the presence of esters; most often the ester group is associated with a fruity odour, except in really high molecular weight compounds, for example, the macrocyclics. The substitution in many chemical entities of a sulphur for an oxygen atom brings an unpleasant odour: hydrogen sulphide and methyl mercaptan are both very unpleasant, but their oxygen analogues, water and methanol are olfactorily innocuous. The introduction of a selenium or a tellurium atom has an even worse effect than sulphur. The chemical similarity of the terpenes and the many likenesses of odour between their different members affords another example.

One of the most interesting suggestions that have come from such researches was made 2,000 years ago by Lucretius; he thought that agreeably odorous substances must be composed of smooth round atoms, and that harsh and unpleasant substances were made of hooked particles. There is still no evidence today of the existence of such hooks, but in the wider sense Lucretius seems to have anticipated the view that odour quality depends on molecular configuration. Perhaps such early views have a still closer link with the recent suggestion of Davies (1965) about the quality of odours. His view is that after adsorption of the odorant molecule on the cell membrane, desorption occurs and that if this is more rapid than the recovery of the membrane to its original position, a tiny hole will exist momentarily in it and will allow an exchange of sodium and potassium ions, thus initiating the nervous impulse. Discrimination between smells might then be explained by differences in speeds of desorption: a slow-moving musk molecule may desorb in 10^{-8} seconds whereas a fast-moving butanol molecule may desorb in 10^{-10} seconds. It must also be postulated that the fluidity of the membranes of the cells varies and that those with the more fluid and more easily penetrated membranes will be those that are sensitive to the fast-moving molecules such as butanol. There is not much evidence for or against it at present.

Minimal differences in configuration

Inevitably one sooner or later realizes that the slightest of differences in structure can make a big difference to the smell.

Stoll (1965) described some of these minimal differences. He had carried out research on substances of relatively high molecular weight. The gist of his argument seems to be that there is an upper limit to the molecular weight of substances that can cause odour perception and that this is about 280; the disappearance of odour at this value is attributed, not to a lower population of odoriferous molecules on the olfactive mucosa, but to blocking of the nervous system by over-adsorption. There are many very different and interesting odours of substances within the molecular weight range of 224 which is that of exaltone, and 274 which is that of the androstenols. Exaltone itself is a macrocyclic compound with a powerful musk odour; its structure is very similar to that of muscone, the essential odorous principle of natural musk:

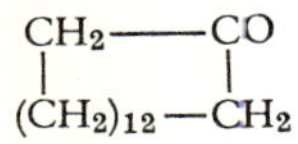

Exaltone

M.W. 224

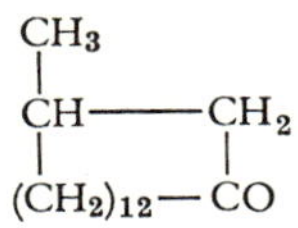

Muscone

M.W. 238

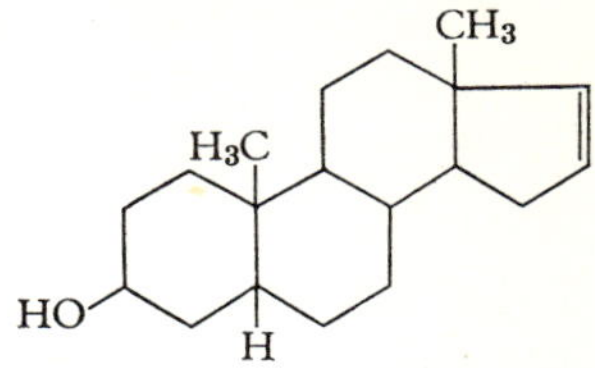

Androstenol ($C_{19}H_{29}OH$)

M.W. 274

Androstenol is a steroid with a completely different structure, all the rings are saturated except for one double bond. It was isolated by Stoll, Hinde, and Ruzicka (1948) from hog testes and was reported to have a pronounced musky odour. According to Stoll sudden changes in odour, often its disappearance or appearance, occur in such high molecular weight compounds as a result of some very slight change in structure; such marked changes in odour are unusual in substances of low or medium molecular weight. Thus, in the medium range, citral and geraniol both have strong odours although they are very different, and so do menthol and menthone; the small structural changes in these molecules of medium size cause considerable changes in the quality of their odours (citral is lemony, whereas geraniol is rose-like), but they neither destroy nor evoke the odorous quality. In the large molecules, on the other hand, slight changes in constitution and even in configuration can bring about the complete disappearance of odour.

Stoll recalls that his co-worker Demole (1964) investigated some terpenylcyclohexanols and found odour only in those which carried the hydroxyl group meta to the terpenyl group, and that of these only the trans (axial) form was odorous. The most striking difference was observed between the two configurations of the meta compound (Fig. 1). The compound with the hydroxyl group of the cyclohexanol in the axial position had a strong odour of sandalwood but its stereoisomer with the hydroxyl group in the equatorial position was odourless. The two compounds illustrated are dihydrocamphenyl-meta-cyclohexanols. As Stoll remarks, it is difficult to imagine receptor sites that by virtue of their specific size and shape would accommodate one of these isomers and not the other. He himself develops a theory that odour perception-discrimination may be regarded as a kind of chromatography in which the receptors provide the stationary phase and the mucus constitutes

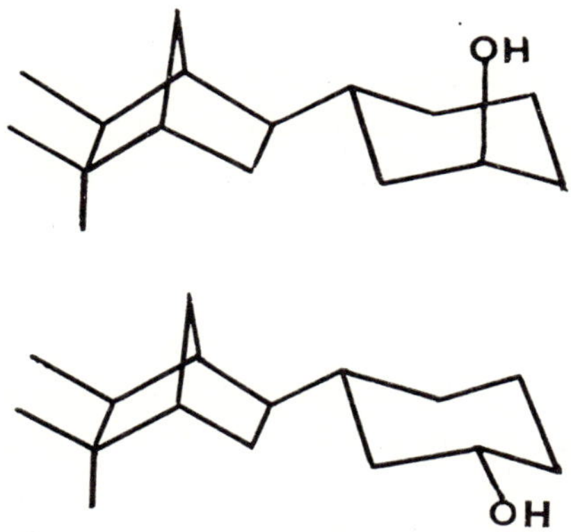

FIG. 1. Stereoisomeric terpenyl-*m*-cyclohexanols. Upper: Axial configuration: strong sandalwood odour. *Lower:* Equatorial configuration: no odour. (After Stoll.)

the moving phase; but the theory raises as many problems as it attempts to solve. However, the pharmacological effects of stereoisomers of drugs such as ascorbic acid, adrenaline, nicotine and testosterone are well known to differ. It should not therefore cause surprise that stereoisomeric forms can have different smells, but it is a finding that most theories of olfactory discrimination find it hard to explain. However, the fact that stereoisomeric forms can have different adsorption characteristics e.g. times of capture, is in itself enough to explain any odour differences. Why stereoisomers should have different adsorption characteristics will of course have to be explained.

The principles relating constitution and odour

After studying the information then available I condensed most of the reported relations between constitution and odour into 62 principles (Moncrieff, 1944b); these were later reproduced almost *in toto* by McCord and Witheridge (1949). Repeated attempts to resolve these sixty-two principles into a few general rules failed; they did not lend themselves to much reduction in bulk. This, of course, was a serious difficulty and indeed, as in the intervening years more information has become accessible, so has the difficulty of including it in these rules grown. The most important fact that they establish is that no single pattern of chemical structure is consistently related to odour properties.

An olfactometer cannot be human

Perhaps the reason for the failure to tie up molecular configuration consistently with odour is partly that our olfactory equipment was designed to be useful in helping us to find food and to keep us in a safe environment; much of what the peripheral receptors report is doubtless lost in the early stages of transmission of the information to the cortex, lost because it has no contribution to make towards keeping the body safe and well. The nose was never designed for use as an olfactometer; it is far too susceptible to adaptation, fatigue, and habituation. As a measuring instrument it is most unsatisfactory, although as a detector it has an unsurpassed sensitivity, and one that is very difficult, sometimes impossible, to equal by instrumental methods. Furthermore, odours are too heavily loaded with emotional associations for us to regard them dispassionately. The way in which our olfactory likes and dislikes change with age illustrates this. Figure 2 shows how the liking for the smell of a fruity flavour (strawberry essence) changes with age. The liking rises to a peak at age 8 or 9, and then falls away except for a short standstill at adolescence. Figure 3 shows how the individual's preferences for oil of lavender

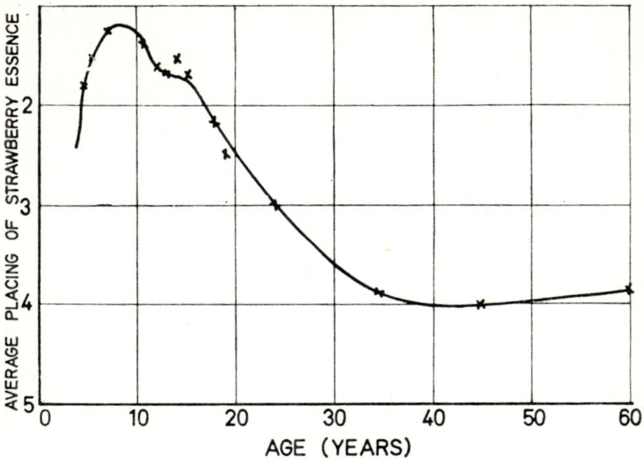

FIG. 2. Changes in liking of strawberry essence odour with age. The higher the curve the greater the liking.

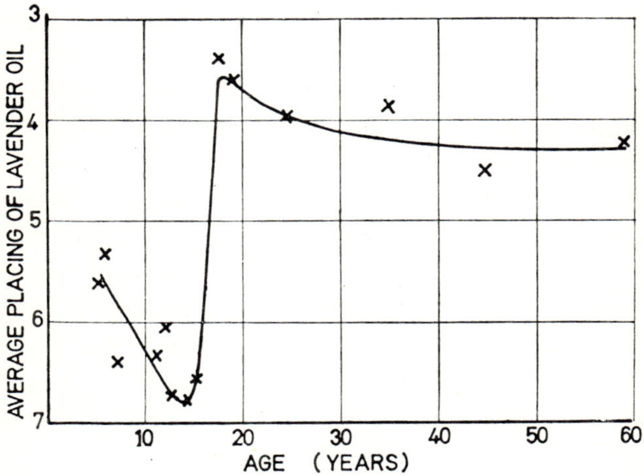

FIG. 3. Changes in liking of French lavender oil with age. The higher the curve the greater the liking.

(French 'Exquisia') change with age; children do not rate it highly but between the ages of 15 and 18 there is a marked and quite sudden increase in liking for it (Moncrieff, 1965).

The way in which likes and preferences for odours change with age is reminiscent of children's greater liking for sweets, and of their lower taste threshold for sugar (Richter and Campbell, 1940). This is due to the wider distribution of taste buds in the child's compared with the grown person's, mouth. For the sweet taste the child has an anatomical advantage which it loses as it grows older; changes in liking for odours of the type shown in Figs. 2 and 3 may well be due to similar anatomical advantages. A child is much fonder of fruity flavours than is an adult, and much less appreciative of flower smells. The changes take place predictably and reliably (Moncrieff, 1966) and emphasize the subjective nature of odours and inevitably point to the difficulty of finding a consistent relationship between odour quality, as assessed by human appreciation, and molecular configuration. The possibility that anatomical changes might explain them is intriguing.

To summarize, the olfactory stimulus is known to be one of continuous adsorption and desorption of the odorant molecules by the olfactory epithelium, and specificity of receptors for some kinds of odorants has been demonstrated, but the underlying reason for this specificity is still debatable. The stimulus for odour perception is almost independent of molecular configuration. Sometimes, as with the large ring compounds of 15–18 ring atoms, the odour is musky irrespective of whether the compound is saturated (muscone) or unsaturated (civettone) and of whether it is a ketone, a lactone, an imine or an ester. Other times, the slightest of differences in configuration, particularly amongst high molecular weight compounds often with musky or sandalwood odours, can banish odour.

In the end we must recognize that molecular configuration is only half the story, and that the other half is the receptor system and brain of the person doing the smelling. The two halves together may sometimes enable us to understand much better what determines the quality of a smell. Modern analytical techniques such as spectrography and nuclear magnetic resonance now enable the shape and size of molecules to be determined precisely and certainly, and knowledge of this kind is rapidly accumulating from the use of these techniques. The neurophysiologists have a more difficult task in trying to unravel what happens between receptor stimulation and its mysterious conversion into sensation. But we need more information of this kind to help resolve some of the anomalies which still beset the subject of odour discrimination.

REFERENCES

Adrian, E. D. (1953). Sensory messages and sensation. The response of the olfactory organ to different smells. *Acta Physiol. Scand.*, **29,** Fasc. 1., 5–14.

Adrian, E. D. (1955). Potential oscillations in the olfactory organ. *J. Physiol.*, **128,** 21P–22P.

Amoore, J. E. (1964). Current status of the steric theory of odor. *Ann. New York Acad. Sci.*, **116,** Art. 2, 457–476.

Bogert, M. T. (1936). Connection between odor and constitution in the benzothiazole group. III. *Amer. Perfumer and Essential Oil Rev.*, **32,** (4), 51.

Davies, J. T. (1965). A theory of the quality of odours. *J. theoret. Biol.*, **8,** 1–7.

Demole, E. (1964). Synthèses et relations entre constitution chimique et odeur dans la série des terpényl-3-cyclohexanols. *Helv. chim. Acta*, **47,** 1766–1774.

Gesteland, R. C., Lettvin, J. Y., Pitts, W. H. and Rojas, A. (1963). Odor specificities of the frog's olfactory receptors. *In* Olfaction and Taste, (ed. Zotterman, Y.) Oxford: Pergamon Press.

Johnston, J. W. (1965). Experiments on the specificities of human olfaction. *In* Surface Effects in Detection. Washington: Spartan Books.

Le Gros Clark, W. (1956). Observations on the structure and organization of olfactory receptors in the rabbit. *Yale J. Biol. Med.*, **29,** 83–95.

Le Gros Clark, W. (1957). Inquiries into the anatomical basis of olfactory discrimination. *Proc. Roy. Soc. B*, **146,** 299–319.

Lucretius, T. C. (47 B.C.), translated by Latham (1951). The Nature of the Universe. Harmondsworth: Penguin.

McCord, C. P. and Witheridge, W. N. (1949). Odors: Physiology and Control. New York: McGraw-Hill.

Moncrieff, R. W. (1944). The Chemical Senses, 1st Edition (a) p. 215, (b) pp. 232–235. London: Leonard Hill.

Moncrieff, R. W. (1951). The Chemical Senses. 2nd Edition, p. 395. London: Leonard Hill.

Moncrieff, R. W. (1955). The sorptive properties of the olfactory membrane. *J. Physiol.*, **130,** 543–558.

Moncrieff, R. W. (1956). The sorptive nature of the olfactory stimulus. *Proc. 2nd International Congress Surface Activity*, **2,** 321–328, London: Butterworth.

Moncrieff, R. W. (1961). An instrument for measuring and classifying odors. *J. appl. Physiol.*, **16,** 742–749.

Moncrieff, R. W. (1964). A physical model of the olfactory apparatus. *Proc. 4th International Congress Surface Activity* B/II. 18 (in the press).

Moncrieff, R. W. (1965). Changes in olfactory preferences with age. *Revue de Laryngologie*, Suppt. Oct. 1965, 895–904.

Moncrieff, R. W. (1966). Odour Preferences. London: Leonard Hill.

Mullins, L. J. (1955). Olfaction. *Ann. New York Acad. Sci.*, **62,** Art. 11, 247–276.

Richter, C. P. and Campbell, K. H. (1940). Sucrose taste thresholds of rats and humans. *Amer. J. Physiol.*, **128,** 291–297.

Ruzicka, L. (1920). Die Grundlagen der Geruchschemie. *Chem. Ztg.*, **44,** 93–94, 129–131.

Stoll, M. (1965). De l'effet important de différences chimiques minimes sur la perception de l'odeur. *La France et ses Parfums*, **8,** 227–232.

Stoll, M., Hinde, M. and Ruzicka, L. (1948). Stéroides et hormones sexuelles. Cycloheptadecane-dione—1, 9. *Helv. chim. Acta.*, **31,** 1176–1178.

Timmermans, J. (1938). Un nouveau état mésomorphe. Les cristaux organiques plastiques. *J. Chim. Phys.*, **35,** 331–334.

Timmermans, J. (1954). Odour and chemical constitution. *Nature*, **174,** 235.

DISCUSSION

King: With regard to Figure 3, what proportion of the sample were women and what were their reading habits before that test was done?

Moncrieff: I can't tell you that, but about half of the 550 subjects were women. I don't quite follow the point about the reading habits.

King: Well, the curve seems to rise about the age of 18. If your sample had had a high proportion of young women in it, their exposure to reading material and to advertising might influence responses to your solutions.

Moncrieff: It is true that one of our sources of subjects was a girls' training college.

Hazelton: When is a bad smell a bad smell? With other mammals one can regard a smell as being unpleasant if the animal avoids it and it is some source of danger, but we highly specialized and trained mammals only regard as nice the things that we are told are nice, and, as nasty, those things that we were told were nasty at the earliest possible age, at about 6 months.

Moncrieff: M. Stein, P. Ottenberg and P. Roulet (*A.M.A. Arch. Neurol. Psychiat.* 1958, **80,** 264), have shown that children up to 4 do not dislike the bad smells that they dislike later. For example, young children of this age tolerate the odours of sweat and faeces well, and Stein and Ottenberg suggest that they probably associate the odour of faeces with a state of abdominal comfort, but the same children when they get to the age of 5 or 6 detest these smells. Possibly this ties up with the suggestion that the distribution of smell receptors changes through life.

There was absolutely perfect agreement among 550 people whom I tested with very bad smells like thiomalic acid, methyl mercaptan and so on. There was good agreement about very pleasant smells like a deep red rose and fresh strawberries, but not so very good as about the bad smells, and in between in the indifferent range there is much more disagreement.

Hazelton: That is very interesting, but it doesn't get us to the source of these opinions. Is the acceptance of smells as being pleasant or unpleasant due to the social training of the human organism from the beginning?

Moncrieff: I don't think that has anything to do with it.

Parkes: How far can the evidence you have given us about the relationship of chemical structure and odour be regarded as reliable in the light of present-day ability to obtain compounds in a high state of purity? I am thinking for example that with the extreme sensitivity of the olfactory organs it is possible that the presence of trace impurities might well give a false odour to the substance and I wonder how much of the evidence has been obtained from materials that have been demonstrated as pure, say by gas chromatography.

Moncrieff: Let me answer that with the example of two terpenyl cyclohexanols, which are identical except for the orientation of the hydroxyl group on the cyclohexanol residue, but of which one is odourless and the other smells of sandalwood. These two substances were made by E. Demole (*Helv. chim. Acta*, 1964, **47,** 1766) at the laboratories of

Fermenich & Co. in Geneva, probably the finest school in the world for the preparation of these organic perfumes; it was built up by Ruzicka and is now directed by Dr. Stoll. I asked Dr. Stoll whether he was absolutely sure of the configuration of these two isomers and he said that with modern analytical techniques such as nuclear magnetic resonance, and chromatography and infrared and ultraviolet spectroscopy, there was no longer room for doubt.

Herxheimer: There is an intriguing parallelism between Davies's theory of the action of odorant molecules on the olfactory cell membrane and Paton's rate theory of drug action (Paton, W. D. M. A theory of drug action based on the rate of drug-receptor combination. *Proc. roy. Soc. B*, 1961, **154**, 21–69). Perhaps an attempt to combine the two theories would be valuable.

THE PHYSIOLOGY AND PSYCHOPHYSICS OF ODOUR

R. Harper

A.R.C. Food Research Institute, Earlham Laboratory, Norwich

1. *Introduction*

Physiology and psychophysics have a common root in the 19th century. Physiology broke away from Medicine to form an independent academic discipline about a generation before Psychology broke away from its ill assorted parents, Physiology and Philosophy. Sensory physiology was an important part of the academic discipline and thus provided one of the roots out of which Psychophysics and Experimental Psychology ultimately grew. I shall mention only four celebrated names. J. Müller (1801–1858) formulated the doctrine of 'specific energies of nerves' according to which the particular qualities experienced by the different senses were attributed to the region of the brain ultimately stimulated. Later writers referred to this as a 'place theory', just as the pitch of a note depends upon the region of the basilar membrane maximally stimulated. This theory is rather typical of the search for uniquely sensitive taste buds and touch spots which characterized some of the major investigations in the late 19th century. This aim is no longer rigorously supported by neurophysiological and other information. Another pioneer of sensory physiology, was Weber (1798–1878). The Weber ratio and the Weber-Fechner 'Law' will be referred to later. Fechner (1801–1877) published in 1860 his 'Elemente der Psychophysik' in which many important psychophysical methods and problems were formulated or anticipated. For more than a generation one of the foremost authorities on the sense of smell was the physiologist Zwaardemaker (1857–1930).

The nature and emphasis of both disciplines has changed during the intervening years. Physiology is taken to refer here to the processes which occur within the organism from the peripheral receptor to the brain. To keep the present discussion within reasonable bounds such topics as the possible effects of humoral transmission, the interaction between the sense of smell and feeding behaviour, the emotions and the interaction between different senses are largely ignored. Psychophysics refers here primarily to the relations between the physico-chemical properties of the olfactory stimulus and observable behaviour and experience. The term 'experience' is deliberately retained since most of the psychophysical studies to be reported are concerned with man. Even if experience is communicated by 'verbal behaviour', as some psychologists would characterize it, the *phenomena* of smell cannot be ignored and require re-examination and re-stating.

In the context of sensory function and drug action Guillot (1956) stressed that the peripheral mechanisms involved when the odorous molecule initiates the first stages of the processes of perception must share many features with those of drug action. Ruzicka (1957) observed that whereas it is usual to apologize for the difficulties involved in studying the sense of smell they are precisely the difficulties generally involved in studying any physiologically active compounds. These he listed as (1) the difficulties of precise measurement; (2) the complex nature of the physiological processes involved, often mistakenly assumed to be unitary; (3) interference by many psychological processes. Many of these psychological processes will form the basis of the psycho-physical data to be considered, although the complications involved are well recognized.

The object of this brief review is primarily to select a few key points from the various fields involved, with special reference to the relation between the properties of the stimulus, the structure and functioning of the olfactory system, and the psychological facts of perception and behaviour.

Since many of the conclusions to be drawn from the investigations reviewed may be interpreted in relation to human responses, a few observations on the human sense of smell are in place here. The sense of smell is remarkably sensitive to certain stimuli; a concentration of a few molecules per cell at the epithelium may suffice. In contrast, differential sensitivity is comparatively poor (about 0·3–0·5 when expressed as a Weber fraction, as compared with a value of about 0·01 for vision). There are comparatively few 'perceptible steps' in odour perception from the threshold to the sharp upper limit of perceived strength. The possible number of different odours is very large, but most ordinary people can identify with precision only a comparatively small number, when required to do this without making direct comparisons. The more trained a person is the more categories or qualities he will be able to distinguish but the upper limit is not really known with certainty, especially for expert subjects. In a laboratory experiment with students as subjects Engen and Pfaffmann (1959, 1960) found an upper limit of about 5 steps with perceived strength and about 16 qualities. Much might depend upon the choice of stimuli and more detailed information about the method is needed than can be considered here (see refs. in original). However, the figures quoted are consistent with studies of the other senses using the methods of information theory and the concept of limited channel capacity. In contrast, experienced perfumers and chemists believe that they can identify quite large numbers of odours; the figure varies from a few hundreds to a few thousands. The challenging inconsistency between this information and the laboratory studies requires further investigation. Jones (in press) has recently provided experimental data from two experienced perfumers which extend the number of odour stimuli identifiable without error to about 150.

Another inescapable topic concerning perception in man is that of descriptive terminology and its functions. Despite continuing search there still exists no satisfactory objective property (or properties) analogous to the wavelength-intensity distribution in light and colour which can provide a rational arrangement of the perceived qualities. Much remains to be learned about available words and their meaning and clustering, a topic which impinges closely upon psychophysical problems. Only very recently have practical steps been taken to determine as precisely as possible how different people describe the same odours and what they mean. Studies along these lines are in progress at The Food Research Institute, Norwich, and will be reported elsewhere (Harper *et al.*, 1966a and in press).

2. *The olfactory stimulus and its properties*

No discussion of the physiology or the psychophysics of odour would be complete without adequate information about the olfactory stimulus itself. This consists of a large number of airborne molecules which, in the case of single substances, must have a minimal molecular concentration of between 10^7 and 10^{19} molecules per ml., depending on the particular stimulus, in order to be perceived. Relevant stimulus properties can be considered from two different points of view: those predominantly associated with stimulus intensity, and those associated with odour quality. Many of these properties may be interrelated (Schutz *et al.*, 1958); they include molecular concentration at threshold; molecular weight, cross-sectional area, molecular structure, spectral characteristics; surface activity (various types), relative solubility in water or fat (lipid), boiling point; polarity; and haemolytic activity.

The 'steric' theory attempts to relate molecular properties to odour qualities and has been discussed by Moncrieff (p. 26). Before referring to it briefly it is worth noting that explanations of perceptual phenomena connected with most other senses have long passed beyond the stage of a search for an exclusively peripheral explanation: spatial and temporal coding within the brain is regarded as important as any unique peripheral structures or processes. Amoore's (1964) approach to the steric theory was to relate the shape of the molecule to the perceived odour quality, basing this upon a frequency analysis of the descriptive terms used in the literature for the odours of over 600 substances of known composition. The top 7 were then postulated as 'primaries'. Earlier Amoore had made it clear that he was concerned with a mechanism capable of discriminating between different qualities and not with the explanation of quality *per se*. The steric theory is closely bound up with the postulation of specific receptor sites, some of whose possible properties are touched upon again later. The theory is currently being modified (Amoore, 1966).

A different approach to the relation between stimulus properties and odour qualities is that of Davies (1965) who plotted the energy of desorption at an oil/water interface against the molecular cross-sectional area of a number of odorants, and then indicated the characteristic odours corresponding to these points. The various qualities were spread out in an interesting way, which has recently been independently confirmed by Self (unpublished), although he found some physical anomalies. But why limit the study to the two chosen properties? A comprehensive study using modern methods of multidimensional scaling or analysis can be conceived in which distinctive clusters of properties and experimentally determined qualities would be examined so as to indicate optimal methods of discriminating qualities through properties.

This review does not refer in detail to the trigeminal features of many odours, which obviously have a special part to play. About four-fifths of all odour stimuli may possess a detectable trigeminal component (Skramlik, 1925).

3. *The peripheral receptors*

In man, the olfactory epithelium has an area of about 4–6 sq. cm. on each side of the nose. To reach the olfactory epithelium the odorant has to traverse a series of tortuous passages during inspiration, or the air may reach the olfactory region via the back of the mouth on swallowing. It used to be thought that a detached eddy formed the basis of the molecular transfer from the main stream to the epithelium, situated in the narrow olfactory cleft.

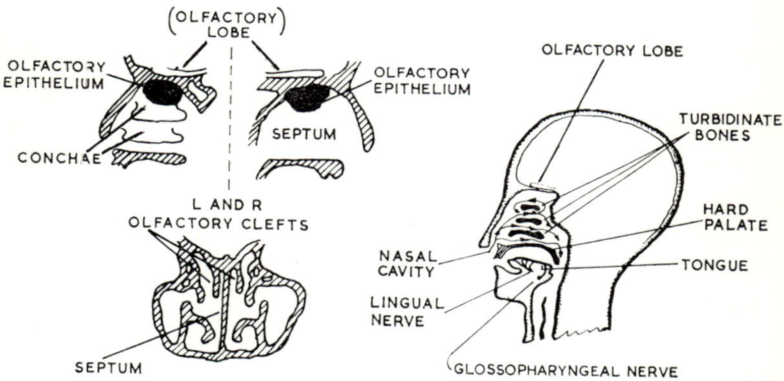

FIG. 1. The olfactory epithelium and its location.

This is now denied by Stuiver (1958) who, by using a flow model, demonstrated that only a few per cent of the inspired air will reach the epithelium on normal breathing. (Hence the value of a sharp sniff.) The matter is further complicated by the vascularity of the spongy tissues.

The olfactory epithelium itself consists of a total of about 8×10^7 free nerve endings in groups of about 10 embedded in supporting structures. Serous glands are located in the submucosa and provide the fluid which covers the external surface of the epithelium. A number of olfactory hairs project from the end of the sensitive receptors into the mucous layer, with the possibility of extensions lying on the surface. Most authorities put the number of hairs at between 10 and 12 per cell, although some think there are many more. These hairs increase the total effective area of the epithelium, and Moulton and Tucker (1964) refer to a 'feltwork'

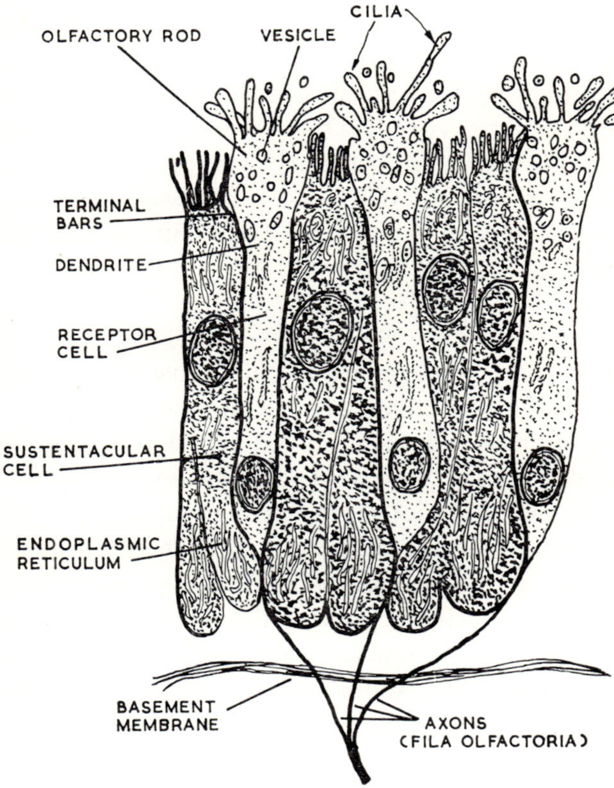

FIG. 2. The structure of the olfactory epithelium (from de Lorenzo, 1963).

whose effective area is greater than that of man's whole body surface.

Davies and Taylor (1959) calculated that a single receptor site might have an area of about 64 sq. Å. Thus a single receptor is not limited to having only a single site, and further calculations suggest that there may be as many as 44,000 'potential sites' on a single receptor. A subtle but unspecified difference in conception seems to be implied between the specific sites of the 'steric theory' and Davies's approach, which involves a small area of penetration. The receptor parts of the olfactory cells are essentially dendritic processes subject to chemical stimulation which is probably converted into the classical 'all-or-none' activity of the primary neurone in two stages (see H. Davis, 1961). The sensitive parts of the receptor cell are thick compared with the olfactory neurones which are short and fine. They pass in bundles through fine holes in the cribriform plate; no synapses occur until the olfactory bulb is reached.

4. *Connections with the olfactory bulb*

A major feature of the olfactory bulb is that of neural condensation of about 1000:1, in which some 5×10^7 primary input neurones connect with some 45,000 mitral cell axons of the main olfactory tract. Basing these calculations upon the work by Allison and Warwick (1949) on the rabbit, the 5×10^7 primary neurones converge in groups of about 25,000 upon some 1,900 glomeruli in the olfactory bulb; these glomeruli are comparatively large structures, visible to the naked eye. The impulses received by each glomerulus pass on through only about 24 mitral cells and 68 tufted cells. Additional fibres which form the anterior portion of the anterior commissure connect the tufted cells of one bulb with several structures in the other, mainly the granular layer, but also the glomerular layer. The axons of the mitral cells also send impulses to the granule layer and these, in turn, reactivate the bulb. This is one of a number of 'feedback loops' which may be important, and it has recently been suggested that the granule layer might be associated with short-term memory. The olfactory tract is believed to contain fibres transmitting impulses from the brain to the olfactory bulb, and these could

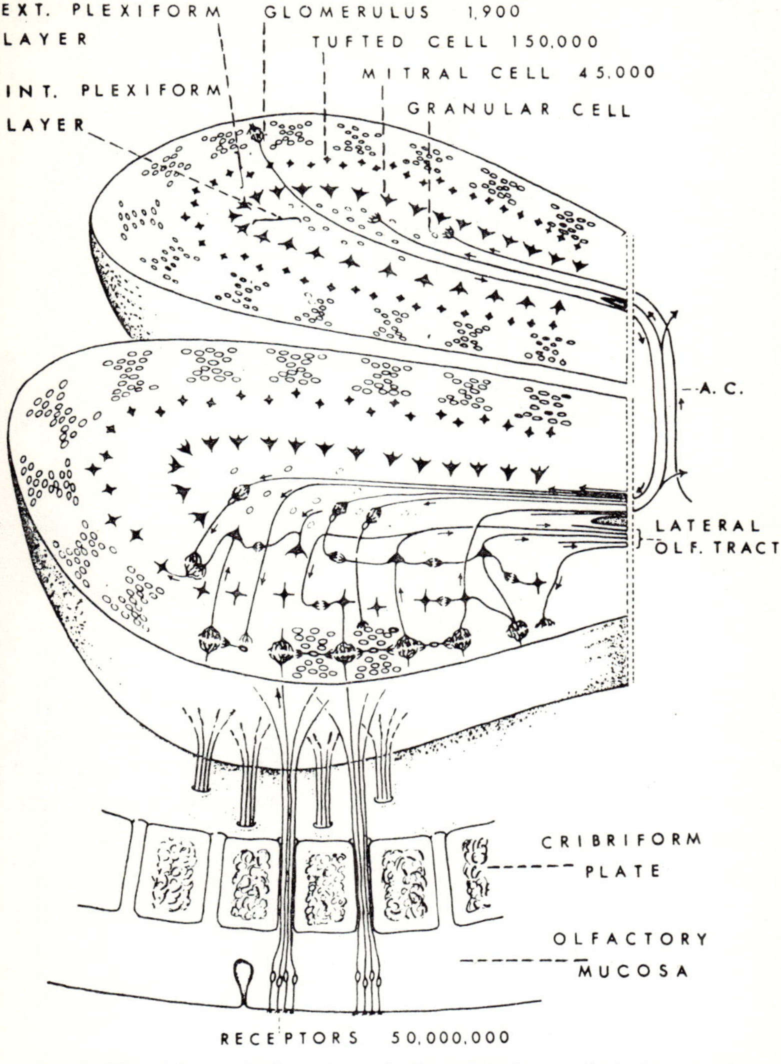

FIG. 3. The olfactory bulb—schematic (from Moulton and Tucker, 1964).

complicate the interpretation of electrical recordings. Moulton and Tucker (1964) indicated that altogether at least five 'feedback loops' and other connections in the olfactory bulb are implied from the available data and that 'there is now electrophysiological evidence that these anatomical paths are functional paths'.

Let us consider briefly some of the implications of neural condensation, in the olfactory bulb and elsewhere. In an important theoretical paper (whose implications have never really been taken further) Hainer *et al.* (1954) examined the quantitative

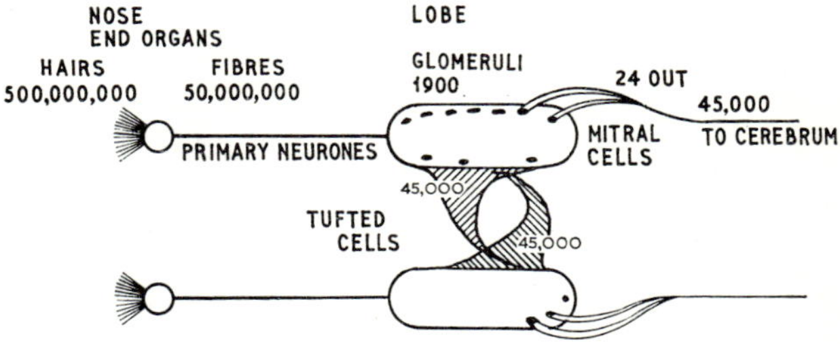

FIG. 4. Neural condensation in the olfactory bulb—schematic (from Hainer *et al.*, 1954).

effects of a structure of the type outlined in the preceding paragraphs. They added the assumptions that discrimination is maintained on the basis of a 'noisy' all-or-none communication system, and that stimulus concentration and perceived strength would be governed by the Weber-Fechner 'law'. The following properties were then deduced:

(1) This model system would involve a strictly limited number of 'just noticeable differences' between threshold and the maximal perceptible strength. Twenty-nine j.n.d.'s (30 levels) were required.
(2) The 29 perceptible steps would involve a range of stimulus concentration of 190,000 to 1.
(3) The required value for the Weber ratio was 0·52.

All these requirements are fairly consistent with what is actually observed in practice. There appears to be a general parallelism between the first two requirements and the decelerating function which relates stimulus intensity to certain forms of electrophysiological response. A similar 'law of diminishing returns' relates increasing stimulus concentration to perceived strength (see below). The calculated value of the Weber ratio is also of the right order of magnitude. These observations provide hypotheses for further elaboration and testing: they admirably illustrate possible relationships between stimulus specification, the structure of the sensory system, and what is perceived.

Hainer also calculated the number of possible odours on the assumption that there might be 24 types of input cells arranged in all possible ways in either state (on or off). This provides for some $2^{24} = 16 \cdot 8 \times 10^6$ separate qualities, which may be many more than actually required, although other model systems could be postulated. Finally, it is well known for other senses that a neural system with convergence has the property of 'sharpening up' output as compared with input. These effects are often discussed in connection with vision and touch, and possibly hearing. Their presence has been noted with odours, but apart from Hainer *et al.* no one seems yet to have attempted to formulate the possible consequences precisely. For example, in vision, Mach's bands have been partly attributed to neural convergence. Punctate tactile or visual stimuli may be sharpened in the output stage more than they are as peripheral stimuli. These phenomena have also been simulated by various computer methods; see, for example, Khanna and Noback (1963), Moray (1965).

5. *Neural connections within the brain*

The mitral cell axons from the olfactory bulb pass via the olfactory tracts to several secondary centres within the brain. Different methods do not give entirely consistent results, but the following details seem to be more or less agreed upon by different authorities. Several major pathways, both afferent and efferent, have been traced. However, the rhinencephalon of classical anatomy is no longer considered to be primarily concerned with olfaction, but rather with emotion, feeding behaviour and other

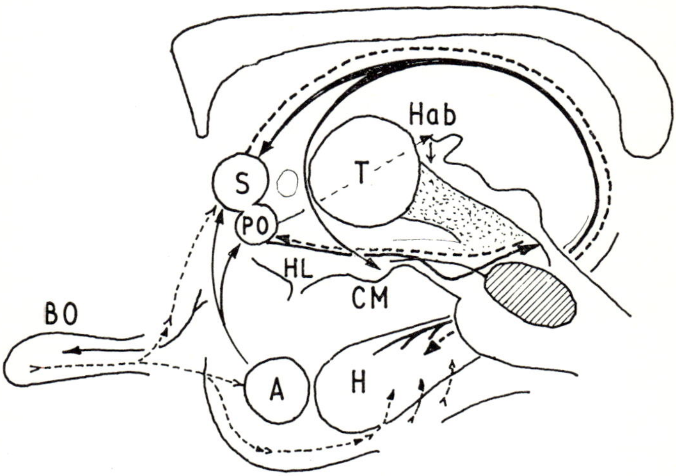

FIG. 5. Some neural connections in the brain (from Passouant, 1965, p. 129).

KEY

BO	Olfactory bulb		
S	Septum	afferent fibres	---->
A	Amygdala		
H	Hippocampus	efferent fibres	——>
T	Thalamus		
HL	Lateral hypothalamus		
PO	Pre-optic region		
CM	Mamillary body		

complex functions. (Brodal, 1947; Green, 1964). Olfactory pathways which have been traced include the afferent connections from the olfactory bulb to the septal region and the amygdaloid complex. Other systems are also involved which tend to form a number of closed loops well illustrated by Passouant (1965). According to Green (1964) electrophysiological data have failed to reveal olfactory activity beyond the piriform cortex. Secondary projection areas involve lateral connections with the prepiriform cortex and the olfactory tubercle. Moulton (1965) stated that another pathway has recently been traced which involves the thalamus, a major relay station for taste and other sensory systems. Information from direct electrical stimulation in man is rare, but according to Penfield and Jasper (1954) only the stimulation of the olfactory bulb itself and the uncus in the temporal lobe induces perception, the quality perceived varying according to the point stimulated. These observations fit in admirably with Hughlings Jackson's views (*c.* 1889) that the uncinate gyrus in the temporal lobe may be involved in the olfactory aurae which precede the fits in some cases of epilepsy. It is interesting that an electro-cortical conditioning technique has been used to determine olfactory thresholds (Riasanov, 1959). These were particularly related to the toxicity of certain substances and it was argued that a concentration which affected the central nervous system without being experienced consciously might be too high for safety.

6. *Some electrophysiological information*

The following main types of electrical activity have been recorded from different regions ranging from the mucosa to within the bulb itself.

(1) The gross electrical activity of the olfactory mucosa which forms the basis of the EOG (Electro-olfactogram) is analogous to certain similar types of activity in other sense organs. This activity is sometimes capable of being differentiated into 'receptor' and 'generator' activity, the latter being concerned with the initiation of the nerve current propogated in the olfactory neurone. Usually the EOG is a slow negative potential, but 'single unit activity' (extra-cellular) may occur superimposed upon the EOG potential.

(2) The 'all-or-none' activity of the olfactory neurones. In view of their fineness it seems rather doubtful whether these have been recorded in the olfactory system, other than extra-cellularly. Modern techniques of electronic averaging may provide 'asynchronous activity' recorded from a bundle of primary neurones.

(3) Slow potentials may be picked up from the olfactory bulb, similar to the EOG but capable of being separated from it. This is most likely to be a form of dendritic activity, probably a generator potential.

(4) Various other types of activity of the bulb which may be recorded from separate points and whose detailed responses depend upon the actual regions sampled.

Adapted from Moulton and Tucker (1964).

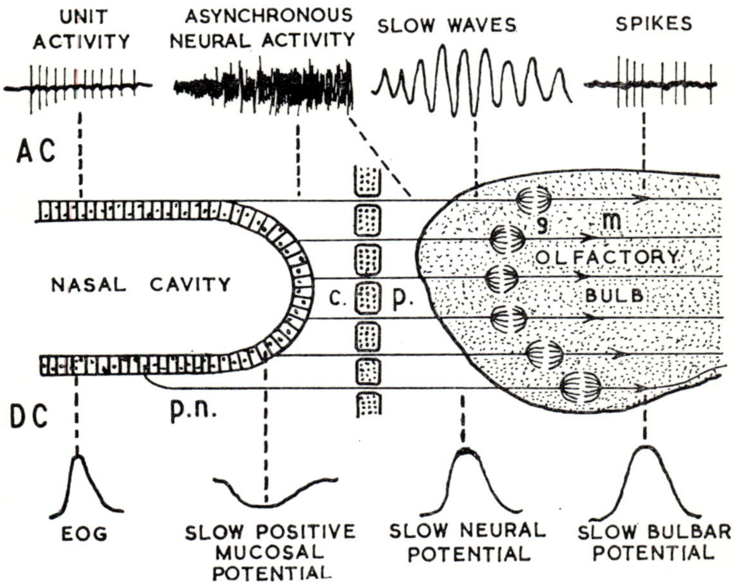

FIG. 6. Major types of electrical activity and their locus (from Moulton and Tucker, 1964).

A few specific examples will now be considered, deliberately moving from the periphery to the bulb. Mucosal potentials were first studied intensively by Ottoson (1956) using an electrode in light contact with the mucosa. A slow negative response was obtained when a puff of odour was directed in the region of the electrode. In some instances Ottoson (1959) found a close parallel between the EOG and the comparable type of activity of the bulb. Ottoson and von Sydow (1964) used this method to obtain information about the olfactory response to the constituents of a complex aroma, but the method requires further consideration, especially in view of the likelihood of species differences. What is required are several indices similar to the trichromatic coefficients and wave-length brightness function in colour perception, but the necessary background knowledge about the rules for olfactory composition is still lacking. More recently Gesteland *et al.* (1965) stressed the need to use moist air and low levels of stimulation. Some degree of regionalized specificity seemed apparent, but the data were not consistent enough under different conditions to demonstrate specific olfactory sites. Gesteland attributed the slow responses to some form of integrated activity of many individual receptors. The 'spike discharges' in recordings from this stage are considered to come from a single cell (extra-cellular). (See also Gesteland, 1966.)

Recordings from the olfactory bulb itself were first made by Lord Adrian, but in view of subsequent developments in technique it is best to attempt to summarize the general implications of these and later studies rather than to follow their historical development (Adrian, 1951, 1953). Recordings from different parts of the bulb tend to give distinctive response patterns, although any currently practicable method of sampling from different parts of the bulb provides a coarse system with comparatively few points. Some degree of differentiated response between the front and rear of the bulb seems to be established. For example, the ratio of A/H (ratio of response to amyl acetate and to heptane, respectively) in the front part of the olfactory bulb exceeds that in the rear (Mozell and Pfaffmann, 1954). These differences cannot be assigned with certainty to differences in sensitivity in different regions of the epithelium, although this could be a contributory factor. More recently, Moulton (1963) used rabbits with electrodes permanently implanted in the olfactory bulb. In one study of 15 odour stimuli, 8 could be distinguished by the electrical responses in 80% of the tests, and the remainder could be assigned to three broad groups. However, compounds yielding similar response patterns in one animal provided distinctive ones in another.

7. *Absolute sensitivity*

More attention has probably been given to determining the absolute sensitivity of the sense of smell than to any other functional relationship. One of the reasons for this lies in the theoretical assumption which dominated early work in both sensory physiology and experimental psychology that the threshold might prove to be a 'fundamental constant' of the human organism. This simple view is no longer held. However, in spite of contemporary reservations about the concept of the threshold, which have come to a head with recent developments in Decision Theory, these are only just beginning to penetrate into the measurement of olfactory thresholds. One of the most important considerations is how to handle in the olfactory situation the problem of the 'false positive' responses following the presentation of 'blank' stimuli. The false positives may be as much as 9% of the total, and since any statistical determination of the threshold is usually based upon that stimulus concentration to which there is a 50% response, the value of the threshold could be greatly affected by these false positives. The false positives are also considerably modified by the relative frequency of stimulus to blank, even for a fixed positive stimulus concentration.

There are many methods of producing odour stimuli, and many methods and arrangements for presenting them to the subject. The particular choice which is made to some extent determines the precise details of appropriate methods of analysis and calculations. Methods of stimulus generation include:

(a) The use of impregnated strips of absorbent paper.
(b) Elsberg's Blast Injection Technique (Elsberg *et al.*, 1935).
(c) Various types of 'Sniff Bottle'.

(d) The use of special chambers which accommodate the subject's head; some are literally 'man-sized'.
(e) Various type of 'flow olfactometer' in which streams of odour-laden gas or air are divided and recombined as required.
(f) Methods involving spraying the stimulus into the mouth.

Particular methods of calculation which should be used in the traditional or 'classical' psychophysical methods are set out in detail in standard texts such as Guilford (1954). Methods in which the subject actually *adjusts* the concentration until he can just detect (or recognize) it are rarely used with the sense of smell. When a regular order of presentation of a series of stimuli with fixed concentrations is used, the ascending series is most common. This method provides a quick and valuable estimate of sensitivity, which may be essential for such purposes as determining the approximate range of stimulus concentration over which to conduct more intensive studies by more precise methods. However, these sequential methods completely ignore the possibility and effect of the false positive responses referred to above. Even with a regular sequential presentation, the threshold value can be determined either by direct interpolation, or by pooling together a number of trials and proceeding by calculation. When random or haphazard orders of presentation are used the threshold can only be determined later by calculation, the implication being that these methods do not allow the investigator to monitor the sensitivity as the data are being collected. One common form is referred to in psychological literature as The Constant Method and was developed by Fechner. This is similar in principle to Probit Analysis used in toxicological studies, which was anticipated by about 70 years.

Many incidental variables are known to affect the value of the threshold but only a few examples will be given by way of illustration. When Komuro (1921) determined thresholds in an 'odourfree' environment he obtained values which represented about a four-fold increase in sensitivity as compared with the 'normal'. The 'recognition threshold' is usually quoted as being about three times the 'detection threshold'. The purity of the stimulus material is a major consideration which could not be dealt with adequately in most investigations carried out more than 10 years ago. Difficulties are greatest with substances of high threshold concentration when minute amounts of low threshold 'impurities' may have considerable effects. Very careful control over these aspects is essential for work of permanent value. Impurities can also have important qualitative effects. Ascending and descending series and random orders of stimulus presentation may give noticeably different threshold values, as shown by the following figures from Pangborn *et al.* (1964):

Stimulus—2-Heptanone
Method—Flow olfactometer

Randomized	$8 \cdot 2 \times 10^{-7}$ mg/ml.
Sequential down	$11 \cdot 2 \times 10^{-7}$ mg./ml.
Sequential up	$4 \cdot 8 \times 10^{-7}$ mg/.ml.

Many forms of systematic bias attributable to the effects of design features and other 'psychological' factors which complicate psychophysical measurements are of the same order of magnitude as the particular measure sought.

Actual methods of specifying the stimulus threshold differ according to the method used, and it is not always possible to state precise conversion factors. Concentration is usually expressed in absolute units (weight or molecules/ml. of air) or as concentration of odorant solution with which the air has come into equilibrium. The first alternative is to be preferred for comparative purposes, but this form of specification is only readily achieved by modern olfactometric techniques, usually involving precise, flow-dilution methods. The second alternative (the odorant in solution) allows easy repetition, but requires calibration procedures to relate solution concentration to absolute vapour concentration. For many substances of interest the data required are lacking and the whole subject warrants a much more comprehensive review. Pfaffmann (1951, p. 1163) stated that different methods put different substances more or less in the same order. However, if satisfactory inter-laboratory comparisons are to be made, it is essential that methods should be standardized *in all respects*. The time is ripe to do this *now* before vast amounts of new data are collected using methods which are not fully satisfactory. The following data are expressed in terms of molecules per ml. They have been obtained from a number of different sources, but experimental details are not given here.

Table 1

Some typical odour thresholds

	Molecules/ml. air	
Ionone	$1{\cdot}6 \times 10^{8}$	(a)
Allyl mercaptan	6×10^{7}	(b)
sec-Butyl mercaptan	2×10^{9}	(b)
Butyric acid	$1{\cdot}4 \times 10^{11}$	(c)
	$6{\cdot}9 \times 10^{9}$	(a)
Pyridine	$3{\cdot}1 \times 10^{11}$	(a)
	$1{\cdot}2 \times 10^{15}$	(a)
	$1{\cdot}5 \times 10^{13}$	(d)
Acetaldehyde	$9{\cdot}6 \times 10^{12}$	(a)
Camphor	5×10^{12}	(c)
	$6{\cdot}4 \times 10^{12}$	(a)
	4×10^{14}	(d)
Trimethylamine	$2{\cdot}2 \times 10^{13}$	(a)
Phenol	$7{\cdot}7 \times 10^{12}$	(a)
	$2{\cdot}6 \times 10^{13}$	(a)
	1×10^{13}	(b)
	$1{\cdot}3 \times 10^{15}$	(d)
Methanol	$1{\cdot}1 \times 10^{16}$	(a)
	$1{\cdot}9 \times 10^{16}$	(a)
Ethanol	$2{\cdot}4 \times 10^{15}$	(c)
	$2{\cdot}3 \times 10^{15}$	(a)
	$1{\cdot}6 \times 10^{17}$	(d)
Phenyl ethanol	$1{\cdot}7 \times 10^{17}$	(e)
Ethane	$1{\cdot}3 \times 10^{19}$	(c)

Sources:

(a) Zwaardemaker (1926) International Critical Tables. Corrected for 100-fold error (Jones, 1953).
(b) Stuiver (1958).
(c) Davies and Taylor (1959).
(d) Skramlik (1948).
(e) Wenzel (1949).

See also recent compilation by Laffort (1963) in which he made composite estimates of *p*.ol (analogous to pH) for 192 pure substances.

These facts may be summarized briefly by stating that reported threshold values for different substances range from about 10^7 to 10^{19} molecules per ml. However, results quoted for the same substances sometimes differ by as much as 100:1. Individual differences between normal persons used to be thought of as small (i.e. not exceeding about 30:1) but recent work by Baker (1963) on odour thresholds in terms of concentration in water reveals individual differences which attain as much as 1000:1, for particular substances (e.g. phenol). The author did not regard these differences as indicative of anosmia; the individual who was least sensitive to one substance might be most sensitive to another. Very careful investigations reveal that a very few molecules of those substances to which the human nose is most sensitive are sufficient to activate a single receptor, and as few as 40 molecules may be sufficient for perception to occur (Stuiver, 1958). Also, the trained human nose may be about 100 times more sensitive to some substances than gas chromatography, the most sensitive detector currently available (Kendall and Neilson, 1964).

8. *Differential sensitivity*

The subject of differential sensitivity can be dismissed quite briefly, although the differential threshold will normally be more tedious to measure than the absolute, except perhaps by the Triangle Test commonly used in the Food and Drink Industries. The differential threshold is usually defined as that change (or difference) in stimulus concentration which can just be detected. Is is a measure of the power of discrimination of the whole sensory system and may conveniently be compared with the resolving power of a physical instrument. Differential sensitivity may be reported in terms of the Weber ratio, defined as $D\Phi/\Phi$ where $D\Phi$ is the change (or difference) in stimulus concentration and Φ is the general level. The symbol Ψ is used to designate the psychological or sensory variable and the symbol Φ the physico-chemical variable (in this case, stimulus concentration). Some investigators have suggested that a small correction should be made to the formula for the ratio in the form:

$$D\Phi/(\Phi + \Phi_0)$$

(Miller 1947; Stone *et al.*, 1965). The main feature of the differential threshold for smell is that it is comparatively large, in direct contrast with the very low, limiting value of the absolute threshold. Relatively few determinations of differential thresholds have been reported in the literature. The figures given in Table 2 give some examples, particularly recent ones.

Table 2

The Weber ratio (selected examples)

Substance	*Weber ratio*	*Investigator*	*Method*
Phenyl ethanol	0·15	Wenzel (1949)	Blast Injection Technique
2-Heptanone	0·23—0·32	Stone *et al.* (1962)	Flow olfactometer
n-Heptanone	0·22—0·24	Stone (1963)	Flow olfactometer
2-Octanone	0·23—0·26	Stone (1964)	Flow olfactometer
n-Heptyl alcohol	0·23—0·31	Stone (1964)	Flow olfactometer
Ethyl-*n*-valerate	0·29—0·57	Stone (1964)	Flow olfactometer
Acetic acid	0·50—0·56	Stone (1964)	Flow olfactometer
Acetic acid	0·28—0·32	Stone *et al.* (1965)	Flow olfactometer
Propionic acid	0·37—0·54	Stone *et al.* (1965)	Flow olfactometer

9. *On perceptual scales*

The subject of perceptual scales is vast and bristles with controversies about the relative merits of different forms of expressing 'perceived strength' in numbers. Practically every method of expression has its own special numerical properties, and it is rarely feasible to test all possible alternatives before selecting a particular one. The simplest possible approach, used in the often quoted studies by Allison and Katz (1919) took the form of five 'categories': Detectable, Faint, Noticeable, Strong, Very Strong. Descriptive terms and the number of steps could each be studied in their own right (see for example Guilford, 1954). As indicated in Hainer's theoretical study the number of perceptible 'steps' of odour strength will not be large, hence a five-point scale is likely to be adequate for most purposes except when likes and dislikes are being considered. In view of the considerable difficulty experienced by some subjects in 'just detecting' or 'just recognizing' odours, some investigators have used the upper parts of such a scale as a means of characterizing the absolute threshold. Thus Stone *et al.* (1962) used 'the percent called high' and estimated the Weber ratio from the slope of the curve relating stimulus concentration on an arithmetic scale to the transformed values of the percentage responses. (This transformation procedure is also used in Probit Analysis.) Another common method of scaling perceived strength is derived from the differential threshold and the Weber-Fechner Law which *assumes* the constancy of the Weber ratio. The Weber-Fechner Law simply takes the familiar form:

$$\Psi = k \log (\Phi)$$

Again Ψ is the psychological variable and Φ the physical variable. Some of the practical and conceptual difficulties can be simplified by using a scale of 'dilution units'. The *number of times* a given stimulus has to be *diluted* until the threshold value is reached is taken as a measure of the strength above thresholds of the original concentration. Since one is normally concerned only with relative rather than absolute units (assuming that Weber's ratio has a constant value) any other arbitrary dilution step can be accepted. Thus in several technological applications the number of dilution steps on the scale of two is widely used and this is often designated the 'Odour Number'. Prince and Ince (1958) used such a dilution device with 32 full steps and odour numbers varying between 6 and 11 were obtained with different observers. These differences may indicate individual differences in threshold sensitivity. (It was found convenient to deal with this range of dilutions by 12 discrete operations of which every *second* one involved a twofold dilution, thus implying effective discrimination in steps of $2\frac{1}{2}$ or an 'equivalent Weber ratio' of approximately 0·41.) Hanson (1964) used a similar method, assuming a value of the differential threshold of 0·30 with an odour-nuisance problem. In order to attenuate an objectionable odour to a tolerable (near threshold) value, a dilution of more than 1000:1 might be required. Merely halving the original concentration has only a slight effect.

Another approach to scaling odour strength which is being increasingly used with the sense of smell is that of Magnitude Estimation, originally proposed by Stevens (1956). In its simplest form this involves the subject using numbers in such a way that if he calls one stimulus 10 it is *perceived as being* 10 times as strong as that which is designated 1 and 1/10 as strong as that designated 100. This method may be used with or without a designated reference standard. In spite of criticisms this method has the advantage of being 'simple and robust' (F. N. Jones, personal communication). A somewhat different theoretical relationship between what is perceived and the stimulus concentration is involved, compared with the Weber-Fechner law. Magnitude Estimation leads to a Power Law rather than to the traditional logarithmic relationship, thus:

(1) Weber-Fechner $\Psi = k \log \Phi$
(2) Magnitude estimation $\Psi = m\Phi^n$
or $\log \Psi = \log m + n \log \Phi$

However, this is not the place to go into the various arguments involved.

The Power Law relationship gives a non-linear function when Ψ is plotted against Φ except when $n = 1$. Values of n which have been obtained with odours are appreciably less than 1, usually ranging from 0·4 to 0·6 (Engen, 1961, 1964; Engen and Lindström, 1963; Jones, 1958a, b; Reese and Stevens, 1960). Engen (1965) obtained two very different values of n for propanol and octanol (0·42 and 0·13, respectively) which fits in well with the fact that octanol seems to decline less rapidly in perceived strength with decreasing concentration than does propanol. (Engen's paper also includes experimental data on the response of the neonate to alcohols having different numbers of carbon atoms.)

We have already seen how the Power Law with $n < 1$ essentially characterizes a system which involves a rapidly decreasing effect of increasing concentration on perceived strength. This fits in well with some of Hainer's observations. It is also basically consistent with the slow response of industrial and other strong odours to the processes of dilution. As Reese and Stevens (1960) have pointed out, the Power Law formulation with $n < 1$ is also consistent with the decreasing rate of growth of the integrated response of the olfactory bulb when the stimulus is increased. However, other theoretical models might also lead to similar conclusions.

10. *The interaction between odours*

The interaction between different odours is a complex subject with many theoretical and practical implications. Neutralization or masking play an important part in odour control, although many of the specific details usually remain trade secrets. The interaction between odours is also of obvious importance both in perfumery and in flavour chemistry, in the production of recognizable and balanced odours and flavours by natural and synthetic means. Much of the subject remains an art rather than a science. Not only is an overall theoretical system lacking, which would enable interactions to be predicted in detail, but also the number of groups of substances actually studied is small. Those examined by different investigators overlap only slightly. Chemical interaction between different odour stimuli is excluded from the present discussion, although it is necessary to ensure that this has not occurred in any particular combination of odour stimuli. The destruction of odours by various methods including the use of ozone or nascent oxygen is one method of odour control; for further details see Summer (1963). It is of interest to note that, according to Zwaardemaker, (1925), before 1888 physiologists took very little interest in odour compensation because they believed it to be due *simply to chemical interaction*. (Zwaardemaker's italics.)

Various terms are used to designate different types of interaction. The terms 'fatigue' and 'adaptation' are practically synonymous, and there is little final evidence about the location of these functions. Part of the renewed interest in detailed information about the interaction between odours lies in the light this may throw on the mechanisms involved and their possible anatomical locus, or the nature of the neural coding-processes involved. In particular, further light should be shed on the subject of specific receptor sites. Other commonly used terms are 'neutralization' or 'compensation', and 'masking', the last term referring to overlaying one odour by another, usually considered to be less undesirable. The masking stimulus itself can come to be regarded as unpleasant by association; perhaps certain specific associations such as that of pine odour, or of *p*-dichlorobenzene with public lavatories represent a case in point.

Methods of studying the main types of interaction between different odours are varied. Some investigators concentrate on measuring thresholds and how these are modified by the presence of additional stimuli (e. g. Zwaardemaker, 1925 p. 124; Cheeseman, 1964; Baker, 1964). Others have studied concentrations well above threshold usually with binary mixtures (e.g. Jones and Woskow, 1964). Still others have investigated qualitative changes and interactions, using procedures comparable with the olfactory analysis of perfumes by successive fatigue with mixtures of progressively identified constituents. Investigations reported by Guillot (1948) and Le Magnen (1948, 1964) fall in this group and were specifically related to partial anosmia and specific receptor sites. Guadagni *et al.* (1963) studied the interaction between a number of important components in flavour complexes. Stimulus concentrations ranging from 1/3 to 5 times the threshold values of the individual constituents were employed. Only one clear instance of synergistic action was claimed. Equal amounts of dimethyl disulphide and 3-methyl butanal (in terms of threshold concentrations) interacted in this way to give an effective sensitivity of 1·37 times that of the consituents, assuming that their effects were simply additive in terms of an equation of the type:

$$\frac{C_1}{T_1}+\frac{C_2}{T_2}=\frac{C_M}{T_M}$$

where C is the stimulus concentration, T the threshold concentration, M the mixture of substances 1 and 2. This exceptional result still requires confirmation, for the error of determining the threshold has to be considered and in any case the difference quoted is still well within the range of the first step from the threshold in terms of the 'just noticeable difference'. The most recent study is that of Kendall and Neilson (1966) in which they examined the combined effects of various binary and quaternary mixtures of four common flavouring agents, in various proportions over the range from 1/100 threshold value to 100 times the threshold. In this case, purely quantitative information about the responses was supplemented by an expert panel's descriptive evaluation.

In view of what has been said about the specificity of current knowledge, there is little point in elaborating further details here. For these the reader must refer to the original sources. The 'Zwaardemaker principle' of neutralization or compensation is still used in commercial practice and one manufacturer reports in his technical literature that well over 1000 specific counteractants are known and are blended together for particular purposes. The formulae for neutralization represent this specific technical knowledge, and procedures have been developed in recent years for incorporating odour pairing agents in a number of commercial products such as plastics and rubber, etc. (Plaistowe, 1966). Summer (1963) drew attention to the fact that a particular mixture functions effectively over a limited range of concentrations, both relative and absolute, and that in everyday conditions the required proportions which have been established in the laboratory may not be maintained. Zwaardemaker (p. 131) himself previously stressed the principle involved here.

Various investigators have described the possible effects of two or more odours upon each other. Zwaardemaker referred to the following possible alternatives: approximate neutralization, a vague and feeble resultant, and rivalry or alternation between the perception of the two odour stimuli. The possibility of new qualities arising, not predictable from a knowledge of the qualities of the original constituents, should be added to this list. Also a number of instances of synergistic interactions between particular stimuli, depending upon the concentrations involved, have been clearly established. In addition to Guadagni's tentative example, Baker reported positive interactions between acetophenone and *m*-cresol, with a pronounced synergism when the mixture contained 75% *m*-cresol. Again, examples of synergism, antagonism and direct additivity were noted. Jones and Woskow's study was entirely concerned with perceived strength above threshold. Contours of 'equal perceived strength' were printed out by computer. In general, the results of mixing were neither simply additive in terms of the functional relationship involved, nor a straightforward average of the (perceived) strength of the constituents. There was one case of enhancement at low intensities (xylene-benzene mixture with benzene as reference standard). Kendall and Neilson reported that geranial was recognizable at 1/100 its threshold value in a mixture containing anethole and geranial in 'equal odour strength combinations', However, insufficient information is given to evaluate the control of psychological variables in this study. Accepting these facts at their face value we may say that they have long been suspected before they have been demonstrated systematically. Perfumers have long been aware of the importance of small quantities of 'impurities' in their raw materials which may modify strength or quality in desirable ways, and it is part of the art of the perfumer, and the flavour chemists, to exploit the emergence of novel qualities.

11. *Some clinical studies*

The term 'clinical' is used here to denote detailed studies about individuals rather than restricting it to abnormal conditions. Several relevant topics have already been touched on; this section draws attention to some of the growing points which might otherwise have been neglected. Several references have already been made to anosmia and its practical and theoretical implications. The need for much more precisely controlled studies has been noted, using stimuli of known and controlled purity. Hardly any of the observations about anosmia have involved precise threshold determinations, which are perhaps too time-consuming for clinical studies. It is customary rather to use a (limited) range of common substances and simply to use the information about whether these can be detected or recognized (i.e. named). Sumner (1962) examined certain features of what psychologists might refer to as the 'item difficulty' represented by the individual items in such a series of common odours. In particular he found that there was little relationship between frequency and desirability of use in clinical practice, and suggested an effective group of stimuli. In a later paper (Sumner, 1964) he discussed various features of 'post-traumatic anosmia' including its incidence, the importance of the period of amnesia and the site of the injury. However, one of the most extensive studies, still using a single stimulus concentration was reported by Patterson and Lauder (1948), who tested over 4000 persons.

On the subject of individual differences a passing reference may be made to preferences and likes and dislikes. Linnaeus (1756) was well aware of these in so far as he divided his seven well-known odour classes into three groups of which the middle one was characterized as 'pleasant to some and unpleasant to others'.

This fact is also familiar in the context of more recent botanical studies. For example, Blakeslee (1918), whose name is much better known in the context of taste blindness, drew attention to the fact that differences in views about the odour of the verbena plant might well reflect actual differences in what is perceived. (We have our own personal experiences of this in the smell of phenyl ethanol, which to one member of the group involved in the studies in Norwich is floral and honey-like, whereas to another it is faecal, or at least it has a 'skatolic' note.) The origin of these and other differences in preference and perception is certainly complex and both biological and social factors may be involved. Thus, for example, Stein *et al.* (1958) were inclined to attribute to socialization processes the fact that, when different age groups are compared, synthetic sweat and synthetic faeces suddenly become disliked (between the ages of 4 and 5) as the child takes on the value judgements of its parents. Foster (1950) also reported a number of differences between different age groups from infancy to the adult stage, and so has Moncrieff (this Symposium p. 32). However, other factors could be investigated.

12. *Summing up*

The sense of smell has been discussed from several different points of view, especially those of physiology and psychophysics. Many interesting topics have been deliberately omitted, and others have received only cursory attention. A few points may be stressed without attempting to recapitulate material that has already been amply condensed. Clearly there is a need for a critical examination of the concept of the specific receptor site from the standpoint of all the disciplines involved. An examination should be made of precisely what properties a set of odour primaries should have and how these could be tested experimentally. The need for careful standardization of quantitative and qualitative methods must be reiterated. Comparatively little has been written here about the effects of drugs on odour perception, since this is touched upon in other contributions to this Symposium. Wenzel and Sieck (1966) included 12 references on this theme in a recent review on olfaction.

New publications continue to appear with increasing frequency, the most recent being the Proceedings of the Second International Symposium on Olfaction and Taste (Hayashi, 1967) in which 17 papers are on odour and olfaction. Such contributions are changing the balance of the literature, but they still tend to be fragmentary rather than integrated. The continued piecemeal accumulation of knowledge is inefficient and strategic problems are raised. Decisions are needed on which approaches are most useful and which problems are the profitable ones to investigate. These decisions should take account of a developing framework of general knowledge as well as specific, factual information, and the importance of the multidisciplinary approach is now self-evident.

Acknowledgements

This review was prepared during the tenure of a Civil Service Principal Research Fellowship, which is gratefully acknowledged. I wish to thank my colleagues, particularly Dr. E. C. Bate Smith, and Dr. D. G. Land for helpful discussions.

REFERENCES

Major Reviews and Texts

Adey, W. R. (1959). The Sense of Smell. *In* Handbook of Physiology, Section 1. Neurophysiology, vol. 1, pp. 535–548. Washington D.C.: American Physiological Society.

Benjamin, R. M., Halpern, B. P., Moulton, D. G. and Mozell, M. M. (1965). *Ann. Rev. Psychol.*, **16**, 381. (230 references).

Hayashi, T. (Ed. 1967). Olfaction and Taste II. Oxford: Pergamon Press.

Miner, R. W. (Ed. 1954), Basic odour research correlation. *Ann. N.Y. Acad. Sci.*, **58**, 13–260.

Moulton, D. G. and Tucker, D. (1964). Electrophysiology of the olfactory apparatus. *Ann. N.Y. Acad. Sci.*, **116**, 380–428.

Wenzel, B. M. (1948). *Psychol. Bull.*, **45**, 231.

Wenzel, B. M. and Sieck, M. H. (1966). Olfaction. *Ann. Rev. Physiol.*, **28,** 381. (262 references).

Zotterman, Y. (Ed. 1963). Olfaction and Taste. Oxford: Pergamon Press.

Other References

Adrian, E. D. (1951). *Année Psychol.*, **50,** 107.

Adrian, E. D. (1953). *J. Laryngol. Otol.*, **70,** 1.

Adrian, E. D. (1953). *Acta Physiol. Scand.*, **29,** 5.

Allison, A. C. and Warwick, R. T. R. (1949). *Brain*, **72,** 186.

Allison, V. C. and Katz, S. H. (1919). *J. ind. eng. Chem.*, **11,** 336.

Amoore, J. E. (1964). *Ann. N.Y. Acad. Sci.*, **116,** 457.

Amoore, J. E. and Venstrom, D. (1966). *J. Food Sci.*, **31,** 118.

Baker, R. (1963). *J. Amer. Water Works Assoc.*, **55,** 913.

Baker, R. (1964). *Ann. N.Y. Acad. Sci.*, **116,** 495.

Blakeslee, A. F. (1918). *Science*, **48,** 298.

Brodal, A. (1947). *Brain*, **70,** 179.

Cheeseman, G. H. (1964). *J. Inst. Packaging*, **10,** 40.

Davies, J. T. (1962). In Biological Receptor Mechanisms. *Soc. exp. Biol.*, **16,** 170. Cambridge University Press.

Davies, J. T. (1965). *J. theoret. Biol.*, **8,** 1.

Davies, J. T. and Taylor, F. H. (1959). *Biol. Bull.*, **117,** 222.

Davis, H. (1961). *Physiol. Rev.*, **41,** 391.

Elsberg, C. A. and Levy, I. (1935). *Bull. Neurol. Inst. N.Y.*, **4,** 5.

Engen, T. (1960). *Percept. and Motor Skills*, **10,** 195.

Engen, T. (1961). Report No. 106, Psychological Laboratory, University of Stockholm.

Engen, T. (1964). *Ann. N.Y. Acad. Sci.*, **116,** 504.

Engen, T. (1965). *J. exp. Psychol.*, **70,** 611.

Engen, T. and Lindström, C. O. (1963). *Scand. J. Psychol.*, **4,** 23.

Engen, T. and McBurney, D. H. (1964). *J. exp. Psychol.*, **68,** 435.

Engen, T. and Pfaffmann, C. (1959). *J. exp. Psychol.*, **58,** 23.

Engen, T. and Pfaffmann, C. (1960). *J. exp. Psychol.*, **59,** 214.

Foster, D. (1950). *Perfumery and Essent. Oil Rec.*, **41,** 244.

Gesteland, R. C. (1966). *Discovery*, **27,** 29.

Gesteland, R. C., Lettvin, J. Y. and Pitts, W. H. (1965). *J. Physiol.*, **181,** 525.

Green, J. D. (1964). *Physiol. Rev.*, **44,** 561.

Guadagni, D. G., Buttery, R. G., Okano, S. and Burr, H. K. (1963). *Nature (Lond.)*, **200,** 1288.

Guilford, J. P. (1954). Psychometric Methods. New York and London: McGraw-Hill.

Guillot, M. (1948). *Compt. rend. Acad. Sci.*, (Paris), **226,** 1307.

Guillot, M. (1956). *In* Actualités Pharmacologiques. (ed. Hazard, R.), 9e series p. 21.

Hainer, R. M., Emslie, A. G. and Jacobsen, A. (1954). *Ann. N.Y. Acad. Sci.*, **58,** 158.

Hanson, S. W. F. (1964). *Fishing News International,* **3,** 171.

Harper, R., Bate Smith, E. C. and Land, D. G. (1966). Odour Description and Odour Classification. A Critical Examination. LTRS Internal Record Memorandum 445—cyclostyled.

Harper, R., Bate Smith, E. C. and Land, D. G. (in press). Odour Description and Odour Classification. London: J. and A. Churchill Ltd.

Jackson, J. Hughlings. (1889, 90). *Brain,* **12,** 346.

Jerome, E. A. (1942). *Arch. Psychol.*, (N.Y.) **39,** No. 274.

Jones, F. N. (1953). *Science,* **118,** 333.

Jones, F. N. (1955). *J. Psychol.*, **40,** 223.

Jones, F. N. (1958a). *Amer. J. Psychol.*, **71,** 305.

Jones, F. N. (1958b). *Amer. J. Psychol.*, **71,** 423.

Jones, F. N. (in press). *In* Theories of Odor and Odor Measurement (ed. Tanyolaç, N.) New York: Spartan Books.

Jones, F. N. and Woskow, M. H. (1964). *Ann. N.Y. Acad. Sci.*, **116,** 484.

Kendall, D. A. and Neilson, A. J. (1964). *Ann. N.Y. Acad. Sci.*, **116,** 567.

Kendall, D.A. and Neilson, A.J. (1966). *J.Food Sci.*, **31,** 268.

Khanna, S. M. and Noback, C. R. (1963). *Trans. N.Y. Acad. Sci., Ser. II,* **25,** 516.

Komuro, K. (1921). *Arch. néerland. physiol.*, **6,** 20.

Kruger, K., Feldzmann, A. N. and Miles, W. R. (1955). *Amer. J. Psychol.,* **68,** 117.

Laffort, P. (1963). *Arch. Sci. Physiol.*, **17,** 75.

Le Magnen, J. (1948). *Compt. rend. Acad. Sci.*, (Paris), **226,** 753.

Le Magnen, J. (1965). *La France et ses Parfums,* **8,** 112.

Linnaeus (Linné, C. von) (1756). Odores medicamentorum (1752). *In* Amoenitates Academicae, 3, 183. Stockholm: Lars Salvius.

McLennan, H. and Graystone, P. (1965). *Can. J. Physiol. and Pharmacol.*, **43,** 1009.

Miller, G. A. (1947). *J. acoust. Soc. Amer.*, **19,** 609.

Moray, N. (1964). Communication to *Brit. Psych. Soc.*, December Conference.

Moulton, D. G. (1963). *In* Olfaction and Taste, (ed. Zotterman Y.) p. 71. Oxford: Pergamon Press.

Moulton, D. G. (1965). *J. Food Sci.*, **30,** 908.

Moulton, D. G. and Tucker, D. (1964). See general reviews.

Mozell, M. M. and Pfaffmann, C. (1954). *Ann. N.Y. Acad. Sci.*, **58,** 96.

Mozell, M. M. (1958). *J. Neurophysiol.*, **21,** 183.

Ottoson, D. (1956). *Acta. Physiol. Scand.*, **35** (supp. 122) 1.

Ottoson, D. (1959). *Acta Physiol. Scand.*, **47,** 149.

Ottoson, D. (1963). *In* Olfaction and Taste (ed. Zotterman, Y.), p. 35. Oxford: Pergamon Press.

Ottoson, D. and von Sydow, E. (1964). *Life Sci.*, **3,** 1111.

Ough, C. S. and Stone, H. (1961). *J. Food Sci.*, **26**, 452.
Pangborn, R. M., Berg, H. W., Roessler, E. B. and Webb, A. D. (1964). *Percept. and Motor Skills*, **18**, 91.
Passouant, P. (1965). *La France et ses Parfums*, **8**, 123.
Patterson, P. M. and Lauder, B. A. (1948). *J. Heredity*, **39**, 295.
Penfield W. and Jasper, H. (1954). Epilepsy and the Functional Anatomy of the Human Brain. Boston: Little Brown.
Pfaffmann, C. (1951). In Handbook of Experimental Psychology (ed. Stevens, S. S.). New York: John Wiley and Sons Inc.
Plaistowe, D. W., Airwick Ltd. (1966). Personal communication.
Prince, R. G. H. and Ince, H. J. (1958). *J. app. Chem.*, **8**, 314.
Reese, T. S. and Stevens, S. S. (1960). *Amer. J. Psychol.*, **73**, 424.
Riasanov, V. A. (1959). Proc. Int. Clean Air Cong. (Lond.), p. 175.
Ruzicka, L. (1957). *In* Molecular Structure and Organoleptic Quality, p. 116. London: Soc. Chem. Ind.
Schutz, H. G., Overbeck, R. C. and Laymon, R. S. (1958). Q.M.F. & C.I. Report (Chicago) Ref. P-1115-Rep + 3.
Skramlik, E. von (1925). *Z. f. Psychol. u. Physiol. d. Sinnesorgane*, **56**, 69.
Skramlik, E. von (1948). *Pflüg. Arch. ges. Physiol.*, **249**, 702.
Stone, H. (1963). *J. exp. Psychol.*, **66**, 466.
Stone, H. (1964). *Ann. N.Y. Acad. Sci.*, **116**, 527.
Stone, H., Ough, C. S. and Pangborn, R. M. (1962). *J. Food Sci.*, **27**, 197.
Stuiver, M. (1958). Biophysics of the sense of smell. Doctoral Thesis. 's-Gravenhage: Uitgeverij Excelsior.
Stein, M., Ottenberg, P. and Roulet, H. (1958). *Arch. Neurol. Psychiat.*, **80**, 264.
Stevens, S. S. (1956). *Amer. J. Psychol.*, **69**, 1.
Summer, W. (1963). Methods of Air Deodorisation. Amsterdam and London: Elsevier.
Sumner, D. (1962). *Lancet*, **ii**, 895.
Sumner, D. (1964). *Brain*, **87**, 107.
Wenzel, B. M. (1949). *J. exp. Psychol.*, **39**, 129.
Wenzel, B. M. (1954). *Ann. N.Y. Acad. Sci.*, **58**, 58.
Zwaardemaker, H. (1925). L'Odorat. Paris: Libraire Octave Doin.
Zwaardemaker, H. (1926). Odoriferous Materials. *In* International Critical Tables, vol. 1, p. 358. London and New York: McGraw-Hill.

EFFECTS OF DRUGS ON RESPONSES IN THE OLFACTORY BULB

G. C. SALMOIRAGHI and R. A. NICOLL

Laboratory of Neuropharmacology (NIMH) at Saint Elizabeth's Hospital, Washington, D.C.

ALTHOUGH this review is primarily concerned with the pharmacology of the olfactory pathway, much of it deals with the anatomy and physiology of the rabbit olfactory bulb. This is justified because even with rather elaborate pharmacological techniques it is often impossible to specify the exact site and mode of action of drugs in the central nervous system. The difficulties of this field of research become still greater when drugs are used as tools for the identification of central synaptic transmitters. Standard routes of drug administration are then undesirable because of the complexity of the synaptic inputs on any given central neurone, the presence of diffusional and enzymatic barriers and the necessity for reducing as much as possible the likelihood of indirect mediation of drug effects. While imperfect, the technique of microelectrophoresis—first introduced for CNS studies by Curtis and Eccles (1958) in an analysis of the pharmacological properties of Renshaw cells, and subsequently extensively used by Curtis *et al.* (1965), Krnjević *et al.* (1965), Bradley and Wolstencroft (1965), Phillis (1965) and in our own laboratory (Salmoiraghi and Stefanis, 1965)—is at present the method of choice for pharmacological studies of central neurones because it restricts drug administration to the immediate surroundings of an individually recorded unit, it bypasses some of the major diffusional barriers and greatly reduces the number of possible indirect sites of drug action. When applied to the study of the responses of the rabbit olfactory bulb neurones to suspected central neurohumoral transmitters, this approach provided evidence of participation of noradrenaline or a close chemical analogue in the mediation of the response in an inhibitory pathway (Bloom *et al.*, 1964; Salmoiraghi *et al.*, 1964). We here review these studies in the light of anatomical, physiological and histochemical evidence, and try to bring out the interpretative difficulties inherent in this field of research and to further elaborate on the possible site or sites of action of noradrenaline in the rabbit olfactory bulb.

Anatomy

Figure 1A, adapted from Cajal (1955) and from Allison (1953), summarizes the major anatomical findings in the rabbit olfactory bulb, including recent histochemical evidence on the distribution of cholinesterase-containing (Shute and Lewis, 1963) and monoamine-containing nerve fibres (Dahlström *et al.* 1965).

Olfactory nerves arise from bipolar cells in the nasal mucosa and spread over the surface of the ipsilateral olfactory bulb, terminating in egg-shaped masses called glomeruli. In addition to some 26,000 olfactory nerve terminals, each glomerulus contains the dendritic tufts of about 100 secondary neurones and of one or two periglomerular neurones (Allison, 1953). The latter are considered to be cells of interglomerular association. The secondary neurones are of two types, mitral cells and tufted cells. The cell bodies of the mitral cells are confined to a narrow layer about 700 μ below the surface of the olfactory bulb, tufted cells being scattered between the glomeruli and the mitral cells. Tufted and mitral cells have two types of dendritic processes—a main dendrite, which terminates in the glomerulus and two or more accessory dendrites which extend laterally forming a dense plexus of fibres in the external plexiform layer, within which lie the cell bodies of tufted cells. Each of the secondary neurones emits one axon—the mitral cell axons form the lateral olfactory tract (LOT) while the axons of tufted cells form the anterior limb of the anterior commissure (AAC). Before forming discrete tracts, the axons of both cell types emit collaterals, of which some end in a rich plexus of fibres beneath the mitral cell layer (internal plexiform layer) and among granule cells, while others double back to end in the external plexiform layer among the accessory dendrites of tufted and mitral cells. The LOT ends in the ipsilateral prepiriform cortex as well as in the central and medial amygdaloid

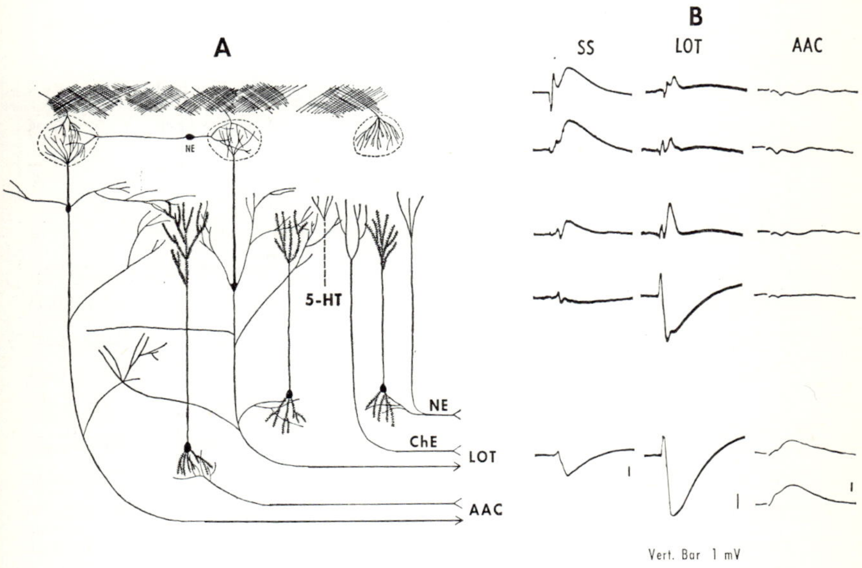

FIG. 1. Diagram of cellular structures and extracellular field potentials at various depths in the rabbit olfactory bulb. *A*. Diagrammatic representation of the interrelationships of major cell types. Symbols: NE indicates fibres and neurones containing noradrenaline; 5-HT and ChE, fibres containing serotonin- and cholinesterase. 1 to 5, layers of the olfactory bulb: (1) layer of olfactory nerves, (2) layer of glomeruli, (3) external plexiform layer, (4) internal plexiform layer, and (5) granular layer. A, B, and C: subdivisions of the external plexiform layer of which C is the layer of mitral cells. *B*. Extracellular field potentials elicited by single-shock electrical stimuli to the surface (SS), the lateral olfactory tract (LOT) and the anterior limb of the anterior commissure (AAC) as recorded in the different layers of the olfactory bulb. Sweep duration for records under SS and LOT, 35 msec; for records under AAC, 170 msec.

nuclei, but it gives off a rich supply of axon collaterals to the olfactory peduncle and to the frontal and temporal cortex as it sweeps over these regions. The AAC ends predominantly in the granule cell layer of the contralateral olfactory bulb, but also bilaterally in the stria terminalis and central amygdaloid nuclei. The deepest layer of the bulb, beneath the internal plexiform layer, contains mostly granule cells whose processes run outward towards the external plexiform layer where they form numerous synapses with the accessory dendrites of tufted and mitral cells, similar to the type II synapses described by Gray (1961), thought to have an inhibitory function (Eccles, 1964). In addition to these, synapses oriented in the opposite direction, i.e. from mitral dendrites to granule cell processes have been described by Hirata (1964), Andres (1965) and Rall *et al.* (1966) and there is anatomical and physiological evidence that these synapses are excitatory.

In addition to the fibre systems leaving the olfactory bulb via the LOT and the AAC, there are centrifugal fibre systems entering the bulb. Cajal (1955) classed these centrifugal fibres into two groups, thick and thin. The thin fibres arise from the tufted cells of the contralateral bulb, are contained in the AAC and then run diffusely through the olfactory peduncle, ending in the granule cell layer. The precise origin of the thick fibres is unclear, but they are thought to arise from the sphenoidal region of the cerebrum, and possibly from the olfactory tubercle. They run diffusely through the olfactory peduncle, some enmeshed in the LOT and the AAC, ending mainly in the granule cell layer but a few extend towards the surface of the olfactory bulb as far as the glomeruli (Cragg, 1962; Powell and Cowan, 1963). From their study of these centrifugal fibres, Powell and Cowan (1963) conclude: 'The finding that the centrifugal fibres in the lateral olfactory tract terminate in relation to the periglomerular cells as well as with the granule cells indicates that the centrifugal control of olfaction may operate at the level of both the first-and second-order neurones, as well as interacting with the commissural fibres from the olfactory bulb of the opposite side.' Recent histochemical studies permit a different classification of centrifugal fibres to the olfactory bulb, but the relationship of these histochemical types of fibres to the thick and thin classification of Cajal (1955) is unclear. Shute and Lewis (1963) traced the cholinesterase-staining olfactory radiation from the lateral preoptic area and olfactory tubercle, which has many cholinesterase-containing neurones, into the olfactory stalk and lateral olfactory tract and from there to the prepiriform cortex and to the glomerular and mitral cell layers of the olfactory bulb. Recently, Dahlström *et al.* (1965) have used histochemical fluorescence techniques to localize nerve fibres and neurones containing monoamines. They found afferent fibres containing noradrenaline (NA) in the olfactory stalk and bulb presumably originating from the brain-stem, and ending principally in the granule cell layer but also in the neighbourhood of mitral cells. In addition, they found nerve terminals containing 5-hydroxytryptamine (5-HT) in the external plexiform layer. With the exception of a few periglomerular neurones containing catecholamines, no other cells in the olfactory bulb appear to contain monoamines. Since the fibres of the periglomerular neurones are restricted to an area adjacent to the glomeruli, the fibres containing NA and 5-HT should be centrifugal. These histochemical findings are paralleled by the pharmacological observations reviewed below.

Physiological studies

Since the olfactory bulb is a laminated structure of concentrically arranged layers, the study of field potentials offers a valuable guide to understanding cellular functions. Figure 1B, adapted from Ochi (1963), shows the relationship of field potentials evoked by single-shock stimuli to the surface of the bulb, the LOT and the AAC respectively to the various layers of the olfactory bulb. With surface stimulation, an initial negative spike followed by a slow negative potential is recorded at the surface some distance away from the stimulating electrode. Inasmuch as the spike is largest in those areas of the bulb containing the most olfactory nerve fibres and it is lost after the nerves have degenerated or when the electrode is advanced into the bulb, the spike is likely to be the compound action potential of olfactory nerve fibres activated by surface stimulation. The slow negative wave which follows the spike is small on the surface, reaches its maximum in the external plexiform layer, decreases to zero near mitral cells and becomes positive below this layer. This observation and the finding that the wave—but not the initial spike—can be inhibited by a conditioning stimulus to the surface or to the LOT suggests that the slow negative potential elicited by surface stimulation is due to the depolarization of the secondary neurones' dendrites (Iwase *et al.*, 1961). With ipsilateral LOT stimulation, similar characteristic changes occur in the field potential as the recording electrode is advanced into the olfactory bulb (Phillips *et al.*, 1963). At the surface, there is an initial positive deflection, followed by a negative wave and then by a second negative deflection of smaller amplitude and longer duration than the first. The positive wave is lost as the electrode penetrates the bulb. On the other hand, the amplitude of the first negative wave progressively increases—while its latency progressively decreases—until the mitral cells are reached. Subsequently, it decreases, but does not disappear, as the recording electrode passes the layer of mitral cells. The second negative wave reaches its maximum in the external plexiform layer and then becomes lost in the large positive deflection which appears suddenly as the recording electrode passes the mitral cells. These findings, along with others, suggest that the first negative wave is generated by the antidromic invasion of mitral cells and their dendrites, while the second negative wave reflects the synaptic driving of tufted and, possibly, mitral cells by direct recurrent collaterals of mitral cell axons (Ochi, 1963). With AAC stimulation, tufted cell axons to and from the bulb are activated, producing mainly a slow negative wave deep in the granule cell layer

(Walsh, 1959; Ochi, 1963). This wave very likely represents the discharge of granule cells but it is unclear whether this is recurrently or centrifugally initiated.

Unit analysis has dealt mainly with the effects of LOT stimulation. In addition to antidromic invasion of mitral cells, single shocks to the LOT cause a prolonged pause of up to 200 msec duration in the spontaneous firing of mitral cells. Since this phenomenon is present also in chronically deafferented bulbs (Green *et al.*, 1962), it should result from the activation of mitral cell recurrent axon collaterals. Both Phillips *et al.* (1963) and Yamamoto *et al.* (1963) were able to record intracellularly from mitral cells and to observe a membrane hyperpolarization of long duration following single shocks to the LOT. Moreover, Yamamoto *et al.* (1963) showed that the same occurred following activation of mitral cells by shocks to the olfactory nerve. Green *et al.* (1962) attributed the suppression of the spontaneous firing of mitral cells by LOT stimulation to direct inhibition by mitral cell recurrent axon collaterals, but the latency and contour of the intracellularly recorded hyperpolarization suggests that an interneurone lies between the recurrent collaterals and the accessory dendrites (Phillips *et al.*, 1963; Yamamoto *et al.*, 1963). This view is supported by the evidence that many recurrent collaterals end among granule cells, some of which send processes to the accessory dendrites, and that granule cells have been found meeting some of the electrophysiological requirements for such an interneurone. These cells fire repetitively following ortho- or antidromic stimulation of mitral cells with a latency comparable to, or shorter than, that of a mitral cell's inhibition. In addition to these effects, LOT stimulation can discharge tufted cells, presumably through direct recurrent collaterals of mitral cells (Green *et al.*, 1962; Shepherd, 1963). Inhibition of mitral and tufted cells also results from antidromic stimulation of tufted cells in chronically deafferented bulbs, via tufted cell recurrent axon collaterals (von Baumgarten *et al.*, 1963). Studying the interaction of LOT and AAC stimulation during intracellular recordings from mitral cells, Yamamoto *et al.* (1963) found the hyperpolarization due to LOT stimulation to be suppressed during AAC induced hyperpolarization. This suggested that AAC stimulation has two separate effects on mitral cells: the production of a hyperpolarizing potential and at the same time the prevention of the hyperpolarization due to activation of the mitral-cell axon collaterals. The first effect was found to be mediated by an inhibitory interneurone while the second apparently results from the inhibition by the AAC of the interneurones mediating the LOT recurrent inhibition (Yamamoto *et al.*, 1963). How far tufted-cell collaterals and centrifugal fibres participate in these phenomena remains to be elucidated. Centrifugal fibre effects are difficult to study owing to their diffuse origin in the CNS and their diffuse distribution through the olfactory peduncle. Such effects are shown by the changes of the olfactory bulb's intrinsic or odour-induced waves (Kerr and Hagbarth, 1955; Arduini and Moruzzi, 1953; Hernández-Peón *et al.*, 1960; Yamamoto and Iwama, 1961), and unit activity (Mancia *et al.*, 1962) observed after stimulation of the rhinencephalon, prepiriform cortex and reticular formation.

Effects of drugs

Pharmacological studies on the olfactory bulb have mainly attempted to elucidate the origin of some parameter of evoked field responses and to identify transmitter substances. Typical of the first group are the studies of Iwase *et al.* (1961) and of Ochi (1963) using topical application of drugs to the surface of the olfactory bulb. In the second group are our own studies using microelectrophoresis to administer drugs directly at the site of extracellular unit recording (von Baumgarten *et al.*, 1963; Bloom *et al.*, 1964; Salmoiraghi *et al.*, 1964).

The surface spike-and-wave complex elicited by surface stimulation is differentially sensitive to topically applied drugs. Procaine and strychnine completely remove the spike and strychnine enhances the slow wave. On the contrary, γ-aminobutyric acid and γ-amino-β-hydroxybutyric acid depress the slow potential but have no effect on the spike, while curarine does not affect either component of the response. Iwase *et al.* (1961) concluded that since the two components of the surface response behave differently to various drugs, the elements responsible for their generation probably differ, a conclusion that accords with other evidence suggesting that the spike represents the compound action potential of olfactory nerve fibres, while the slow negative wave reflects dendritic depolarization. Though curarine did not affect the surface response (Iwase *et al.*, 1961), it abolished the second negative wave of the LOT response when applied to the surface of the bulb (Ochi, 1963) and abolished the slow negative wave resulting from contralateral bulb stimulation when given into the carotid artery (Walsh, 1959). Dihydro-β-erythroidine, however, and strychnine—given intravenously—have no apparent effect on the inhibition of mitral cells produced by LOT stimulation (Green *et al.*, 1962).

Many of the problems of interpreting the responses related to blood-brain barrier permeability, to drug-induced vascular effects, or to primary drug effects upon distant neurones are excluded when the drugs are administered electrophoretically into the immediate external environment of the recorded nerve cell. Using this technique to study units in the rabbit olfactory bulb, von Baumgarten *et al.* (1963) obtained direct evidence for the presence of neurones sensitive to acetylcholine (ACh), noradrenaline (NA) and 5-hydroxytryptamine (5-HT). Further studies by Bloom *et al.* (1964) and Salmoiraghi *et al.* (1964) have established certain pharmacological points of reference for the characterization of transmitters in the olfactory bulb. These studies can be summarized as follows.

A small proportion of olfactory neurones in decerebrate rabbits respond to ACh by increasing their discharge rate. However, most of the responsive units decrease their discharge rate when tested with ACh, although these responses are seldom dramatic or intense. Physostigmine prolonged but usually did not potentiate the unit's response to ACh and frequently depressed the spontaneous activity of test units regardless of their sensitivity to ACh. Similar depressant effects, seemingly unrelated to ACh sensitivity, were also observed with dihydro-β-erythroidine, atropine, hexamethonium, chlorisondamine (Ecolid) and dimethylpiperazinium (DMPP); nevertheless all of these drugs, except DMPP, were shown to block ACh responses reversibly. Dihydro-β-erythroidine, moreover, consistently blocked the ACh response without interfering with responses to either 5-HT or NA. Responses to 5-HT and NA always consisted of a depression of the unit's rate of spontaneous discharge in the unanaesthetized decerebrate rabbits, but in rabbits anaesthetized with pentobarbitone facilitatory effects of NA have occasionally been observed. Decreased rates of discharge are also produced by tyramine and metaraminol but neither of these drugs affected subsequent responses to NA nor caused tachyphylaxis. NA responses could be blocked by Dibenamine and by phentolamine given between 0·5 and 15 minutes before NA, but not by dichloroisoprenaline. For some cells, the electrophoretic administration of Dibenamine caused a biphasic effect: the NA response was enhanced either before the onset of NA blockade or during the period of recovery from Dibenamine. Prolonged Dibenamine treatment often caused a sustained, moderate increase in spontaneous discharge rate for the duration of the NA blockade. In no case did Dibenamine affect ACh or 5-HT responses. The same was not true for blockade of 5-HT responses by lysergide (LSD) and bromolysergide (BOL-148): 5-HT blockade never occurred without prior or concurrent blockade of responses to NA. The ability of ACh, NA or 5-HT to decrease unit activity was qualitatively unchanged 1—4 hours after intravenous injection of 1 mg./kg. of reserpine to deplete brain stores of NA, 5-HT and dopamine. Similarly, unit responsiveness to ACh, NA or 5-HT was present in rabbits 7—11 days after intravenous injection of 100 mg./kg. of α-methyl-meta-tyrosine (MMT) at which time brain stores of 5-HT and dopamine had presumably returned to normal values while NA stores were still depleted (Gessa *et al.*, 1962). These findings in reserpine and MMT-treated rabbits, therefore, suggest that the effects of electrophoretically administered ACh, NA and 5-HT do not depend upon intact brain stores of NA, 5-HT and dopamine.

We also studied the effects of ACh, NA and 5-HT blockers on the pause caused by shocks to the LOT in the spontaneous discharge of the mitral cells. Some of the cells investigated were identified as mitral cells by the antidromic spike discharge occurring within 2 milliseconds after electrical stimulation of the ipsilateral LOT. Other spontaneously active cells not exhibiting the antidromic spike response were included in the study only if the shape of the field potential evoked by LOT stimulation (Fig. 1B) indicated that the tip of the 5-barrelled micropipette was within the mitral cell layer. Most of the units studied were from the ventral mitral layer (presumably mitral cells), yielded action potentials of not less than 150–200 μV, and had a rate of discharge sufficiently high (20/sec. or more) during continuous 1/sec. stimuli to the LOT to show a clear inhibitory response for stimuli suprathreshold for the production of a maximal field response. For the sake of brevity, the 40–160 msec. pause in the rate of spontaneous discharge of these units following the electrical stimulus will be called here, as in the original paper (Salmoiraghi *et al.*, 1964), 'LOT inhibitory response' bearing in mind, however, that the LOT stimulus probably included, in addition to mitral cell axons, also the afferents described by Powell and Cowan (1963) and perhaps other afferents and efferents as well.

The duration of the LOT inhibitory response was not significantly affected during blockade of ACh responses by hexamethonium, chlorisondamine and dihydro-β-erythroidine (Fig. 2), or by administration of strychnine. On the other hand, all units in which Dibenamine blocked the NA response, also showed a shortening of the LOT inhibitory response. In some cases, however, Dibenamine reduced the LOT inhibitory response when either the cell was not responsive to NA or the NA effect was not

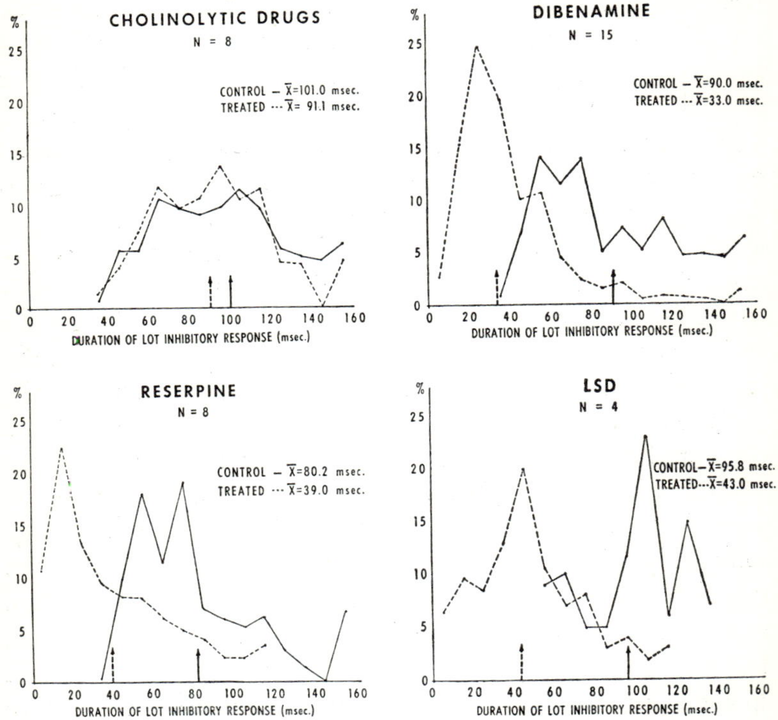

FIG. 2. Effects of drugs on the duration of the LOT inhibitory responses. Each plot constructed from filmed records obtained from several units (N) before (solid line) and after (broken line) drug administration. Ordinate: percent of occurrence of LOT inhibitory responses; abscissa: duration of LOT inhibitory responses grouped in 10 msec classes. $\overline{x}$: means. Solid and broken vertical arrows: means before and after the drug. P less than 0·001% (chi-square) for all except the results with cholinolytic drugs.

reduced. Reduction of the LOT inhibitory response was obtained also with lysergide and bromolysergide. However, it was difficult to control the spontaneous outflux of lysergide and bromolysergide from the tip of the electrode, despite the large retaining currents used to minimize spontaneous drug diffusion. When one of the barrels of the electrode contained lysergide, most units showed very short LOT inhibitory responses. Furthermore about two-thirds fewer NA-sensitive units were found while the proportion of 5-HT-sensitive units found was unchanged. This finding and all other observations on the blocking actions of lysergide and bromolysergide suggest that these drugs antagonize NA more powerfully than 5-HT in the rabbit olfactory bulb. In addition to Dibenamine, phentolamine, lysergide and bromolysergide, reserpine also reduced the LOT inhibitory response within 1 hour of intravenous injection or following its administration by pressure at the site of recording from a reserpine-filled barrel of the electrode. All the above observations were made using each unit as its own control before and after drug administration. The effects of MMT, on the other hand, had to be compared using units from different groups of rabbits since it is not technically possible to record the response of the same cell during the several days required for MMT to produce the desired selective biochemical change. Nevertheless, the mean LOT inhibitory response recorded from units in MMT-treated rabbits was significantly shorter than the response exhibited by an equal number of cells in untreated rabbits, using identical parameters of LOT stimulation.

Taken individually, none of these findings proves unequivocally that NA participates in olfactory bulb activity but in total the data offer strong pharmacological evidence for the existence of an adrenergic synapse in the rabbit olfactory bulb. Admittedly not all the criteria required for transmitter identification (Paton, 1958; Eccles, 1964) have been satisfied but the recent histochemical findings of Dahlström *et al.* (1965) support this hypothesis. It is when we try to fit the pharmacological data to the anatomy and physiology of the bulb that difficulties arise. Since the noradrenaline-containing fibres have been found medial to the LOT, it must be concluded that the stimulus used to elicit the 'LOT inhibitory response' included fibres other than those in the LOT. This is not surprising in view of the ever-present danger in the CNS of current spread from the point of stimulation and the possibility of small errors in electrode placement using stereotaxic coordinates. A greater difficulty arises when attempting to specify the postulated adrenergic synapse. According to Dahlström *et al.* (1965) the fibres containing NA appear to end predominantly in the granule cell layer, though some have been traced to the neighbourhood of mitral cells. This would suggest that although the micropipette was recording in the mitral cell layer, the drugs may have exerted their effects indirectly by diffusing into the granule cell layer. The synaptic arrangements within the olfactory bulb are so complex and so little is known about the functional organization of the units in the granule cell layer, that this postulated adrenergic synapse cannot at present be localized with any precision. Furthermore, it would be premature to state whether NA is excitatory or inhibitory for it.

Lastly, the observation that some neurones in the rabbit olfactory bulb are sensitive to ACh and/or 5-HT acquires added interest in the light of the histochemical studies by Shute and Lewis (1963) and Dahlström *et al.* (1965) showing the presence in the olfactory bulb of cholinesterase-containing and 5-HT-containing fibres respectively. These studies and the findings of Ochi (1963) and Walsh (1959) on the effects of curarine on components of the field potentials evoked by LOT and contralateral bulb stimulation, suggest that both ACh and 5-HT may eventually be found to be transmitters in the rabbit olfactory bulb. Nevertheless, if the experience gained in the studies on NA is any indication, it will be as difficult to establish the exact location and function of these hypothetical cholinergic and serotoninergic synapses.

Conclusion

The rigorous interpretation of pharmacological results in the central nervous system must be based on a thorough understanding of anatomy and physiology. Much remains to be learned about the functional organization of the olfactory bulb, but what is already known about its anatomy, physiology and histochemistry makes it relatively convenient for pharmacological studies. None of the pharmacological procedures now in use, however, gives unequivocal results. In each case, assumptions have to be made that are difficult to verify. The microelectrophoretic approach, being the most direct, is particularly valuable but it also has limitations. Nevertheless, the available pharmacological and histochemical evidence indicates that the rabbit olfactory bulb contains adrenergic synapses which ultimately cause inhibition of mitral cells.

REFERENCES

Allison, A. C. (1953). The structure of the olfactory bulb and its relationship to the olfactory pathways in the rabbit and rat. *J. comp. Neurol.*, **98**, 308–353.

Andres, K. H. (1965). Der Feinbau des Bulbus Olfactorius der Ratte unter besonderer Berücksichtigung der synaptischen Verbindungen. *Z. Zellforsch.*, **65**, 530–561.

Arduini, A. and Moruzzi, G. (1953). Sensory and thalamic synchronization in the olfactory bulb. *EEG clin. Neurophysiol.*, **5**, 235–242.

Bloom, F. E., Costa, E. and Salmoiraghi, G. C. (1964). Analysis of individual rabbit olfactory bulb neuron responses to the micro-electrophoresis of acetylcholine, norepinephrine and serotonin synergists and antagonists. *J. Pharm. exp. Therap.*, **146**, 16–23.

Bradley, P. B. and Wolstencroft, J. H. (1965). Actions of drugs on single neurones in the brain stem. *Brit. med. Bull.*, **21**, 15–18.

Cajal, S. Ramon y (1955). Histologie du Système Nerveux de l'Homme et des Vertébrés. Paris: Maloine, 1911, **2**. Reprinted, Madrid, Consejo Superior de Investigaciónes Cientificas.

Cragg, B. G. (1962). Centrifugal fibers to the retina and olfactory bulb and composition of the supraoptic commissures in the rabbit. *Exp. Neurol.*, **5**, 406–427.

Curtis, D. R. (1965). Actions of drugs on single neurones in the spinal cord and thalamus. *Brit. med. Bull.*, **21**, 5–9.

Curtis, D. R. and Eccles, R. M. (1958). The excitation of Renshaw cells by pharmacological agents applied electrophoretically. *J. Physiol.*, **141**, 435–445.

Dahlström, A., Fuxe, K., Olson, L. and Ungerstedt, U. (1965). On the distribution and possible function of monoamine nerve terminals in the olfactory bulb of the rabbit. *Life Sci.*, **4**, 2071–2074.

Eccles, J. C. (1964). The Physiology of Synapses, p. 316. New York: Academic Press.

Gessa, F. L., Costa, E., Kuntzman, R. and Brodie, B. B. (1962). On the mechanism of norepinephrine release by α-methyl metatyrosine. *Life Sci.*, **1**, 353–360.

Gray, E. G. (1961). Ultrastructure of synapses of the cerebral cortex and of certain specializations of neuroglial membranes. *In* Electron Microscopy in Anatomy (ed. Boyd *et al.*), pp. 54–73. London: Edward Arnold.

Green, J. D., Mancia, M. and von Baumgarten, R. (1962). Recurrent inhibition in the olfactory bulb. I. Effects of antidromic stimulation of the lateral olfactory tract. *J. Neurophysiol.*, **25**, 467–488.

Hernández-Peón, R., Lavin, A., Alcocer-Cuarón, C. and Marcelin, J. P. (1960). Electrical activity of the olfactory bulb during wakefulness and sleep. *EEG clin. Neurophysiol.*, **12**, 41–58.

Hirata, Y. (1964). Some observations on the fine structure of the synapses in the olfactory bulb of the mouse, with particular reference to the atypical synaptic configuration. *Arch. Histol. Okayama*, **24**, 293–302.

Iwase, Y., Uruha, M., and Ochi, J. (1961). Analysis of the olfactory bulb response induced by direct electrical stimulation in the rabbit. *Jap. J. Physiol.*, **11**, 507–519.

Kerr, D. I. B. and Hagbarth, K. E. (1955). An investigation of olfactory centrifugal fibre system. *J. Neurophysiol.*, **18**, 362–374.

Krnjević, K. (1965). Actions of drugs on single neurones in the cerebral cortex. *Brit. med. Bull.*, **21**, 10–14.

Mancia, M., Green, J. D. and von Baumgarten, R. (1962). Reticular control of single neurones in the olfactory bulb. *Arch. ital. Biol.*, **100**, 463–475.

Ochi, J. (1963). Olfactory bulb response to antidromic olfactory tract stimulation in the rabbit. *Jap. J. Physiol.*, **13**, 113–128.

Paton, W. D. M. (1958). Central and synaptic transmission in the nervous system (pharmacological aspects). *Ann. Rev. Physiol.*, **20**, 431–471.

Phillips, C. G., Powell, T. P. S. and Shepherd, G. M. (1963). Responses of mitral cells to stimulation of the lateral olfactory tract in the rabbit. *J. Physiol.*, **168**, 65–88.

Phillis, J. W. (1965). Cholinergic mechanisms in the cerebellum. *Brit. med. Bull.*, **21**, 26–29.

Powell, T. P. S. and Cowan, W. M. (1963). Centrifugal fibres in the lateral olfactory tract. *Nature*, **199**, 1296–1297.

Rall, W., Shepherd, G. M., Resse, T. S. and Brightman, M. W. (1966). Dendrodendritic synaptic pathway for inhibition in the olfactory bulb. *Exp. Neurol.*, **14**, 44–56.

Salmoiraghi, G. C., Bloom, F. E. and Costa, E. (1964). Adrenergic mechanisms in rabbit olfactory bulb. *Am. J. Physiol.*, **207,** 1417–1424.

Salmoiraghi, G. C. and Stefanis, C. N. (1965). Patterns of central neurons responses to suspected transmitters. *Arch. ital. Biol.*, **103,** 705–724.

Shepherd, G. M. (1963). Neuronal systems controlling mitral cell excitability. *J. Physiol.*, **168,** 101–117.

Shute, C. C. D. and Lewis, P. R. (1963). Cholinesterase-containing systems of the brain of the rat. *Nature*, **199,** 1160–1164.

von Baumgarten, R., Bloom, F. E., Oliver, A. P. and Salmoiraghi, G. C. (1963). Response of individual olfactory nerve cells to microelectrophoretically administered chemical susbtances. *Pflüger's Arch. ges. Physiol.*, **277,** 125–140.

von Baumgarten, R., Green, J. D. and Mancia, M. (1962). Recurrent inhibition in the olfactory bulb. II. Effects of antidromic stimulation of commissural fibers. *J. Neurophysiol.*, **25,** 489–500.

Walsh, R. R. (1959). Olfactory bulb potentials by electrical stimulation of the contralateral bulb. *Am. J. Physiol.*, **196,** 327-329.

Yamamoto, C. and Iwama, K. (1961). Arousal reaction of the olfactory bulb. *Jap. J. Physiol.*, **11,** 335–345.

Yamamoto, C., Yamamoto, T. and Iwama, K. (1963). The inhibitory system in the olfactory bulb studied by intracellular recording. *J. Neurophysiol.*, **26,** 403–415.

DISCUSSION

Wade: Dr. Harper, can you say whether there is any particular molecular configuration which makes a smell detectable at very great dilutions?

Harper: I think that these are the very tiny molecules that according to Davies' theory would easily penetrate the olfactory hair.

Feldberg: Did I understand you right, Dr. Salmoiraghi, you were surprised to obtain the same effect whether you used acetylcholine, noradrenaline or 5-HT?

Salmoiraghi: Not all mitral cells respond to acetylcholine and I would doubt that all of them would respond to 5-HT. Most of those we studied responded to noradrenaline; those that responded to acetylcholine, noradrenaline and 5-HT—always responded in the same direction in unanaesthetized animals.

Herxheimer: Did you try any smells on your preparation?

Salmoiraghi: No, we did not, because, according to the experience of Baumgarten and Green, the same smell can produce all sorts of different effects on neurones of the same histological type, depressing some and exciting others. We did not want to rely for our study on a stimulus which had a potentially uncertain effect.

Blane: Dr. Salmoiraghi, you have suggested that a noradrenergic mechanism is involved in at least one of the olfactory sensory pathways. If this is so, one would have thought that there would be reports of altered sensations of smell in patients treated with drugs which modify adrenergic function. I have in mind, of course, particularly reserpine which depletes brain monoamines, including 5-HT. You also mentioned 5-HT in the context of neurohumours involved in olfactory perception. Do you know of any such reports?

Salmoiraghi: This is a very well taken point. However, Green et al. (*J. Neurophysiol.*, 1962, **25**, 467) could not modify the LOT response with intravenous Dibenamine, presumably because it does not penetrate the blood-brain barrier in sufficient quantity to produce an effect. I do not know of any report relevant to your question.

Feldberg: Adrenaline i.v. does not pass the blood-brain barrier. Noradrenaline, 5-HT and 5-HTP occur in the olfactory bulb, and this indicates that they are concerned there with transmission processes.

Kosterlitz: We know from work on the peripheral autonomic system that Dibenamine and phenoxybenzamine antagonize adrenaline and noradrenaline; their action, however, is not specific since they may occupy all kinds of other receptors. How specific is their action in the CNS?

Salmoiraghi: I would not like to claim any specificity for blocking agents in the CNS, whether cholinergic, adrenergic or tryptaminergic. I can only report empirical observations which indicate that in the mitral cells responding to pairs of drugs, i.e. NA and Ach, or Ach and tryptamine, or NA and tryptamine, we could never block both drugs with the antagonist of one of the two. This is not true for lysergide (LSD) and bromolysergide (BOL), which seem to be particularly good at blocking both NA and 5-HT responses of mitral cells.

Herxheimer: It is difficult to analyse the effects of drugs like noradrenaline and reserpine on smell, because they have a very prominent effect on the nasal mucosa. Noradrenaline and adrenaline are powerful decongestants, whereas reserpine commonly causes nasal obstruction from vasodilation in the mucosa, and can prevent patients from smelling anything at all. These vascular effects will be difficult to disentangle from any effects such drugs may have on olfactory neurones.

AMPHETAMINES AND SMELL THRESHOLD IN MAN

PAUL TURNER

Department of Medicine, St. Bartholomew's Hospital, London

THE smell threshold is one of the least satisfactory of human sensory functions to study quantitatively. This is due primarily to the marked variation between subjects and in the same subject in ability to perceive odours. A recent study by Sumner (1962) emphasizes this, and also shows how difficult it may be for a subject to identify a perceptible odour when he has had no previous experience of it. The measurement of smell is made difficult particularly because of the location of the end-organ, the olfactory mucosa, which is readily covered with mucus secreted by the glandular epithelium of the surrounding region, and which varies according to changes in blood flow induced by temperature and humidity, by infectious diseases and by allergic states.

This difficulty in measuring the olfactory threshold is, perhaps, reflected in the fact that it was not until 1935 that a satisfactory method was introduced by Elsberg and Levy. Most of their work was concerned with pathological conditions of the nose and brain, and they claimed that the method was of value in localizing intracranial lesions. Schneider and Wolf (1955) criticized it on several grounds, and devised an elaborate 'walk-in' type of olfactorium, but this in itself introduced problems, particularly of the time taken to establish thresholds which made it unsuitable for acute pharmacological experiments. They were able to demonstrate, however, the importance of hormonal influences on olfaction, by an increased acuity during oestrogen administration and a decrease during androgen administration to hypogonadal women (Schneider, Costiloe, Howard and Wolf, 1958). These effects were probably due to changes in vascularity of the olfactory mucosa induced by these agents (Mortimer, Wright and Collip, 1936).

Apart from a limited amount of work on the effect of topical application of drugs into the nose (Skouby and Zilstorff-Pedersen, 1954; Zilstorff-Pedersen, 1965), most of the studies on the effects of drugs on smell in man have been concerned with the amphetamine drugs. This followed the claim by Goetzl and Stone (1947, 1948) that olfactory acuity increased significantly before meals and decreased with satiety. They further claimed that amphetamine not only abolished this increase, but that it produced a decrease in olfactory acuity if taken instead of a meal, and suggested that the anorectic action of the drug might be attributable to its depressant effect on olfactory acuity. Although Guild (1956) claimed to confirm these observations, the experimental detail and statistical analyses of the various investigations are hard to assess and controlled placebo trials seem to be lacking.

The validity of these results was challenged by Janowitz and Grossman (1949) and Zilstorff-Pedersen (1964) who failed to demonstrate any significant difference between times of day, and particularly any pre-cibal increase and post-cibal decrease in acuity. This naturally called in question the results with amphetamine, and it seemed reasonable to reassess the action of this and similar drugs on the olfactory threshold.

The method used was based on that of Elsberg and Levy (1935) in which increasing volumes of odorised air were released from a bottle into the subject's nose while he held his breath, and decided whether or not the odour could be perceived (minimum perceptible odour). In preliminary experiments we studied several odours and found that xylol gave the most definite sensation, and therefore used it in this experiment. Certain modifications were introduced in an attempt to eliminate variables which could contribute to the variations previously observed, and these are described in more detail elsewhere (Turner and Patterson, 1966). Two determinations of threshold were made at any one time, with an interval of 5 minutes between. Increments of 1 ml. were used, starting below threshold and increasing until an odour was perceived. Thirty seconds elapsed between each delivery of odorized air to the nose. The smell threshold was defined as the smallest volume (ml.) of odorized air in which the odour could be perceived. The subjects were members of the staff of the Medical Professorial Unit at St. Bartholomew's Hospital, who were experienced in the technique. They were of both sexes, their ages ranging from 20–40 years.

Dexamphetamine sulphate 10 mg. was compared with a appetite-depressant mixture containing phenmetrazine theoclate 30 mg. and phenbutrazate hydrochloride 20 mg. (Heine and Turner, 1963), and with a placebo in a double-blind procedure, the order of administration being based on a Latin Square design. Six subjects were studied on three separate days with an interval of 3–7 days between each treatment. Two measurements of smell threshold were made before and at 60, 120 and 180 minutes after administration. The subjects fasted during this time and abstained from smoking. The results were subjected to analysis of variance (Table 1) and considered significant if their *P* values were equal to or less than 0·05.

As expected, there was a highly significant difference between subjects, and in the second order interactions subjects-by-drugs and subjects-by-times. The overall difference between times, however, was not significant. The difference between treatments was significant, and the order effect of two determinations was on the border of significance at the 5% level.

Table 2 shows the changes in mean first and second thresholds before and at 60, 120 and 180 minutes after administration of the three treatments. The second determinations are higher than the first in almost all instances, the mean difference being 0·54 ml.

(S.E. = 0·171). Although this effect barely reaches significance in the analysis of variance, we have found it consistently with xylol (Turner and Patterson, 1966), and when 5 determinations were

Table 1

Analysis of variance of results comparing dexamphetamine, a phenmetrazine preparation and placebo on smell threshold in six subjects

S.V.	*D.F.*	*S.S.*	*M.S.*	*F*	*P*
Subjects (S)	5	549·54	104·91	+++	<0·001
Drugs (D)	2	32·10	16·50	5·75	<0·01
Times (T)	3	4·58	1·53	—	—
Order (O)	1	10·57	10·57	3·68	0·1/0·05
S×D	10	426·07	42·61	+++	<0·001
S×T	15	103·38	6·84	2·40	<0·025
D×T	6	36·57	6·10	2·13	0·1/0·05
S×D×T	30	99·59	3·32	1·16	—
D×O	2	0·37	0·19	—	—
T×O	3	2·01	0·67	—	—
D×T×O	6	9·30	1·55	—	—
Residual	60	172·25	2·87		

Table 2

Mean first and second olfactory thresholds (ml.) in six subjects before and at 60, 120 and 180 minutes after administration of a placebo, dexamphetamine sulphate and the phenmetrazine theoclate preparation (see text)

		Time after administration (min.)			
Drug	*Determination*	0	60	120	180
Placebo	1	4·2	4·2	4·3	5·5
	2	5·3	4·5	4·8	6·2
Dexamphetamine	1	5·8	4·3	5·3	4·7
	2	5·7	5·0	6·2	5·5
Phenmetrazine	1	4·2	3·7	4·7	3·3
	2	4·2	5·5	4·7	3·2

S.E. of mean = 0·69
5% crit. diff. between means of each 1st and 2nd determinations = 1·37

made at any one time, it was highly significant ($p < 0·001$, Turner, 1965). In experiments with coffee it has not been present, and it may therefore represent a transient toxic depression of the sensory cells of the olfactory mucosa by xylol. On the other hand, it may be associated with adaptation of the sense organs, for although the olfactory receptors are not easily fatigued by weak stimuli (Adrian, 1950), Ottoson (1956) has shown that strong stimuli markedly reduce the response.

When mean thresholds are compared between times, there is considerable random variation, and the changes after amphetamine throughout the three hours are not significant at the 5% level. There is, in fact, no significant change in the three treatments for two hours, but between 120 and 180 minutes, a rise in threshold, or fall in acuity occurs after the placebo which does not occur after amphetamine, and there is a significant fall in threshold, or increase in acuity, after phenmetrazine.

The significance of the rise following the placebo is uncertain. It may reflect a diurnal variation in the six subjects studied, but has not been shown in other normal subjects in experiments not concerned with drug testing (Turner and Patterson, 1966), or when using coffee rather than xylol. In fact, with coffee we have failed to demonstrate any overall change between times of day, confirming the findings of Janowitz and Grossman (1949) and Zilstorff-Pedersen (1964). We feel that this is more likely to be a fatigue effect related to the xylol and to the experimental situation requiring fasting and abstinence (Schneider and Wolf, 1960), as it developed just before lunch, and at 4–5 hours after a light breakfast. This would be compatible with its absence after amphetamine and its reversal by the phenmetrazine preparation. It may also be relevant that the difference between first and second determinations is absent at 2 and 3 hours after phenmetrazine, although the interaction drugs-by-order was not significant. This, of course, presupposes that these drugs are having a central rather than a peripheral action. While a local effect on the blood vessels of the mucosa cannot be ruled out, the time relationship is consistent with that of a central action, for in studies of these two drugs on a visual function, the critical flicker fusion frequency, we have found the maximum action of both phenmetrazine and amphetamine to be at 2–3 hours (Turner, 1965; Smart and Turner, 1966); phenmetrazine also produces a more significant increase in the critical flicker fusion frequency than does dexamphetamine (Turner, 1965).

These results suggest that amphetamines may enhance rather than depress olfactory acuity, and this is in keeping with the demonstration by Myznikov (1958) of increased olfactory sensitivity in dogs produced by such central stimulant agents as caffeine. In man, however, the olfactory threshold is an unsatisfactory measure because uncontrolled variations of between 10 and 20% mean that changes greater than this must be induced before significant effects can be recognized. Zilstorff-Pedersen (1965) selected for study only those subjects in whom variations in resting threshold were less than 10%. The necessity for such a selection is undesirable, however, when the effects of a drug on a population are to be investigated.

In summary, therefore, a randomized, double-blind, within-subjects trial failed to demonstrate a pre-cibal increase in olfactory acuity for xylol, but rather was there a decreased acuity in the subjects studied. This did not occur after dexamphetamine and was reversed by a phenmetrazine preparation. The mechanism of these effects is uncertain.

Acknowledgement

I thank J. V. Smart and D. S. Patterson for their invaluable assistance.

REFERENCES

Adrian, E. D. (1950). *Electroenceph. clin. Neurophysiol.*, **2**, 377.
Elsberg, C. A. and Levy, I. (1935). *Bull. Neurol. Inst. New York*, **4**, 5.
Goetzl, F. R. and Stone, F. (1947). *Gastroenterology*, **9**, 444.
Goetzl, F. R. and Stone, F. (1948). *Gastroenterology*, **10**, 708.
Guild, A. A. (1956). *J. Laryngol.*, **70**, 408.
Heine, B. E. and Turner, P. (1963). *Brit. J. clin. Pract.*, **17**, 529.
Janowitz, H. D. and Grossman, M. I. (1949). *J. appl. Physiol.*, **2**, 217.
Mortimer, H., Wright, R. P. and Collip, J. B. (1936). *Canad. med. Ass. J.*, **35**, 615.
Myznikov, N. M. (1958). *Zl. vyss. nerv. Deyat. Pavlova*, **8**, 742.

Ottoson, D. (1956). *Acta physiol. scand.*, **35,** 1.
Schneider, R. A. and Wolf, S. (1955). *J. appl. Physiol.*, **8,** 337.
Schneider, R. A., Costiloe, J. P., Howard, R. P. and Wolf, S. (1958). *J. clin. Endocrin.*, **18,** 379.
Schneider, R. A. and Wolf, S. (1960). *J. appl. Physiol.*, **15,** 914.
Skouby, A. P. and Zilstorff-Pedersen, K. (1954). *Acta physiol. scand.*, **32,** 252.
Smart, J. V. and Turner, P. (1966). *Brit. J. Pharmacol.* **26,** 468.
Sumner, D. (1962). *Lancet,* **ii,** 895.
Turner, P. (1965). The changes in critical flicker fusion frequency induced by some physiological procedures and by drugs, together with observations on the reliability of olfactory testing. M.D. Thesis. University of London.
Turner, P. and Patterson, D. S. (1966). *Acta otolaryngol.* **62,** 149.
Zilstorff-Pedersen, K. (1964). *Arch. Otolaryngol.* (*Chic.*), **79,** 412.
Zilstorff-Pedersen, K. (1965). *Arch. Otolaryngol.* (*Chic.*), **82,** 53.

DISCUSSION

Fox: Did the subjects regard xylol as a pleasant odour and do you think that the effect that you get with a drug like amphetamine might possibly depend on whether you used a pleasant or unpleasant odour?

Turner: In experiments with descending thresholds, when they were exposed to very high levels initially, some subjects complained of a trigeminal component or a pain, but below threshold and up to threshold no unpleasantness was complained of.

McIlwain: There is at least some structural similarity between xylol and amphetamine: both are simple aromatic compounds. On the other hand, the odour of xylol may be remote from that of foodstuffs. Are these factors likely to influence the relevance of your findings to the question of food selection which was initially posed?

Turner: Yes, I think we must emphasize that we were not using food substances for this experiment, but an artificial non-food substance.

Arden: Have you tried to make sure that the threshold dose is of the same concentration as xylol in the nose?

Turner: This is uncertain but it is possible to place the nosepiece in a standard position to try to minimize differences. Before each examination we breathe in and out in order to try and clear the nose of any previous xylol which may be present. We also put a clamp across the nosepiece to try and prevent the diffusion of the xylol mixture in and out of the air.

Land: One problem is that although the methods are published in the pharmacological and medical literature, the critical reviews are published elsewhere.

Turner: In studying drug effects we need methods that are fairly easy for subjects to use, and with this one we have obtained good cooperation, but the great variations that one finds indicate that it is not a satisfactory method for this type of work.

Arden: Did you consider doing the type of experiment in which you cycle up and down across the threshold?

Turner: Yes, we did. We practised these experiments by doing ascending and descending and randomized thresholds and we found no significant difference between the results. For that reason we simply used an ascending threshold. It may be that because we are using such large increments of 1 millilitre we are not detecting these subtler changes, but the fact that we have to use such large changes is an indication that the method is unsatisfactory.

Moncrieff: There is one point about the use of xylol: some earlier work from Edinburgh suggested that the smell of xylol was more acceptable to women than to men (Kenneth, J. H. A few odour preferences and their constancy. *J. exp. Psychol.*, 1928, **11**, 56.)

Turner: We did not find this.

Land: You said that you tested a number of different odorants and settled on xylol as being the one that gave the most reproducible results. I wonder whether you discarded any of the substances which may have a somewhat lower threshold than xylol.

Turner: We looked mainly at substances such as coffee, citron oil and almonds, and found that many subjects gave very irregular thresholds to them. We felt that these were substances they met every day, and their smell might be affected by psychological factors; most of the subjects had little to do with chemicals such as xylol and we felt that this lack of association with them was helpful.

Herxheimer: I'd like to ask Dr. Harper about the use of logarithmic and arithmetical scales in threshold determinations as in Dr. Turner's experiments. He was using an arithmetical scale by using the same increment in the volume of stimulus air—was this the best thing in the circumstances?

Harper: It particularly affects the choice of discrete concentrations for use in testing exercises, and in view of what I said about the order of magnitude of the differential threshold, shall we say about 30%, a geometric scale with an appropriate multiple is a convenient way of getting 5 or 6 stimuli of various concentrations covering a useful range.

The question of whether straightforward arithmetic scales or logarithmic scales should be used for olfactory studies cannot be answered dogmatically from actual evidence. If the Weber-Fechner law is assumed to be true (i.e. Sensation level is proportional to log stimulus) then the logarithmic transformation is appropriate. There is a good deal of evidence with *taste* thresholds that a logarithmic concentration will give an approximately normal distribution. Sufficient data are not available about the distribution of olfactory thresholds positively to support the same contention, but I would favour such a logarithmic form of stimulus specification (i.e. a geometric series of concentrations). However, different methods of quantifying 'perceived intensity' lead to somewhat different functional relationships, which ideally should be determined experimentally.

Herxheimer: Yes, what one really wants are steps of equal subjective discriminability.

Arden: I calculated these errors of threshold determination to be about 0·2 of a unit on the scale used in visual thresholds. The point about using the logarithmic scale is that, if you say it quickly, 0·3 logarithms sounds rather small, but if you say 5–12 it sounds huge, that is I think the only difference, and it is trivial. The distribution of many of these thresholds is according to the statistical theory of signal noise and is a Poisson distribution. For analysis one needs to use statistical methods to determine the true threshold; I don't think it makes much difference in the subsequent analysis whether one initially uses logarithmic or arithmetical units.

Crawford: We have worked for many years on the measurement of threshold sensations and similar quantities. There seem to be two fairly good reasons for using the logarithmic scale. One is that a good deal of information can be put on one piece of paper, spread out in a more or less intelligible way, because as the quantities get smaller they are spread out towards minus infinity. This avoids losing a lot of information at the bottom or at the sides of the graph simply because it is on too small a scale. The use of the logarithmic scale is also linked with the observation that in many psychophysical experiments a measure of sensation is approximately proportional to the logarithm of the stimulus. For example, if a subject is asked to divide the range from white to black into approximately equal steps, he could do this by selecting bits of grey paper. When the selected grey papers are measured for their reflectivity, they are found to be approximately, though not exactly, a logarithmic scale. I think those are two practical reasons for using the logarithmic presentation.

Harper: I agree perfectly with Dr. Crawford about the spreading-out, but the olfactory data, by virtue of the lower differential sensitivity, will be less spread out naturally than the visual data on the same scale. If you *assume* the Weber-Fechner law, the use of logarithmic concentrations automatically follows. Towards the end of my paper I mentioned the Stevens' magnitude estimation relationship (Reese & Stevens, 1960). This is another possible alternative which becomes a straight line, not when you take the log stimulus of concentration alone, but when you take log of both the C-*sensation* magnitude and the log of the stimulus concentration. I will not pursue this any further but obviously there are many possible varieties of quantifications and one has got to look at the properties of each in relation to the task in hand.

DRUG EFFECTS ON TASTE, OLFACTION, AND FOOD INTAKE*

SEBASTIAN P. GROSSMAN

Department of Psychology, University of Chicago

Effects of local anaesthetics and gymnemic acid on taste and olfaction

DRUG-INDUCED modifications of olfactory or gustatory sensations first aroused scientific interest in the course of early investigations of cocaine. This alkaloid was synthesized by von Niemann in 1859 and received extensive experimental and clinical testing around the turn of the century because of its practical importance as a local anaesthetic.

Many of the early investigators (Anrep, 1880; Knapp, 1885; Shore, 1892) reported that local applications of cocaine to the tongue produced a general, long-lasting inhibition of all taste sensations. Variations in the concentration of the cocaine solution and/or the frequency of its application were reported to produce quantitative but not qualitative differences in the drug's inhibitory action on gustatory sensations. Similarly non-specific effects on olfactory as well as other sensory thresholds were soon reported (see early reviews by Anrep, 1880; Kiesow, 1894) and provide the experimental basis for the drug's clinical application as a local anaesthetic.

The cocaine effects are of particular interest in the present context because subsequent studies demonstrated a most interesting selectivity for specific gustatory modalities. Aducco and Mosso

* Supported by grant number MH-10130-02 from the National Institutes of Health, United States Public Health Service.

(1886) showed that low concentrations of cocaine selectively affected the taste for bitter substances. Subsequent investigations confirmed this observation and demonstrated a second, selective effect on the threshold for sweet tasting substances. Kiesow (1894) reported, for instance, that the local application of a 0·5% cocaine solution did not affect the threshold for sodium chloride, and dulled the gustatory sensitivity for sour only slightly after repeated applications. The thresholds for bitter and, to a less extent, sweet substances were dramatically raised even after a single application of this low concentration of the drug. The selective effects persisted at higher concentrations. Complete ageusia for bitter tastes was achieved at a cocaine concentration of only 2%. Other gustatory sensations, particularly salt and sour, disappeared only after repeated applications of a 5% solution. The taste for salty and sour substances recovered to normal levels within only 2 to 3 hours, whereas the sensitivity for bitter and sweet substances was impaired for as long as 12 to 24 hours. An interesting and potentially useful by-product of these investigations is the observation that cocaine affected gustatory receptors within a much shorter period (about 3 minutes) than touch or pressure receptors (about 20 minutes).

Subsequent investigations showed that a number of other local anaesthetics such as eucaine hydrochloride (Fontana, 1902) and amydricaine hydrochloride (Ponzo, 1909) produce similarly selective effects on the threshold for bitter and sweet tastes. These observations suggest a relatively uninteresting interpretation of the apparent specificity of the cocaine effect in terms of a differential response of the bitter and sweet receptors to all anaesthetics—a peculiarity which might be related to such factors as size or myelination of the receptors or associated fibres.

However, detailed observations of the effects of the local anaesthetic amylocaine (stovaine) by Mario Ponzo (1909) suggest that the specificity of the cocaine effect may be related to a more complex receptor affinity. Amylocaine hydrochloride was first synthesized by Fourneau in 1904 and has been used extensively as a local anaesthetic since Launoy and Billon (see Fourneau, 1904) showed that the toxicity of this drug was reliably less than that of cocaine and related substances. Amylocaine selectively and completely eliminated the taste for all salty substances (which are least affected by cocaine) at concentrations which raised the threshold for other taste modalities only little or not at all. At higher concentrations, the salt and bitter thresholds were immediately and drastically affected; the sweet and sour thresholds showed smaller and delayed effects. The depressant effects of amylocaine persisted with diminishing effectiveness for approximately 90 to 120 minutes.

A detailed analysis of the time course of the amylocaine effects demonstrated, furthermore, that this drug produced not only inhibitory effects. During the first few minutes after the local application of amylocaine, a marked and selective lowering of the threshold for salty tastes occurred, at a time when the threshold for all other gustatory stimuli increased rapidly. This facilitatory effect may be due to a selective central action of the drug, these effects being obscured under normal conditions by its peripheral anaesthetic properties. This interpretation is suggested by experiments showing (a) a long-lasting lowering of the salt threshold on the left side of the tongue following applications of amylocaine to the right side (which consequently showed a selectively raised salt threshold) and (b) a selective facilitation of the salt receptors when amylocaine was ingested in a capsule or injected into the thigh muscle. Local applications of the drug produced also a marked lowering of the salt threshold *after* the primary anaesthesia had disappeared. It is not known whether this third phase of the amylocaine effect is related to peripheral or central actions of the drug.

In view of earlier reports by Ferrari (1905) that the anaesthetic effect of cocaine on taste receptors appeared to be preceded by a transient hyperaesthesia, particularly for bitter tastes, Ponzo replicated his amylocaine experiments with cocaine. This drug produced a marked initial lowering of the thresholds for bitter and sweet substances (as well as a selective subsequent depressant effect) but no hyperaesthesia for salty (or sour) substances.

It is notable that the reflex secretion of saliva in response to the application of foodstuffs to a cocainized buccal cavity remains intact even after taste sensations have been completely eliminated. Most surprising, perhaps, is the observation (Birjukov, 1938) that the secretory response to sweet and acid compounds is actually increased under such circumstances whereas the response to bitter and acid appears slightly decreased, suggesting that the salivary glands can respond selectively to specific taste stimuli even after the conscious appreciation of all taste sensations has been eliminated.

Skramlik (1963) has recently compared the effects of 15 local anaesthetics on taste sensations in man and concluded that most anaesthetics selectively affect bitter and salt sensations while sour and particularly sweet appeared relatively less affected. The individual substances differed markedly with respect to their efficacy in suppressing specific taste modalities, but the general pattern of effects (bitter > salt > sour > sweet) was only rarely modified ('anaestheform', amethocaine, *iso*cocaine, and tropacocaine exerted selective effects on sweet sensations; eucaine, and *iso*-amylhydrocupreine preferentially affected sour sensations). In contrast to earlier observations Skramlik failed to observe a selective cocaine effect on sweet sensations. Relatively high dosages may have obscured other selective effects in this study, since for example amethocaine totally obliterated all taste sensations in the concentrations used.

An interesting feature of Skramlik's results is the demonstration of apparently modality-specific facilitatory effects which result in brief periods of supersensitivity. Benzocaine, for instance, selectively facilitated the sour receptors, amydricaine and amethocaine the bitter receptors. None of the substances tested produced hyperaesthesia to sweet or salty substances.

Locally applied cocaine or amydricaine appear to affect gustatory receptor responses on the frog's tongue in ways which do not fit with the human data. Kusano (1958, 1959) reported, for instance, that cocaine selectively inhibited the response to sucrose, while quinine (bitter) and acid (sour) were only little affected. The response to potassium chloride (salt) was not changed at lower concentrations of the anaesthetic. Local applications of *d*-tubocurarine or urethane did not basically modify the response of gustatory receptors in this interesting series of experiments, although the rate of adaptation to specific substances such as water or sucrose was reliably affected. The author suggests that the receptors for monovalent salts may have developed mechanisms of excitation which are basically different from those of other gustatory sensations, but this does not account for all the apparent differences between the human and frog data.

The apparently selective action of some drugs on specific gustatory receptors is not a unique property of local anaesthetics. Observations by Ferrari (1905) and others suggest that the admixture of alcohol selectively lowers the threshold for sweet substances and Gardella (1904) reported some selective facilitatory effects of carbonic acid. Quite dramatic inhibitory effects have been observed following the local application of gymnemic acid, a substance which can be purified from the leaves of *Gymnema sylvestre*. Shore (1892) discovered that even brief contact of this substance with the tongue and buccal mucosa completely and selectively abolished all sweet sensations, and this observation has been verified by many other investigators (Kiesow, 1894; Power and Tutin, 1904; Mhaskar and Caius, 1930). Kiesow (1894) and others have reported that during the 2–24 hours of complete and selective ageusia for sweet substances, sugar or saccharin solutions acquire an unpleasant metallic taste which is not like any normal gustatory sensation. Gymnemic acid acts primarily on the taste receptors which mediate sweet sensations. However,

Kiesow (1894) and others (Shore, 1892; Belletrud and Mercier, 1904) have reported smaller inhibitory effects on bitter taste thresholds and, following repeated applications of high concentrations of the drug, even some effects on the thresholds for sour tastes. Only the salt receptors are apparently completely exempt from the inhibitory effects of gymnemic acid. (Touch and temperature sensations are also unaffected.) Yerba Santa, an extract of the leaves of *Eriodicyton californicum* is said to produce effects similar to those of gymnemic acid.

The differential action of gymnemic acid on sweet receptors has also been demonstrated electrophysiologically. Hagerstrom (1957) found that the electrical response of the chorda tympani nerve to sweet (but not salt) stimuli was reliably depressed 10 minutes after the application of gymnemic acid to the tongue.

Lovell *et al.* (1961) have recently reported an interesting differential effect of a gymnemic decoction on the acceptability of nutritive and non-nutritive sweet substances. Normal rats show a marked preference for sweet fluids regardless of the nutritive value of the sweetener. In a preference experiment, the concentrations of the sweetener can be adjusted such that the preference for nutritive and non-nutritive sweet solutions is roughly equal. Lovell *et al.* found in such a situation that pretreatment with a gymnemic decoction significantly lowered the acceptability of saccharine solutions but increased the acceptability of sucrose. These results are puzzling in view of earlier observations which show that gymnemic acid raises the threshold for sucrose as well as saccharin (Shore, 1892; Kiesow, 1894) and that equal sweetness matches remain unchanged by this drug (Warren and Pfaffmann, 1960). Lovell *et al.* suggest that the increased sucrose ingestion may have occurred in response to a fall in blood sugar induced by gymnemic acid, but this, together with the marked depression of saccharin intake, would seem to require a surprising acuity of gustatory sensations for such a preparation. The reflex secretion of saliva in response to sweet substances appears to be unaffected by gymnemic acid treatments which completely obliterate the sensation of sweetness (Birjukov, 1938).

Le Magnen (1953) has reported a possibly related observation of the effects of insulin on the voluntary intake of nutritive and non-nutritive sweet substances. Insulin injections increased the preference for sweet substances but completely obliterated the discrimination between nutritive (5% sucrose) and non-nutritive (0·037% saccharin) solutions.

The depressant effects of local anaesthetics on olfactory thresholds are, as already mentioned, apparently non-specific and hence of little interest in the present context. However, transient phases of hyperosmia often precede and follow the primary anosmia. Transient facilitatory effects were mentioned in many of the initial studies of the effects of cocaine on olfactory acuity (Zwaardemaker, 1895; Reuter, 1900) and were further investigated by Ponzo (1909). Local applications of amylocaine into one nasal cavity produced a transient hyperosmia for apparently all odours, followed by a prolonged and complete anosmia. The recovery of olfactory acuity followed an interesting pattern which suggested a differential drug effect on specific olfactory receptors. The threshold for some odours returned to normal levels long before any sensitivity to other substances reappeared and some deficits, notably for the smell of rubber, remained for several months. The nasal cavity treated with amylocaine showed complete anosmia for several hours. The other, untreated nasal passage, showed a concurrent lowering of all olfactory thresholds, which persisted for up to 24 hours. That this facilitatory effect may be the result of a central action of the drug is suggested by the observation that a persistent bilateral hyperosmia could be induced by intramuscular injections of amylocaine.

It may be appropriate to mention here the apparently specific effects of methylpentynol on the acceptability of alcohol. Methylpentynol is not an anaesthetic but a sedative (Margolin *et al.*, 1956; Halpern, 1956), which appears to have a direct action on the hypothalamus and midbrain reticular formation (Halpern and Lehmann, 1956). This drug specifically increases the acceptability of alcohol solutions (20%) which are normally unacceptable to the rat (Dicker, 1958). Though an interpretation of this effect is complicated by other effects such as general hypodipsia, a marked rise of the taste threshold appears to be the most likely explanation.

The apparent specificity of the local anaesthetics and gymnemic acid derivatives cannot, as is commonly assumed, be based on a selective affinity of certain classes of taste receptors. This is most clearly demonstrated by studies of evoked potentials (see Pfaffmann, 1959) which have shown that individual receptors respond to salt as well as sugar. This suggests that gymnemic acid and low concentrations of the local anaesthetics selectively block the receptor sites for specific tastes rather than the entire gustatory receptor. Such a selective chemical affinity for specific portions of a single receptor suggests that taste modalities may be coded pharmacologically as well as anatomically.

The role of metabolic factors

Taste sensations are peculiarly dependent on the chemical composition of the internal environment. The details of this relationship are only poorly understood at present, but some interesting factors are worth discussing.

The postnatal development of the human taste organs occurs in three phases: (a) a period of rudimentary growth during the first year of life, (b) complete differentiation about puberty, and (c) involution and gradual atrophy beginning about age 45 to 55 (Allara, 1939). The development and regression of the gustatory receptors appears to parallel sexual maturation and decline. Furthermore, castration in male as well as female cats caused a gradual atrophy of the taste organs (Allara, 1952a, b), which was reversed by sex hormone substitution therapy. The effects were particularly marked when castration occurred before puberty. Allara (1952a) concluded from his studies that the structure and function of the taste receptors must be significantly determined by the level of circulating sex hormones. The implications of this conclusion for taste thresholds in the normal organism have not yet been followed up.

On a more functional level, it has been shown that rats and mice of different strains (Yunikura, 1955a, b) and metabolic patterns (Mori, 1957) vary significantly in the acuity of their gustatory receptors. A specific relationship with melanin metabolism (which determines such strain characteristics as fur color) has not been demonstrated (Hoshishima *et al.*, 1962).

Some interesting effects have been reported following selective interference with specific metabolic processes. Richter (1938) showed that adrenalectomy specifically lowered the preference threshold for salt-selection in rats. This phenomenon has been observed in several more recent preference studies (Pfaffmann and Bare, 1950; Radomski *et al.*, 1950; Pfaffmann, 1957; Nachman, 1963) and correlates nicely with the marked salt-hunger of patients with Addison's disease—the clinical counterpart of this condition (Wilkins and Richter, 1940). Mice, however, do not seem to show this compensatory adjustment (Hoshishima *et al.*, 1962). Richter's studies (Richter and Eckert, 1937; Richter and Schmidt, 1941; Richter, 1942) also showed that: (a) Removal of the parathyroid glands caused a sharp and specific increase in the animals' preference for calcium solutions. Implantation of a parathyroid gland reversed this effect reliably. (b) Removal of the pancreas sharply decreased the normal preference for sugar and increased olive oil consumption. This pattern of preference changes was also seen after experimentally induced vitamin B deficiency. (c) Repeated insulin injections (which lowered the insulin content of the pancreas and induced transitory diabetes) sharply increased the acceptability of sugar. (d) Riboflavin deficiency caused a rejection of casein and rise in sugar consumption.

Recent work by Hoshishima *et al.* (1962) suggests that mice react somewhat differently to these drastic changes in metabolic conditions. Adrenalectomy produced a sharp increase in the threshold for acetic acid. The hypoaesthesia was at least partially reversed by DOCA administration. Hypofunction of the thyroid gland brought about by injections of I^{131} raised the threshold for sweet (saccharin), bitter (phenylthiocarbamate), and sour (acetic acid) substances but did not affect salt consumption. An almost identical pattern of effects was observed following chemically (carbon tetrachloride administration) or surgically induced hepatic hypofunction.

Richter (1939) demonstrated that adrenalectomized rats did not show the usual change in salt preference when the glossopharyngeal, chorda tympani, and lingual nerves were cut. He concluded from his observations that the adrenalectomy-induced lowering of the preference thresholds must reflect a primary change in the sensory threshold of the salt receptors. This interpretation has been widely accepted and has led to an uncritical acceptance of preference data as indices of sensory threshold changes. Although the two measures may correlate in individual cases, alternative interpretations cannot be ruled out, a priori. Pfaffmann (Pfaffmann and Bare, 1950; Pfaffmann, 1955) demonstrated, for instance, that adrenalectomy-induced changes in salt preference are due to a change in acceptability rather than sensory thresholds. Recordings of the afferent nerve discharge of the chorda tympani showed that the preference threshold of normal rats lies much above the concentration at which a distinct discharge of the salt receptors can be detected—i.e., normal animals can taste the salt at low concentrations but show no preference for the weak solutions. Adrenalectomized animals, on the other hand, ingest salt whenever they can taste it—the neural and preference thresholds coincide.

Adrenalectomy also fails to lower the behavioural preference threshold in forced discrimination situations (Carr, 1952; Harriman and MacLeod, 1953).

De Wardener and Herxheimer (1957) reported that in man excessive water consumption lowered the taste threshold for sodium and, to a less extent glucose. The threshold changes were not accompanied by a significant change in plasma osmolarity but plasma sodium concentrations were increased. Yensen (1958a, b) subsequently demonstrated that the taste threshold for sodium chloride in man is also lowered by sodium deprivation but raised by water deprivation. These observations suggest that the salt thresholds might be related to the concentration of sodium in the intracellular fluid compartment or, alternatively, the transfer of sodium from bone and cells to the extracellular fluids. Herxheimer and Woodbury (1960) have tested this hypothesis by lowering the intracellular concentration of sodium by chronic administration of deoxycortone (DOCA) to rats. Their experiments demonstrated a marked and apparently specific lowering of the salt-preference threshold following the implantation of DOCA pellets into the backs of rats. This agrees well with earlier observations that DOCA increases salt intake in rats (Rice and Richter, 1943). The results are not readily reconcilable with the finding that adrenalectomy increases salt-preference (though not physiological or psychophysical sensory thresholds) and that DOCA appears to reverse this effect (Richter, 1941).

An interference with thyroid function may be responsible for the prolonged and complete ageusia which is occasionally seen after repeated treatment with thiouracil compounds. These drugs are widely used in the treatment of hyperthyroidism. One of the first clinical studies of thiouracil (Leys, 1945) mentioned that one patient complained of a temporary ageusia. Schneeberg (1952) and Grossman (1953) have published extensive clinical observations of the side-effects of thiouracil on gustatory and olfactory sensibilities which permit the following generalizations: (a) All gustatory modalities are apparently concurrently and equally affected, causing a general flattening and eventual disappearance of all taste sensations. (b) Sweet substances tend to acquire a novel and highly unpleasant bitter taste during the initial stages of the thiouracil effect and during recovery. (c) Gustatory sensations are typically affected long before a change in olfactory thresholds can be noted but prolonged treatments may affect both chemical senses. (d) After discontinuation of thiouracil treatment the sensation of salty tastes recovers most rapidly—that for sweet most slowly.

The compounds of the thiouracil group are of interest in the present context for still another reason. Most chemical substances have taste thresholds which follow a normal (Gaussian) distribution. However, the ability to taste phenylthiourea (PTC) and related compounds is bimodally distributed, i.e., there are 'tasters' and 'non-tasters' of this interesting substance. Cohen and Ogdon (1949) showed that a 'taster' could be converted into a 'non-taster' by removing his saliva before each test. In later work Fischer and associate (Fischer and Griffin, 1961a, b, 1964; Fischer *et al.*, 1962, 1963, 1965) found that saliva was required not only for the bitter taste of thiouracil compounds but also for the normally distributed bitter taste of quinine. Sensitive 'tasters' could not detect propyluracil or quinine in high concentrations when their tongue was rinsed with distilled water or saliva from a 'non-taster'. Fischer found that the saliva of 'non-tasters' has a much higher oxidation rate than that of 'tasters' (a difference which may be related to the concentration of hydrogen peroxide) but suggested that this cannot account for all of the difference in taste thresholds. He also reported that 'tasters' have a significantly higher salivary catalase activity than 'non-tasters' but the intriguing question why one's own saliva is necessary for the taste of bitter substances is not yet answered.

Kuhn and Zilliken (1950) have reported that the ability to taste *p*-acetamino-benzaldehyde-thiosemicarbazone is bimodally distributed in exactly the same way as thiouracil and its derivatives. A subsequent investigation by Knüchel (1950) demonstrated that 'tasters' of this drug cannot tolerate its repeated administration whereas 'non-tasters' report few unpleasant side-effects. Perhaps the process which results in harmful metabolites of this drug also liberates a substance into the salivary secretions which sensitizes the taste receptors. This facilitatory effect appears to be specific to bitter tastes.

Possibly related to these observations are studies by Ehrenberg and Güttes (1949) which demonstrate that the threshold for sweet tastes was reliably lowered by the addition of sulphates (particularly potassium sulphate) to the saccharin solution but reliably raised by the addition of rhodanides (potassium sulphothiamide) which are normally found in saliva. The taste threshold for a bitter substance (quinine hydrochloride) showed directly opposite effects—a marked lowering after the addition of rhodanide, and a smaller but apparently reliable increase when sulphate was added.

Effects of aminoacids on taste sensations

The effects of aminoacids on gustatory sensations have been studied in some detail because the selection of specific dietary components in response to metabolic needs may be explained by a selective response to some of these simple structural elements of organic matter. Halpern *et al.* (1962) have extensively investigated this problem.

In a simple aminoacid/water preference situation, rats were found to prefer low concentrations of DL- and L-alanine and glycine and reject high concentrations of DL-methionine, DL-alanine, DL-valine, and glycine. D-, L-, and DL-tryptophan and low concentrations of DL-methionine were accepted in about equal proportions to water. Electrophysiological recordings from the chorda tympani showed that neural activity increased when aminoacid solutions 0·01 M or above passed over the tongue and that the response magnitude for concentrations close to the individual solubility limits was: DL-methionine < DL-tryptophan < DL-valine < DL-alanine < glycine < 0·1 M sodium chloride.

Aminoacid administration to the tongue also significantly reduced the chorda tympani response to sodium chloride. The inhibition of the response to NaCl began about 1 hour after the aminoacids had been applied and was still present after 20 hours. Recent experiments by Rapuzzi, Ricagno and Ventura (1963) have shown that the inhibitory effect of aminoacids is not specific to sodium chloride. Various aminoacids severely depressed the electrical response of the frog's taste receptors to calcium chloride. At high concentrations (2 to 3 M) all aminoacids tested produced a roughly equal (approximately 75%)inhibition of neural activity. However, at concentrations of 10 mM some interesting differential effects became apparent. β-Alanine was one of the most effective inhibitors, causing almost 50% depression of neural activity, whereas α-alanine produced slight facilitation. Similarly β-aminobutyric acid significantly inhibited the receptor response to $CaCl_2$, and α-aminobutyric acid did not. γ-Aminobutyric acid caused an interesting intermediary effect. Valine and glycine produced small inhibitory effects comparable to those seen after γ-aminobutyric acid. Leucine resulted in intense inhibition similar to that seen after β-alanine and β-aminobutyric acid.

Miscellaneous drug effects on taste and olfaction

A review of the clinical literature suggests that a number of drugs are potentially capable of interfering with taste and olfactory sensations in man. However, these 'side-effects' occur only rarely and are therefore difficult to interpret or even replicate under controlled conditions. In view of these difficulties, only a few examples will be cited here.

One of the more common gustatory side-effects reported in the clinical literature is a marked rise in the subjective threshold for sweet substances (sometimes accompanied by a lowering of the threshold for bitter-tasting foods) which occurs during a prolonged period of amphetamine treatment. Although several clinical observers have reported statistically significant effects (Ahokas *et al.*, 1950; Mata, 1963), others (Janowitz and Grossman, 1949) have failed to observe a consistent change in either sweet or bitter thresholds. A closer look at the data suggests that some patients reliably report large and apparently repeatable changes in one or both thresholds whereas others show no effect at all or complain of diametrically opposed symptoms. These differential effects must be related to a drug-receptor interaction which depends on a chemical reaction that is not common to all individuals. Just what that reaction might be is unfortunately not yet apparent. It seems unlikely, in any case, that the appetite-depressant action of the amphetamines could be due to their effect on the sweet taste threshold as has been suggested by Ahokas and her associates.

Less commonly reported abnormalities include:

(a) an apparently selective and complete ageusia for sweet substances, accompanied by a distortion of salt-related taste sensations, following prolonged insulin therapy (Cazzola, 1952).

(b) Complex alterations in taste perception have been produced by treatment with dinitrophenol, which was used as an appetite depressant until its toxicity for the central nervous system was fully appreciated. Prolonged dinitrophenol treatment was frequently accompanied by a gradual disappearance of all salt sensations, often accompanied by a general modification of taste perception such that all substances acquired a marked bitter and unpleasant taste quality. Some patients even reported a complete loss of taste for sweet, salt and acid substances, only bitter remaining intact and even intensified (Bogaert, 1935). Concurrent modifications of visual and auditory perception suggest that general, central effects are involved rather than a selective effect on gustatory receptors or pathways.

(c) Intravenous injections of some drugs at times elicit unusual taste and olfactory sensations. Occasionally, it is reported that individuals have salt or sweet sensations following intravenous injections of hypertonic sodium chloride or glucose solutions but the role of suggestion has not been adequately ruled out in the few cases on record. More adequately documented are some unusual taste and olfactory sensations following the administration of drugs of unknown direct effect on taste or olfactory receptors. A nice example of such an indirect stimulating effect has been reported by Kraupa-Runk (1961). Some patients given neoarsphenamine injections reported strange olfactory sensations which appeared similar to those elicited by ether, and gustatory sensations which were unlike any normal taste. In some cases these disturbances persisted for several hours.

Interaction of taste stimuli

So far in our discussion we have largely neglected the fact that some of the drugs which have been used to modify the response of the taste receptors are themselves capable of eliciting specific taste sensations. That these sensations may themselves be at least partly responsible for the observed changes in threshold is suggested by the fact that some taste receptors are capable of responding to more than one basic taste modality. Subjective interaction effects are nicely demonstrated in studies which are concerned with the effects of compound taste stimuli.

Because of its obvious practical implications for the food industry, this problem has a long and complex history. Some of the earlier experiments (Zuntz, 1892; Kiesow, 1984) demonstrated that the presentation of sucrose in a slightly salty solution increased the apparent sweetness of the mixture. This effect was reversed when the salt concentration of the solution was increased above some minimum. More recently, Cragg (1937) reported that sucrose decreased the apparent sourness of hydrochloric acid whereas sodium chloride admixtures had no effect. Komm and Lammer (1940) replicated these experiments and reported that the sourness of organic acids in sugar solution varies as a function of the sugar concentration.

The effects of subthreshold concentrations of taste substances on the intensity of other tastes were studied by Fabian and Blum (1942). Sodium chloride in subthreshold concentrations consistently reduced the sourness of acids, the response to lactic, malic, and tartaric acid being preferentially affected. Sodium chloride also increased the sweetness of all sugars. The magnitude of this effect was maltose > lactose > fructose > dextrose > sucrose when the comparison was based on concentration by weight of sugar. All acids (except hydrochloric acid) in subthreshold concentrations increased the saltiness of sodium chloride and increased the sweetness of sucrose. The sweetness of fructose, on the other hand, was reduced by all acids except hydrochloric and citric acids. These two acids were found to reduce the sweetness of dextrose which was unaffected by any of the other acids. All sugars consistently reduced the saltiness of sodium chloride and the sourness of all acids. The effect of sodium chloride and sugars on the sourness of acids could not be correlated with changes in the phosphate buffer titration or with changes in pH.

Beebe-Center *et al.* (1959) have more recently reported that suprathreshold concentrations of sodium chloride (in relatively weak solutions) enhanced the sweetness of sugars and masked all other taste sensations. Kamen *et al.* (1961; see also Pilgrim, 1961) have reported a more extensive investigation of the effects of suprathreshold solutions of some substances. Caffeine (bitter) did not reliably affect the sensation of saltiness or sweetness but significantly enhanced the sourness of citric acid. Suprathreshold concentrations of sodium chloride did not reliably affect the bitterness of caffeine but slightly masked sweetness. The sour taste of citric acid was enhanced by sodium chloride. Sugar reduced the bitterness of caffeine, as well as the sourness of citric acid but produced no reliable effect on the perception of salt. Citric acid markedly enhanced the taste of bitter, salty, and sweet substances, the largest effect being recorded on the bitterness of caffeine. These differential effects contrast with an earlier report by Pangborn (1960) which demonstrated only mutually inhibitory effects of subthreshold, threshold, and suprathreshold concentrations of sodium chloride, caffeine, citric acid, and sucrose.

These subjective interactions are difficult to reconcile with electrophysiological evidence which indicates only an algebraic summation of the neural response to mixtures. Andersson *et al.* (1950) reported, for instance, that the electrical response of single taste fibres to citric acid/sugar mixtures (which provide the most marked and consistent mutual masking of subjective taste sensations in man) was a simple algebraic addition of the neurone's response to citric acid and to sugar alone. Halpern (1959) observed a similar additive relationship between the chorda tympani response to acetic acid and sucrose. The additive effects were most clearly demonstrated when the two compounds, individually, produced approximately equal neural responses. Similar recordings from the solitary nucleus in the medulla (the first relay nucleus of the taste pathways) continued to show some additive effects but the response to the acetic acid/sucrose mixture was not nearly as large as the sum of the response to the individual substances.

The effect of drugs on food intake

The control of appetite and food intake has become a major medical problem in our affluent society. Drug houses all over the world have been experimenting with anorexigenic agents and a number of these appetite depressants have been given extensive clinical tests. A large and often contradictory literature has attempted to describe their effectiveness and mode of action.

One approach to the problem of appetite control has relied on an interference with peripheral mechanisms (such as an inhibition of gastric motility or secretion) or the substitution of non-nutritive bulk at mealtime. By and large, this technique has not been successful, and its use has shed little light on specific pharmacological mechanisms that might be involved in the control of food intake.

The use of centrally acting appetite depressants has contributed much more to our understanding. The anorexigenic effects of the amphetamines have been extensively studied in the past 20 years (see recent reviews by Fazekas, 1961; Fazekas *et al.*, 1958; Gelvin *et al.*, 1958). More recently, attempts have been made to modify the structure of amphetamines to maximize the appetite depressant effects while minimizing some of their undesirable effects. The most notable results of this research have been the drugs phenmetrazine, diethylpropion, and phenylpropanolamine (Berneike, 1954; Spiegelberg, 1954; Thomä and Wick, 1954; Gelvin *et al.*, 1956).

Some of the earlier investigators (Melchionna *et al.*, 1952; Parson and Crispel, 1952) of the sympathomimetic amines could not convince themselves that the drugs produced significant effects above and beyond a 'placebo' effect ascribable to suggestion or other 'psychological' factors. It is now quite well established that these drugs can serve as a significant aid in a comprehensive programme of weight control (Feldman *et al.*, 1957; Barnes, 1958; Fineberg, 1961). However, most clinical studies indicate that obese patients cannot sustain an acceptable rate of weight loss (1 pound per week) when the drug therapy is not supported by a low calorie diet (Gelvin and McGavack, 1949; Gelvin *et al.*, 1953, 1954, 1956; Barnes, 1958). Moreover, the reaction of individuals varies widely. Almost all clinical investigators report that some patients (usually between 20 and 30%) do not respond at all. Others lose a significant amount of weight but the effect is no larger than that observed following the administration of a completely harmless placebo. However, 40 to 50% of the obese patients respond promptly and markedly to the sympathomimetics, losing up to 3 or 4 pounds per week and reporting such a marked effect on subjective appetite sensations that interspersed placebo treatments are immediately recognized. Usually, it is the younger and less obese patients who respond best to the anorexigenic agents, perhaps because the motivation to lose weight is stronger in the young and the abnormal tendency to overeat less well developed in the moderately obese. A closer look at the many clinical studies suggests, however, that these obvious factors explain only a small fraction of the variance between patients, suggesting that the drug effects on food intake and appetite are complex, and still poorly understood.

It is widely assumed that the sympathomimetic appetite depressants depress food intake because of a direct action on central mechanisms that regulate the organism's energy balance (Fazekas, 1961). Various pharmacological mechanisms have been proposed to account for this central effect, among them: (a) an inhibition of the depressant effects of tyramine and other amines on cerebral oxidative metabolism, (b) a depression (or alternatively excitation or facilitation) of central adrenergic receptors, (c) a preservation of central noradrenaline stores because of a competitive inhibition of amine oxidase activity, and (d) indirect central effects due to peripheral stimulating or inhibiting effects of the drug.

If the anorexigenic effects of the sympathomimetic amines are, in fact, centrally mediated, our search for a target organ can be narrowed to a relatively small core portion of the brain since a number of studies have shown that these substances cross the blood-brain barrier only in the region of the brain-stem and hypothalamus (Vogt, 1954; Carlsson *et al.*, 1958; Weil-Malherbe *et al.*, 1959). On purely logical grounds, this would make some sense since distinct 'feeding' and 'satiety' centers have been demonstrated in the hypothalamus of rats, cats, goats, and monkeys. Electrical stimulation of the lateral hypothalamic feeding centre elicits food intake in sated animals (Bruegger, 1943); its destruction results in complete though perhaps not permanent aphagia (Anand and Brobeck, 1951; Teitelbaum and Stellar, 1954). Stimulation of the more medial satiety centre reduces or stops food intake (Anand and Dua, 1955) and its destruction leads to marked hyperphagia (Hetherington and Ranson, 1939). The behavioural as well as electrophysiological arousal effects of the sympathomimetics (Dell *et al.*, 1954; Rothballer, 1956) which constitute the most troublesome effects of the appetite depressants have been ascribed to a direct action of the drugs on cells in the mesencephalic reticular formation (Dell, 1960).

A group of experiments from our own laboratory (Grossman, 1960, 1962a, b, 1964a, b, 1966a, b; Grossman and Grossman, 1966) have provided some information which may help us understand some of the mechanisms involved. Double-walled cannulas, permitting repeated applications of chemicals to the same site in the brain were stereotaxically implanted into the medial, lateral, and anterior hypothalamus; midbrain reticular formation; and several limbic system structures. After recovery from surgery, various chemicals were injected into each of these areas.

The local application of minute quantities of sympathomimetic amines, notably adrenaline and noradrenaline, directly to the lateral hypothalamic 'feeding' centre, elicited food intake in completely sated animals. For approximately 30 to 50 minutes the animals ate all available nutritive and even non-nutritive substances and worked a lever to obtain bits of food. When the injections were given to hungry (24-hour food deprived) animals, their feeding behaviour became frantic and reliably exceeded normal levels. These injections also lowered the animals' activity, and, in larger doses, induced sleep. Similar injections into the immediately adjacent medial 'satiety' centre did not influence the food consumption of sated or hungry animals. Local applications of drugs suspected of a sympatholytic (i.e., blocking) action with respect to adrenergic mechanisms (phenoxybenzamine, ethoxybutamoxane) to the lateral feeding centre specifically reduced the food intake of hungry animals and blocked the noradrenaline-induced feeding effect. Systemic injections of these adrenergic blocking agents also selectively interfered with food intake.

More recently, we have found that local injections of adrenergic substances into a variety of limbic system structures (the amygdala, hippocampus, and anterior hypothalamus), which are known to contribute to the regulation of food intake, also elicit or facilitate feeding. Micro-injections of noradrenaline or adrenaline into the mesencephalic reticular formation were found to have excitatory or facilitatory effects on locomotor activity, electrophysiological arousal, and the animals' behaviour in various standard psychological test situations.

These observations suggest that the central mechanisms which regulate food intake may be selectively stimulated by catecholamines, and the question arises why the systemic administration of these drugs produces apparently inhibitory effects. One possibility is that the amphetamines and related sympathomimetics act as 'false' transmitters and block the action of endogenous noradrenaline in the neural pathways which regulate feeding behaviour. Such an interpretation seems to be contradicted by the observation that systemic injection of adrenaline (Russek and Tina, 1962) and noradrenaline (Miller, 1965) produces anorexia in cats and rats. However, the inhibitory or depressant effects of systemically administered noradrenaline and adrenaline are not at all specific to food intake. Miller (1965) observed that systemic noradrenaline injection depressed water as well as food intake and concluded that these effects might be due to some general peripheral sympathetic disturbance such as a sudden increase in blood pressure.

The hypothesis that the amphetamines may act as false transmitters in the CNS and block rather than excite activity in adrenergic mechanisms is also supported by the drugs' peculiar effects on behavioural and electrophysiological arousal. All anorexic agents produce marked facilitatory or stimulating effects. However, intrahypothalamic injections of noradrenaline or adrenaline depress the general level of activity and may induce sleep or coma. Preliminary observations indicate that the amphetamines (unlike noradrenaline) do not produce an alerting reaction when applied directly to the mesencephalic reticular formation. These findings suggest that the excitatory effects of the anorexic agents may be due to blockade of an inhibitory mechanism which may be part of the reticular arousal system or modify its activity indirectly. However, alternative interpretations in terms of a direct stimulating effect on specific aspects of the brain-stem arousal system cannot be ruled out until the effects of locally applied amphetamines have been studied in greater detail.

The suggested interpretation of the anorexic effects of catecholamines also receives some support from the observation that systemic injections of monoamine oxidase inhibitors such as iproniazid (which increase the central catecholamine stores) increase food intake, whereas reserpine which depletes the brain of catecholamines reduces food consumption. However, it is difficult to make much of these observations, since both drugs affect a bewildering variety of central and peripheral functions.

REFERENCES

Aducco et V. Mosso. (1886). *Giornale della Acc. di Med. di Torino.*

Ahokas, A. J., Payne, J. G. and Goetzl, F. R. (1950). *Permanente Foundation Medical Bulletin*, **8**, 107.

Allara, E. (1939). *Arch. Ital. Anat. & Embriol.*, **42**, 506.

Allara, E. (1952). *Rivista di Biologia (Perugia)*, **44**, 209.

Allara, E. (1952). *Boll. Soc. Ital. Biol. sper.*, **28**, 68.

Anand, B. K. and Brobeck, J. R. (1951). *Yale J. Biol. & Med.*, **24**, 123.

Anand, B. K. and Dua, S. (1955). *Indian J. med. Res.*, **43**, 113.

Andersson, B., Landgren, S., Olsson, L. and Zotterman, Y. (1950). *Acta physiol. scand.*, **21**, 105.

Anrep, B. (1880). *Pflüg. Arch. ges. Physiol.* **21**, 38.

Barnes, R. H. (1958). *J. Amer. med. Assoc.*, **166**, 898.

Beebe-Center, J. G., Rogers, M. S., Atkinson, W. H. and O'Connel, D. H. *J. exptl. Psychol.*, **57**, 231.

Belletrud, M. and Mercier, M. (1907). *L'Encéphale*, Paris, **2**, 251.

Berneike, K. H. (1954). *Med. Klin.*, **49**, 478.

Birjukov, D. A. (1938). *Fiziologicheskii Zhurnal SSSR. Imeni, I. M. Sechenova*, **25**, 119.

Bogaert, L. van. (1935). *Bull. Mém. Soc. Méd. Hôp. Paris*, **51**, 1393.

Carlsson, A., Lindqvist, A., Magnusson, T. and Waldeck, B. (1958). *Science*, **127**, 471.

Carr, W. J. (1952). *J. comp. physiol. Psychol.*, **45**, 377.

Cohen, J. and Ogdon, D. P. (1949). *Science*, **110**, 522.

Cragg, L. H. (1937a). *Roy. Soc. Canada*, **31**, 7.

Cragg, L. H. (1937b). *Proc. roy. Soc. Canada*, **31**, 131.
Dell, P., Bonvallet, M. and Hugelin, A. (1954). *EEG clin. Neurophysiol.*, **6**, 599.
Dell, P. (1960). *In* Ciba Found. Symp. Adrenergic Mech. (ed. Wolstenholme, G. E. W. and O'Connor, M.), p. 393. London: Churchill.
de Wardener, H. E. and Herxheimer, A. (1957). *J. Physiol.*, **139**, 53,
Dicker, S. E. (1958). *J. Physiol.*, **144**, 138.
Ehrenberg, R. and Güttes, H. J. (1949). *Pflüg. Arch. ges. Physiol.*, **251**, 664.
Fabian, F. W. and Blum, H. B. (1943). *J. Food. Sci.*, **8**, 179.
Fazekas, F. (1961). *New England J. Med.*, **264**, 501.
Fazekas, J. F., Ehrmantraut, W. R. and Kleh, J. (1958). *Am. J. med. Sci.*, **236**, 692.
Feldman, R., Alberton, E. C. and Craig, L. (1957). *Cal. Med.*, **87**, 408.
Ferrari, P. (1905). *Arch. Ital. Biol.*, **42**, 411.
Fineberg, S. K. (1961). *J. Amer. med. Ass.*, **175**, 680.
Fischer, R. and Griffin, F. (1961a). *J. Neuropsychiat.*, **3**, 98.
Fischer, R. and Griffin, F. (1961b). *Experientia*, **17**, 36.
Fischer, R. and Griffin, F. (1964). **14**, 673.
Fischer, R., Griffin F. and Mead, E. L. (1962). *Med. exptl.*, **6**, 177.
Fischer, R., Griffin, F. and Kaplan, A. R. (1963). *Lancet*, **i**, 393.
Fischer, R., Griffin, F. and Pasamanick, B. (1965). *In* Psychopathology of Perception, (ed. Hoch, P., and Zubin, J.), p. 129. New York: Stratton.
Fontana, A. (1902). *Zeitschrift für Psychologie und Physiologie der Sinnesorgane*, **28**, 253.
Fourneau, M. (1904). *Comptes Rendus*, **138**, 766.
Fourneau, M. (1905). Recueil des principaux mémoires concernant la stovaine. Paris: Challamel.
Gardella, E. (1904). *Archivio di Fisiologie*, **1**, 398.
Gazzola, G. (1952). *Arch. di. Psichol., Neurol. & Psichiat.*, **13**, 104.
Gelvin, E. P. and McGavack, T. H. (1949). *N.Y. State J. Med.*, **49**, 279.
Gelvin, E. P. and McGavack, T. H. (1956). *Am. J. digest. Dis.*, **1**, 155.
Gelvin, E. P., McGavack, T. H. and Kenigsberg, S. (1953). *Am. J. digest. Dis.*, **20**, 307.
Gelvin, E. P., McGavack, T. H. and Kenigsberg, S. (1954). *N.Y. State J. Med.*, **54**, 1340.
Gelvin, E. P., McGavack, T. H. and Kenigsberg, S. (1956). *J. dig. Dis., New Series*, **1**, 155.
Gelvin, E. P., McGavack, T. H. and Kenigsberg, S. (1958). *Amer. Pract. & Digest Treat.*, **9**, 2008.
Grossman, S. (1953). *N. Y. State J. Med.*, **53**, 1236.
Grossman, S. P. (1960). *Science*, **132**, 301.
Grossman, S. P. (1962a). *Am. J. Physiol.*, **202**, 872.
Grossman, S. P. (1962b). *Am. J. Physiol.*, **202**, 1230.
Grossman, S. P. (1964a). *J. comp. physiol. Psychol.*, **57**, 29.

Grossman, S. P. (1964b). *J. comp. physiol. Psychol.*, **58,** 194.
Grossman, S. P. (1966a). *J. Physiol. & Behav.*, **1,** 1.
Grossman, S. P. (1966b). *J. comp. physiol. Psychol.* **61,** 42.
Grossman, S. P. and Grossman, L. (1966). *J. comp. physiol. Psychol.* **61,** 333.
Halpern, B. N. (1956). *Comptes Rendus, Soc. Biol. (Paris)*, **150,** 1152.
Halpern, B. N. and Lehmann, A. (1956). *Comptes Rendus, Soc. Biol. (Paris)*, **150,** 1863.
Halpern, B. P. (1959). Ph.D. Thesis, Brown University.
Halpern, B. P., Bernard, R. A. and Kare, M. R. (1962). *J. gen. Physiol.*, **45,** 681.
Harriman, A. and MacLeod, R. B. (1963). *Amer. J. Psychol.*, **66,** 465.
Herxheimer, A. and Woodbury, D. M. (1960). *J. Physiol.*, **151,** 253.
Hetherington, A. W. and Ranson, S. W. (1939). *Proc. Soc. exptl. Biol. Med. N.Y.* **41,** 465.
Hoshishima, K., Yokoyama, S. and Seto, K. (1962). *Am. J. Physiol.*, **202,** 1200.
Janowitz, H. D. and Grossman, M. I. (1949). *J. appl. Physiol.*, **2,** 217.
Kamen, J. M., Pilgrim, F. J., Gutman, N. J. and Kroll, B. J. (1961). *J. exptl. Psychol.*, **62,** 348.
Kiesow, F. (1894). *Philos. Stud.*, **9,** 510.
Knapp, H. (1885). *Arch. f. Augenheilkunde*, **15,** 398.
Knüchel, W. (1950). *Neue Medizinische Welt*, **1,** 1487.
Komm, E. and Lammer, H. (1940). *Ztschr. f. Untersuch. d. Lebensmtl.*, **79,** 541.
Kraupa-Runk, M. (1916). *Münchener med. Wschr.*, **63,** 46.
Kuhn, R. and Zilliken, F. (1950). *Naturwiss.*, **37,** 167.
Kusano, K. (1958). *Kumamoto Med.*, **11,** 174.
Kusano, K. (1959). *Kumamoto Med.*, **12,** 236.
Launoy e Billon. (1905). Cited by Fourneau.
Le Magnen, J. (1953). *Compt. Rendus Soc. Biol., Paris*, **147,** 1753.
Leys, D. (1945). *Lancet*, **i,** 461.
Lovell, M. R. C., Gross, C. G. and Weiskrantz, L. (1961). *Animal Behaviour*, **9,** 31.
Margolin, S., Perlman, P., Villani, F. and McGavack, T. (1951). *Science*, **114,** 384.
Mata, F. (1963). *J. Neuropsychiat.* **4,** 315.
Melchionna, R. and Ferguson, F. (1952). *Am. J. med. Sci.*, **13,** 478.
Mhaskar, K. S. and Caius, J. F. (1930). *Br. Ind. med. Res. Mem.*, **16,** 1.
Miller, N. E. (1965). *Science*, **148,** 328.
Mori, A. (1957). *Nippon Chikusangaku Kaihô*, **28,** 21.
Nachman, M. (1963). *Am. J. Physiol.* **205,** 219.
Pangborn, R. M. (1960). *J. Food Sci.*, **25,** 245.
Parson, W. and Crispell, K. R. (1952). *Med. Clin N. Amer.*, **36,** 385.
Pfaffmann, C. (1955). *J. Neurophysiol.*, **18,** 429.
Pfaffmann, C. (1959). *In* Handbook of Physiology (ed. Field, J., Magoun, H. W. and Hall, V. E.), Section 1, volume I, p. 507, Baltimore: Williams and Wilkins.

Pfaffmann, C. and Bare, J. K. (1950). *J. comp. physiol. Psychol.*, **43**, 320.
Pilgrim, F. J. (1961). *In* Physiological and Behavioral Aspects of Taste (ed. Kare, M. R. and Halpern, B. P.) Chicago: Univ. Chicago Press.
Ponzo, M. (1909). *Arch. ges. Psychol.*, **14**, 385.
Power, F. B. and Tutin, F. (1904). *Pharm. J.*, **73**, 234.
Radomski, J. L., Fuyat, H. W., Nelson, A. A. and Smith, P. K. (1950). *J. Pharmacol. exp. Therap.*, **100**, 429.
Rapuzzi, G., Ricagno, G. and Ventura, U. (1963). *Boll. Soc. Ital. Biol. sper.*, **39**, 1853.
Reuter, S. (1900). Thesis, University of Utrecht, Holland.
Rice, K. K. and Richter, C. P. (1943). *Endocrinology*, **33**, 106.
Richter, C. P. (1936). *Am. J. Physiol.*, **115**, 155.
Richter, C. P. (1939). *Trans. Amer. Neurol. Assoc.* **65**, 49.
Richter, C. P. (1941). *Endocrinology*, **29**, 115.
Richter, C. P. (1942), *Am. J. Physiol.*, **135**, 781.
Richter, C. P. and Eckert, J. F. (1937). *Endocrinology*, **21**, 50.
Richter, C. P. and Schmidt, E. (1941). *Endocrinology*, **28**, 179.
Rothballer, A. B. (1956). *EEG clin. Neurophysiol.*, **8**, 603.
Russek, M. and Tina, S. (1962). *Nature (Lond.)*, **193**, 1296.
Schneeberg, N. G. (1952). *J. Amer. med. Ass.*, **149**, 1091.
Shore, L. E. (1892). *J. Physiol.*, **13**, 191.
Skramlik, E. von. (1963). *In* Olfaction and Taste, (ed. Zotterman, Y.), p. 125. Oxford: Pergamon Press.
Spiegelberg, U. (1954). *Nervenarzt*, **25**, 276.
Teitelbaum, P. and Stellar, E. (1954). *Science*, **120**, 894.
Thomä, O. and Wick, H. (1954). *Arch. exper. Path. Pharmak.*, **222**, 540.
Vogt, M. (1954). *Brit. med. Bull.*, **13**, 166.
Weil-Malherbe, H. Axelrod, J. and Tomchick, R. (1959). *Science*, **129**, 1226.
Wilkins, L. and Richter, C. P. (1940). *J. Amer. med. Ass.*, **114**, 866.
Yensen, R. (1958a). *Nature (Lond.)*, **181**, 1472.
Yensen, R. (1958b). *Nature (Lond.)*, **182**, 677.
Yumikura, T. (1955a). *Med. J. Osaka. Univ.*, **7**, 409.
Yumikura, T. (1955b). *Med. J. Osaka Univ.*, **7**, 415.
Zuntz, N. (1892). *Arch. f. Anat. u. Physiol. Physiol. Abt.*, p. 556.
Zwaardemaker, H. (1895). Physiologie des Geruchs, p. 147. Leipzig: W. Engelmann.

DISCUSSION

Wade: The effect of amphetamine on food intake has always seemed to be a very complex matter. Clinicians try to persuade fat people to reduce in weight, but giving them these tablets makes them feel they no longer need use will-power.

Grossman: That may be the trouble. If you give amphetamine to normal animals or people who have a normal craving for food, quite drastic changes in food intake typically occur. The questionable effect of amphetamines may result from a masking of the amphetamine effect by a pathological desire for food. Just how that arises and why it is not affected by amphetamine is another question. Psychiatric information suggests that the over-eating, at least in many cases, may not be due to a primary disturbance of the organism's energy balance, but be secondary to other, perhaps emotional factors. Amphetamines may not be able to overcome such influences.

Harper: How definite are the effects of one's own saliva? Washing the tongue with distilled water could lead to subsequent stimulus dilution. In contrast, however, Pfaffmann found that the threshold for salt could be lowered about 100-fold by washing the tongue with distilled water. However, this was attributed to the effect of sodium ions in the saliva.

Grossman: The original studies with thiouracil show that this is essentially an all-or-none effect. With respect to the work of Fischer and his associates on quinine, the effect is specific to bitter, and is not quite as all-or-none as with thiouracil.

Chadwick: I was most interested in the selective effect of cocaine on the threshold of taste for bitter substances and wonder whether anything similar happens with smell. In my surgical practice I prepare noses for operation by instilling a solution containing cocaine hydrochloride 2·5% and adrenaline 1 part in 4,000. On a number of occasions following this procedure, patients have subsequently remarked upon a diminution in their sense of smell, which seems to persist indefinitely. Since the field of operation does not involve the olfactory area, this anosmia seems to be due to a permanent toxic effect on the olfactory receptors or nerves. I should like your comments.

Grossman: Cocaine has effects on olfactory acuity, but as far as I know these are not specific. A number of studies suggest that the effect is general, and is very long lasting, particularly with respect to some odours, such as 'burnt rubber'. The cocaine effect lasts for days and even weeks or months, indicating structural damage.

Collier: Some years ago J. R. Vane showed that amphetamine acted like 5-hydroxytryptamine rather than adrenaline on the rat stomach strip (*Brit. J. Pharmacol.*, 1957, **12**, 344–349). In my laboratory, Schneider (unpublished) likewise found that several substituted tryptamines had anorectic activity of about the same order as amphetamine in the rat.

Grossman: We have injected tryptamine and a number of related substances into the hypothalamus with equivocal results. I didn't mention the fact that amphetamine itself when injected into one side of the hypothalamus does not seem to affect food intake. That may mean merely that unilateral interference with the feeding mechanism produces no changes and I don't have the obvious data that one would want, namely what happens after bilateral injection.

Turner: Anorexia is a prominent feature of depression, and depression may be produced by reserpine, after which your animals took less food. Recent work suggests that imipramine selectively improves appetite in depression. Have you studied this drug in animals? Do you feel that the anorexia in the depressive syndrome is due to a specific amine depletion in the appetite centres or a general result of the depressive syndrome?

Grossman: I think the answer to both questions is no. The iproniazid effects that I mentioned might be explained in the way you suggest, though this drug is probably less specific than the drugs you mentioned.

Gray: I wonder whether Dr. Grossman's hypothesis as to how amphetamine depresses food intake would account for some curious features of the behaviour which occurs not only with amphetamine but also with other stimulants. It has been reported several times that animals given such drugs stop taking or eating the food available in a situation in which they are performing a response ostensibly for a food reward, but nevertheless produce the response at a much greater intensity or rate. I have observed this myself with pipradrol (Gray, J. A. The effects of pipradrol hydrochloride and sodium amylobarbitone on operant responding in a discrimination situation. *Psychopharmacologia*, 1964, **6**, 417–434), and it has been reported with methylphenidate (Faidherbe, J., Richelle, M. and Schlag, J. Non-consumption of the reinforcer under drug action. *J. exp. Anal. Behav.*, 1962, **5**, 521–524), and I think amphetamine as well.

Grossman: A number of drugs produce general facilitatory effects on the central nervous system which may be reflected in an apparently specific facilitation of behavioural reactions which are 'dominant' because of previous training or innate response tendencies. If the animal is in a situation where he previously has worked a lever to obtain food, such a drug may produce an apparently specific increase in the rate of lever-pressing. The same drug may, however, facilitate avoidance responses in a double-grill box or merely increase random locomotion in a novel environment.

Feldberg: May I also ask you a question Dr. Grossman? Years ago, we found that small doses of anaesthetics, pentobarbitone sodium or chloralose, injected into the cerebral ventricles of the cat produced hyperphagia: adrenaline similarly injected did not do so although it produced a sleep-like condition. Now the fact that anaesthetics produce hyperphagia can't be fully explained by their action on the medial hypothalamus, which has an inhibitory influence on the more laterally located feeding centre, because the same effect is obtained with small doses of pentobarbitone sodium given intravenously.

Grossman: We found that injections of noradrenaline into the lateral hypothalamus induced sleep, or reduced arousal or alertness.

Feldberg: But you also obtained an increased food intake?

Grossman: Yes, it did elicit feeding in sated animals or raised the food intake of hungry animals, but also reduced activity, and, in larger doses, induced sleep.

Feldberg: We could never obtain this effect, but we may only have reached the medial hypothalamus.

Grossman: I think the explanation might be related to species differences. You were doing this work in cats and the adrenaline would have to diffuse quite a way into the hypothalamus before it could affect the lateral hypothalamus. All our studies were done in rats where the absolute distance is much smaller. However, we have not been able to obtain sleep or even a reduction in locomotor activity from medial placements in the rat, so I don't quite know what the answer is.

Feldberg: I am glad, because I don't either.

Bradley: What you have just said suggests that the anorexic effects of these compounds is unrelated to their effects on wakefulness and sleep.

Grossman: I never intended to imply that the same population of neurones might be responsible for both, the feeding and the sleep effects. Sleep, coma, or a reduction in arousal can be elicited from a much larger portion of the lateral and ventral hypothalamus than the feeding effect. It seems that two populations of neurones overlap sufficiently for the depression to accompany the feeding effect fairly often, if not always.

Land: In studying amphetamine depression of appetite the cat, a carnivore, is probably less analogous to man than omnivorous animals and will certainly be quite different from herbivores.

Feldberg: That is a good point. Nevertheless the cat is a very useful animal!

AMPHETAMINE AND TASTE IN MAN

ANDREW HERXHEIMER

Department of Pharmacology, London Hospital Medical College

THAT the taste of food and drink is an important determinant of intake is clear from everyday experience and from many animal experiments (e.g. Richter, 1939; Herxheimer and Woodbury, 1960; Teitelbaum and Epstein, 1962). It is therefore worth asking whether depression of appetite by amphetamine is associated with any effects of the drug on taste. Conceivably the drug might indirectly depress appetite by altering the intensity of tastes. It might for example weaken the subjective intensity of some or of all tastes, so making food less attractive. Or if amphetamine intensified some taste sensations, less food than usual might satisfy the desire for it. An obvious approach to this problem is to examine the effect of amphetamine on taste thresholds. The results so far published on sucrose (Janowitz and Grossman, 1949; Ahokas, Payne and Goetzl, 1950) and on quinine taste thresholds (Mata, 1963) are conflicting and the experimental designs used were rather unsatisfactory.

However, threshold measurements concern only very low intensities of taste sensation which can only be marginally relevant to eating or drinking behaviour. Taste sensations that influence such behaviour are usually far above threshold intensity. A promising method for investigating subjective intensities of taste above threshold has been developed by Beebe-Center (1949) and his collaborators (Beebe-Center, Rogers and Atkinson, 1955). They showed that it is possible to make consistent judgements of the relative taste intensities of solutions that taste qualitatively different. For example, one salt solution tastes consistently weaker than a particular sugar solution; another salt solution tastes consistently stronger. One can in fact construct series of salt and sugar solutions of matching taste intensities—so-called hetero-qualitative taste intensity matching. The intensity of a taste corresponds to the brightness of a light, or the loudness of a sound; taste quality corresponds to colour or pitch. Brightness and loudness can however be measured objectively, whereas the intensity of a taste remains obstinately subjective. That is probably why it has been so long neglected. Psychophysical scaling methods for measuring subjective intensities in various sensory modalities have been reviewed by Stevens (1958).

Because Beebe-Center's matching technique can show whether a drug alters the relative intensity of two different taste qualities, I have investigated amphetamine with it; in the same experiment I also re-examined the effects of amphetamine on taste thresholds.

Six volunteers aged 19–20 (5 men, 1 woman) were each given three treatments under double-blind conditions: a placebo, dexamphetamine sulphate 7·5 mg and dexamphetamine sulphate 15 mg. The order of administration was balanced in a Latin square design; at least 48 hours elapsed between successive sessions for each subject. The drug was taken as a flavoured solution in the mid-afternoon. Testing was begun one hour later and occupied about one hour. Before the first experimental session each subject was given a practice session to acquaint him with the procedure.

Taste thresholds to sucrose, sodium chloride and tartaric acid were determined first, and this was followed by taste intensity matching of solutions of sucrose and sodium chloride. Table 1 lists the solutions used. For the first three subjects all solutions were made with tap-water, for the other three with distilled water. Differences between these two groups of subjects have been ignored, since they were no greater than differences within the groups.

Table 1

Solutions used in the experiments

Concentrations are expressed in G solute per 100 ml. solution

(a) *Solutions used for intensity matching (after Beebe-Center, 1949)*

Sucrose		Standard A 7·87				Standard B 24·3			
Sodium chloride	solution no.	1	2	3	4	5	6	7	8
	concentration	0·298	0·456	0·700	1·11	1·99	3·80	7·31	15·14

Solutions 1–7 were compared with standard A, and solutions 2 to 8 with standard B.

(b) *Solutions used in taste threshold determinations*

Sucrose	solution no.	1	2	3	4	5	6	7	8	9	10	11	12
	concentration	0·125	0·175	0·25	0·35	0·5	0·7	1·0	1·4	2·0	2·8	4·0	5·6
Sodium chloride	solution no.	1	2	3	4	5	6	7	8	9	10		
	concentration	0·0125	0·0175	0·025	0·035	0·05	0·07	0·10	0·14	0·20	0·28		
Tartaric acid	solution no.	1	2	3	4	5	6	7	8	9	10		
	concentration	0·0025	0·0035	0·005	0·007	0·010	0·014	0·020	0·028	0·040	0·056		

In the *matching procedure* the subject compared the taste intensity of a standard sucrose solution with that of each of 7 comparison solutions of sodium chloride. Each comparison stimulus in turn was presented with the standard and was tasted first. After each solution had been tasted the mouth was rinsed with water. After each comparison the subject reported whether the salt solution tasted weaker or stronger than the sweet standard. The comparison solutions were presented in random order. In each session four series of comparisons were made, two with each of two sucrose standards.

Taste thresholds were determined by presenting series of solutions in ascending concentration; the subject was asked to report what he tasted. The concentration increased by a factor of 1·4 from one step to the next. The starting concentration of the series was varied between occasions. At each session three series were presented, one for each of the tastes under test, the order being balanced with respect to both treatments and subjects. Determination of the specific taste threshold to tartaric acid proved unreliable because some subjects could not distinguish between bitter and acid taste. The results obtained with tartaric acid are therefore not reported. Confusion of bitter and acid tastes is said to be common (Pangborn, 1961), but the phenomenon is not widely known.

Intensity equivalents and taste thresholds were estimated from the individual observations by an interpolation procedure suggested by Dr. M. H. Quenouille; it is best made clear by an example. When a series of salt solutions, 1 to 7, is compared with a standard sweet solution, suppose the results to be as follows: solution 1, weaker (*w*); 2, of equal strength (*e*); 3, *w*; 4, stronger (*s*); 5, *w*; 6, *s*; 7, *s*. Each judgement is given a score (*w* scores 0, *e* scores 1, *s* scores 2) and all the transition points from one score to another are tabulated. Between solutions 1 and 2, i.e. at $1\frac{1}{2}$, there is a transition from 0 to 1; between 2 and 3, at $2\frac{1}{2}$, a transition from 1 to 0, i.e., -1; at $3\frac{1}{2}$ a transition of $+2$; at $4\frac{1}{2}$ a transition of -2; at $5\frac{1}{2}$ a transition of $+2$. The mean transition point is calculated by summing the individual products (transition point × difference across transition point) and dividing by 2 (because at the required mean transition point there is a change of $+2$). In the example given the steps are: $(1\frac{1}{2}\times 1)+(2\frac{1}{2}\times -1)+(3\frac{1}{2}\times 2)+(4\frac{1}{2}\times -2)+(5\frac{1}{2}\times 2)=8$. The mean transition point is therefore 4, and this is taken as the intensity equivalent. The procedure for calculating taste thresholds is similar, but simpler because only two types of response can be made for any solution: either the specific taste is detected (score 1) or it is not (score 0). The summed products are therefore not divided by two.

The taste intensity equivalents were unaffected by the treatments (Table 2), indicating that dexamphetamine did not change the relative taste intensity of sucrose and sodium chloride solutions at concentrations above the taste thresholds. The intensity equivalents were consistent and agree closely with those found by Beebe-Center *et al.* (1955), which were more accurate than the earlier estimates (Beebe-Center, 1949).

Table 2

Taste intensity equivalents

The means and their standard error are expressed in terms of the solution numbers given in Table 1a; these numbers are proportional to log gusts. One gust is defined as the subjective strength of a 1% solution of sucrose (Beebe-Center, 1949).

Treatment		*Placebo*	*Dexamphetamine 7·5 mg*	*Dexamphetamine 15 mg*	*Standard error of means*
Sucrose standard	A	3·75	3·2	3·4	±0·21
	B	5·4	5·25	5·6	

Analysis of variance

Source	*d.f.*	*Sum of squares*	*Mean square*	*F*	*p*
Treatments	2	12·72	6·36	1·54	>0·2
Subjects	5	115·11	23·02	5·57	<0·01
Standards	1	469·44	469·44	113	⩽0·001
Residual	27	111·61	4·13		
Total	35	708·88			

The taste thresholds also seemed unaffected by the drug, but the variation was very great, and I therefore repeated the experiment in a further 3 volunteers, determining each taste threshold in triplicate instead of only once on each occasion. The combined results for all 9 subjects show no consistent changes that can be attributed to dexamphetamine (Table 3), though with this small number of subjects it cannot be proved that the drug has no effect.

Table 3

Specific salt and sweet taste thresholds

The means and their standard errors are expressed in terms of the solution numbers given in Table 1b; these numbers are proportional to the log concentrations of the solutes. The standard errors of the means have been calculated from analyses of variance.

Treatment	*Placebo*	*Dexamphetamine 7·5 mg*	*Dexamphetamine 15 mg*	*Standard error of means*
Sodium chloride	6·4	7·5	6·3	±0·50
Sucrose	5·8	4·2	4·2	±0·50

These observations have failed to demonstrate an effect of dexamphetamine on taste, and such an effect seems unlikely to play a part in the depression of appetite caused by the drug. Perhaps an effect on the subjective intensity of odours might be expected to affect appetite more than one on taste. However, the experiment illustrates that the method of taste intensity matching can be used to study any effects on taste.

Acknowledgements

I am grateful to Dr. M. H. Quenouille for suggesting the method of analysing the observations; to Mr. C. H. Sykes, M.B.E., F.P.S. for preparing the treatments; and to the subjects for their conscientious co-operation.

REFERENCES

Ahokas, A. J., Payne, J. G. and Goetzl, F. R. (1950). The influence of amphetamine sulfate upon the acuity of taste for sucrose and upon the sensation of appetite and satiety. *Permanente Found. med. Bull.* **8,** 107–112.

Beebe-Center, J. G. (1949). Standards for use of the gust scale. *J. Psychol.,* **28,** 411–419.

Beebe-Center, J. G., Rogers, M. S. and Atkinson, W. H. (1955). Intensive equivalence for sucrose and NaCl solutions. *J. Psychol.,* **39,** 371–372.

Herxheimer, A., and Woodbury, D. M. (1960). The effect of deoxycorticosterone on salt and sucrose preference thresholds and drinking behaviour in rats. *J. Physiol. (Lond.),* **151,** 253–260.

Janowitz, H. D. and Grossman, M. I. (1949). Gusto-olfactory thresholds in relation to appetite and hunger sensations. *J. appl. Physiol.,* **2,** 217–222.

Mata, F. (1963). Effect of dextro-amphetamine on bitter taste thresholds. *J. Neuropsychiatry*, **4**, 315–320.
Pangborn, R. M. (1961). Discussion *in* The physiological and behavioural aspects of taste. Ed. M. R. Kare and B. P. Halpern, p. 72. Chicago University Press.
Richter, C. P. (1939). Sodium chloride and dextrose appetite of untreated and treated adrenalectomized rats. *Endocrinology*, **29**, 115–125.
Stevens, S. S. (1958). Measurement and man. *Science*, **127**, 383–389.
Teitelbaum, P. and Epstein, A. (1962). The hypothalamic syndrome: recovery of feeding and drinking after lateral hypothalamic lesions. *Psychol. Rev.*, **69**, 74–90.

DISCUSSION

Herxheimer: Does anyone feel that there is any point in investigating the effect of amphetamine on taste thresholds further?

Grossman: It would seem to me that anything that is done with amphetamine and apparent thresholds, and I am using that word advisedly, would have to take into account the general excitatory effect that the drug has. We speculate that this is related to an effect on the reticular formation. If that is true it might conceivably remove an inhibitory effect or produce direct stimulation of the reticular formation which might be reflected in a general rather than a specific lowering of thresholds, similar to what has been reported in some studies following electrical stimulation of the reticular formation. So I think if anybody wants to persist in looking for changes in taste threshold, I would urge that he also look for changes in other sensory thresholds.

Wilson: I was interested in what Dr. Grossman said about preference versus acceptability. I feel that this is a semantic point. Richter showed that there were different taste thresholds for different substances in his rats. Now whatever the mechanism of this was, whether we call it taste thresholds or preference or acceptability, he did show that rats selected various substances at differing concentrations. The only mechanism which we know will enable them to do this is the sensation in their mouth or in their nose. Now, is it not possible that the electrophysiological methods and the methods for testing taste sensitivity, which we are at present using, are not sensitive enough to pick up differences between levels of acceptability for these substances? I think we need more sensitive methods, such as Dr. Herxheimer has been trying to find, for measuring taste subjectively because we have not yet found an objective way of doing it. Do you agree?

Grossman: It depends on how you define a sensory threshold. There is no argument if you are unwilling to accept the electro-physiological definition which states that a receptor has its threshold exceeded when it generates and propagates an action potential. The work of Pfaffmann and his associates quite clearly shows that normal animals do not show a preference for a salt solution which they definitely can taste (as determined by electrophysiological methods), whereas in the adrenalectomized animal the detection and preference thresholds coincide almost exactly. The coincidence of the electrophysiological and behavioural threshold under stress conditions is the best argument for the electrophysiological thresholds. The test subject in many preference experiments may be perfectly capable of discriminating distilled water from the very weak salt solution or whatever is being tested, but he may be unwilling to make an extra effort in order to get some of it. Preference thresholds are to a large extent a question of motivation. Cortical damage produces an apparent increase in sensory thresholds. If you look at the behaviour of these animals a little more carefully—and I have done that to satisfy my own curiosity—it turns out that the thresholds rapidly return to normal levels if you make it worth the animal's while to respond, by punishing incorrect responses. What has changed in this preparation is the willingness to co-operate, to go to the trouble of making the difficult discrimination near the difference threshold, not the sensory ability to make the discrimination. We have relied to a great extent on animal data which are based on the assumption that the animal is perfectly willing to do what we are asking it to do and that may not be true in all cases. In all animal work a marked lowering of sensory thresholds can be demonstrated when incorrect responses are punished or better rewards are offered.

Herxheimer: I found how crucial motivation can be when I tried to discover what a seal could taste, by presenting it with its usual food, dead herrings, in solutions of various substances. The seal was supposed to learn to take the herrings from solutions it liked rather than from those it disliked, but it evidently disliked the whole procedure, and got very angry even when the herrings were presented in salt water.

Watson: Dr. Grossman, in view of the fact that a reduction in food intake can be achieved by causing food to remain longer in the alimentary canal, for example by increasing the proportion of protein or fat, to what extent is the anorexia caused by amphetamine attributable to its effect on gastric motility?

Grossman: That problem was extensively investigated in the late thirties (e.g. Myerson, A. and Ritvo, M. *J. Amer. med. Ass.*, 1936, **107,** 24; Smith, O. N. and Chamberlin, G. W. *Radiology*, 1937, **29,** 676) and I think the general conclusion is that the effect on gastric motility or acid secretion is not large enough to account for any change in food intake or absorption.

Silverstone: Animal studies concerning the effect of amphetamines are perhaps not directly relevant to human clinical pharmacology in that the dose required to suppress food intake in animals is much larger than that ever given to patients. I have recently assessed both food intake and subjective hunger responses after varying doses of d-amphetamine sulphate in normal subjects. I found that at least 10 mg. of amphetamine was required to affect hunger—but the suppression of hunger and food intake was not nearly as large as that produced by a meal.

Hinchcliffe: I was interested in Dr. Herxheimer's extension of psychophysical methods to encompass supra-threshold measurements. By analogy with what is known to occur for another sense modality, hearing, a comparison of shifts in sensory threshold with shifts in the subjective magnitude of supra-threshold stimuli might indicate whether an effect is produced at the end-organ or elsewhere. Thus where the particular stimulus parameters have been found to produce a threshold impairment, the experiments should be repeated and cross-qualitative or cross-modality intensity matches made to assess whether there is any change in the subject magnitude of supra-intensity stimuli also.

Session III

Hearing

Chairman: R. Hinchcliffe

OTOTOXIC DRUGS

JAN WERSÄLL and P.-G. LUNDQUIST

Department of Otolaryngology, Karolinska Hospital, Stockholm

OTOTOXIC drugs are substances which, in therapeutic dosage, may affect hearing or equilibrium functions in humans. Quinine and salicylic acid have long been recognized as ototoxic. Thus tinnitus and varying degrees of depression of hearing were observed in patients treated with high dosages of aspirin or other salicylates. McCabe and Dey (1965) in controlled experiments in man found strong evidence for locating the site of action of salicylic acid in the cochlea, and considered mechanical disturbances of the hair cells or metabolic changes in the cochlear duct to be the most likely cause of the disturbances.

Covell (1936), and Rüedi *et al.* (1952) reported that degenerative changes, due to systemic administration of quinine, began in the outer hair cells of the cochlea. Hinohara (1961) considered the changes to be more severe in the inner hair cells.

The effect of ototoxic antibiotics on the inner ear has been studied in the last twenty years, since Hindshaw and Feldman (1945) demonstrated vestibular disturbances in a large series of patients treated with high doses of streptomycin. The constant trend to produce more and more effective antibiotics has over the years resulted in the introduction of a number of new antibiotics, even more ototoxic than streptomycin. At present the most important of the ototoxic drugs are streptomycin, dihydrostreptomycin, neomycin, kanamycin, vancomycin and viomycin. Recently both ristocetin and gentamicin have also been described as ototoxic. Patterson and Gulick (1963) have described disturbances in cochlear responses after administration of chloramphenicol. This has also been indicated by Koide *et al.* (1966). Most ototoxic antibiotics in current use belong to the group of antibiotics produced by various strains of streptomyces (Table 1).

Table 1—*Effects of commonly used ototoxic antibiotics on the inner ear*

	Vestibular damage	*Cochlear damage*	*Renal damage*
Streptomycin	+++	+	
Dihydrostreptomycin	++	++	
Neomycin	++	++++	+++
Kanamycin	+	++++	++
Viomycin	++	++	+
Vancomycin		++	

Already at an early stage streptomycin and dihydrostreptomycin were found to be ototoxic (Hindshaw and Feldman, 1945; Berg, 1951; Hawkins and Lurie, 1952; Duvall and Wersäll, 1964), streptomycin affecting mainly the vestibular system, and dihydrostreptomycin the vestibular system and, unfortunately, even more the acoustical system. The enthusiasm for dihydrostreptomycin, when this drug was found to cause less vestibular disturbances than streptomycin, soon turned to tragedy when dihydrostreptomycin was found to cause hearing disturbances not only during the period of treatment but also after treatment had ceased (Shambaugh *et al.* 1959).

Neomycin was discovered in 1949 and as early as 1950 Carr *et al.* reported that four out of a group of six patients treated with neomycin showed partial, but irreversible, loss of hearing after 4–6 weeks' treatment with a dose of 0·5 to 2 g. daily. Neomycin can cause both vestibular and acoustical disturbances but clinically hearing disorders dominate the picture.

Kanamycin was discovered in 1957 by Umezawa. The first experiments in mice gave no signs of ototoxic action. However, reports by Finegold *et al.* in 1958 showed ototoxic reactions in 22 patients out of 146 treated with kanamycin for various diseases.

Kanamycin ototoxicity resembles that of neomycin, whose structure is close to that of kanamycin. It thus causes severe disturbances in hearing, but has little vestibular action.

Vancomycin was introduced in 1956, and its ototoxic action was described by Geraci and his collaborators in 1958, with severe perceptive loss of hearing as a typical sign of its ototoxic action.

Viomycin was introduced in 1950 and has been used extensively in the treatment of tuberculosis. According to Hackney *et al.* (1953) the first signs of ototoxicity occur in the acoustical system. Recently, Daly and Cohen (1965) described a series of controlled cases receiving 1 g. a day of viomycin with regular controls of vestibular and hearing functions. Both vestibular and acoustic toxic reactions developed, but the vestibular reaction dominated the early picture. According to Daly and Cohen viomycin is more toxic than streptomycin in therapeutic doses.

The clinical signs of vestibular damage are ataxia, dizziness and, in severe cases, vomiting. Early symptoms of damage to the sense organ of hearing are a feeling of fullness in the ear, tinnitus, and loss of hearing. Several authors have pointed out that the signs of vestibular disturbances may not appear until the patient gets up. Frequently, minor disturbances in vestibular function are not observed until controlled studies are made with cupolometry and electronystagmography including rotation and caloric testing.

The site of action of ototoxic antibiotics has been disputed since it was first demonstrated. Early signs of degeneration of the sensory cells in the vestibular end organs were detected by Berg (1951). Several authors have claimed, however, that the ototoxic action is mainly due to disturbances in the ganglia and vestibular and cochlear nuclei in the brain. By combining electrophysiological testing with histological methods, Hawkins and his group have, however, produced convincing evidence of early damage to the sensory epithelia in the labyrinth. Further evidence was produced when it became possible to use electron microscopy for studying changes caused by antibiotics in these sensory epithelia. We have thus been able to prove that selective degeneration occurs in the sensory epithelia of the vestibular part of the labyrinth when experimental animals are given high doses of streptomycin sulphate.

When large doses of streptomycin sulphate are injected into guinea-pigs subcutaneously or intramuscularly for a period of time, irreversible changes occur in the sensory cells, with degeneration of the mitochondria, and changes in the cell membrane causing fusion of the sensory hairs and bulging of the cell surface towards the endolymph. The remnants of the cells ultimately disappear into the endolymph of the ampulla. The final result will be completely degenerated sensory cells throughout the sensory areas of the vestibular part of the labyrinth (Figs. 1–3). The epithelium of the maculae of the utricle and saccule is slightly less sensitive than that of the cristae ampullares. The efferent nerve fibres may remain long after the disappearance of the sensory cells (Wersäll and Hawkins, 1963; Duvall and Wersäll, 1964).

These studies suggested that streptomycin might be concentrated in the endolymph, there destroying the sensory cells. Wersäll and Flock (1964) were able to show that the normal microphonic potentials, produced by the receptors in the lateral-line-canal organ in fish—which are equivalent organs to the crista in the labyrinth—are inhibited by concentrations of streptomycin as low as 1/100,000 in the endolymph. This early effect of streptomycin could be counteracted by rinsing the organ with fresh endolymph or Ringer solution with added potassium to give a concentration equivalent to that in the normal endolymph, i.e. about 40 mEq/l. solution. It seems reasonable to assume that streptomycin is secreted into the endolymph from the blood, but is only slowly reabsorbed. High concentrations of streptomycin in the blood, or low concentrations kept constant for a long time, would thus cause a slowly rising concentration of streptomycin in the endolymph.

Hawkins has shown unequivocally that kanamycin and neomycin cause severe degeneration of the sensory cells in the organ of Corti when the drugs are given in high doses to various animals; at the same time, the typical potentials normally produced in the organ of Corti during stimulation with sound could no longer be elicited (Hawkins, 1959).

With the aid of electron microscopy Lundquist and Wersäll (1966) have followed the early degeneration of the sensory cells in the organ of Corti in guinea-pigs. The early changes appeared in the nuclei and ribosomes of the outer hair cells in the basal coil, and progressed upward in the cochlea during the treatment (Figs. 4–7). These initial changes in the nuclei and in the ribosomes of the cells indicate an inhibition of RNA synthesis in the sensory cells. Kanamycin also inhibits RNA synthesis in bacteria.

The early reversible changes are followed by a later stage with changes in the mitochondria and degeneration of the cell membrane. The hairs and cuticles remain until the last stage of degeneration (Fig. 6). The inner hair cells are less sensitive to the destructive agent. Ganglion cells and efferent nerve fibres can also be observed long after the outer hair cells have degenerated. The upper part of the cochlea and the first row of outer hair cells are more sensitive to the drug than the outermost rows.

The experimental findings thus indicate that the primary effect of ototoxic antibiotics is seen in the hair cells of the sensory epithelia in the labyrinth. This does not show, however, why antibiotics differ in their effect on the vestibular and cochlear sensory cells.

The fact that the ototoxic antibiotics are slowly reabsorbed from the endolymph once they have been secreted into it explains why the concentration of an antibiotic in the blood, and its rate of excretion through the kidney are two important factors in the toxicity of an antibiotic in a patient. None of the ototoxic antibiotics is destroyed within the body: all have to be excreted through the kidneys. When renal function is normal, most anti-

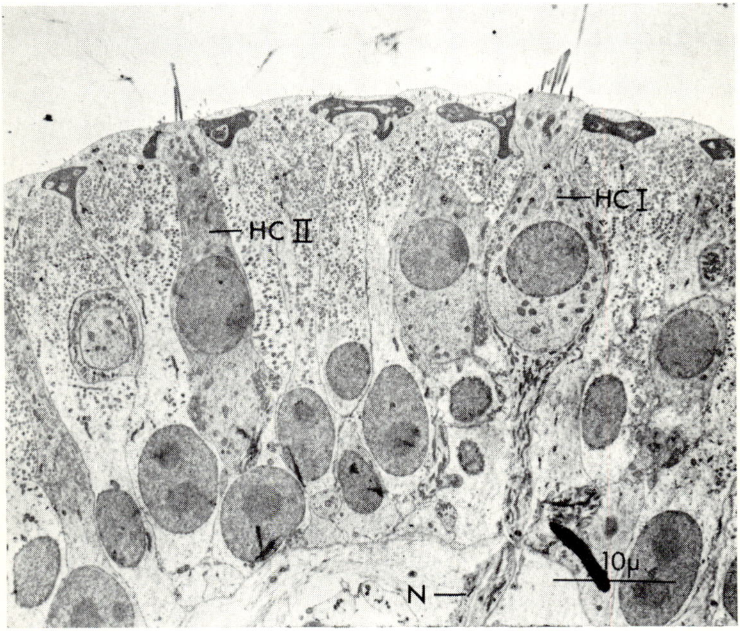

FIG. 1. Normal sensory epithelium from the crista ampullaris in the guinea-pig. HC I: Hair cell of type I. HC II: Hair cell of type II. N: nerve fibre to a hair cell type I.

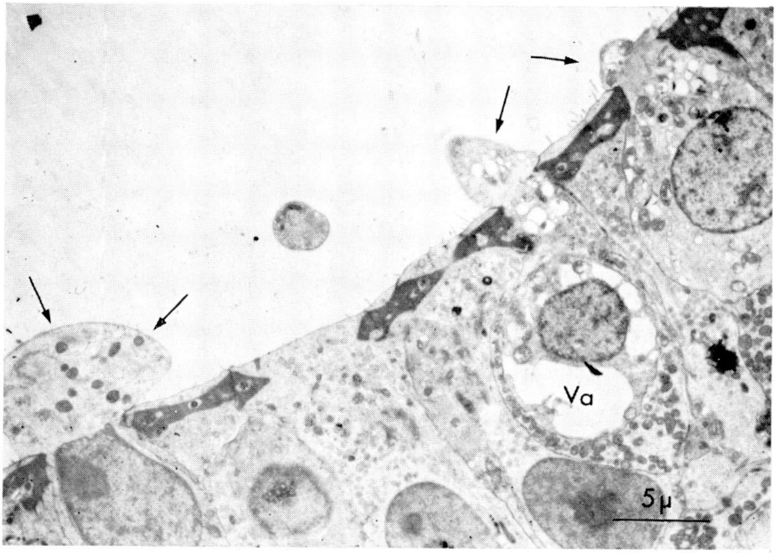

FIG. 2. Survey of sensory epithelium from the crista ampullaris of a guinea-pig treated with streptomycin 300 mg./kg. per day for 18 days. The sensory hairs have disappeared and the sensory cells are bulging out over the epithelial surface (arrows). Va: Vacuoles in a degenerating hair cell.

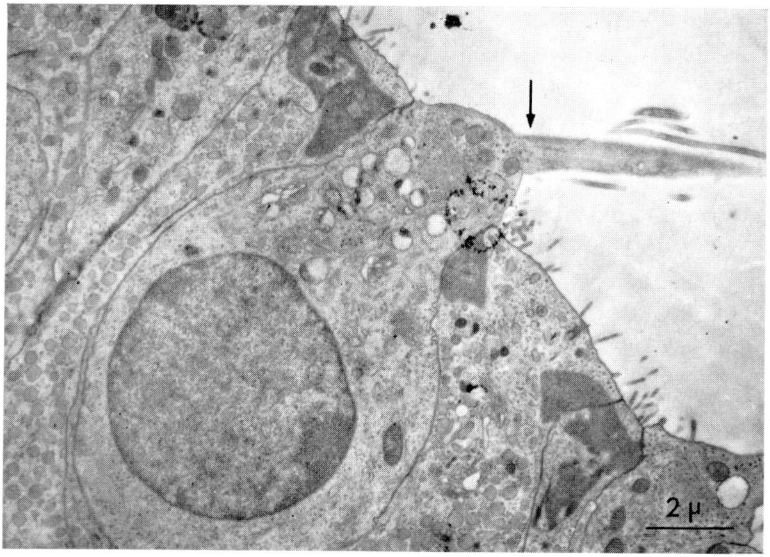

FIG. 3. Upper part of sensory cell in the epithelium of crista ampullaris in guinea-pig after streptomycin intoxication, demonstrating the destruction of sensory hairs (arrow) and vacuolization of cell body.

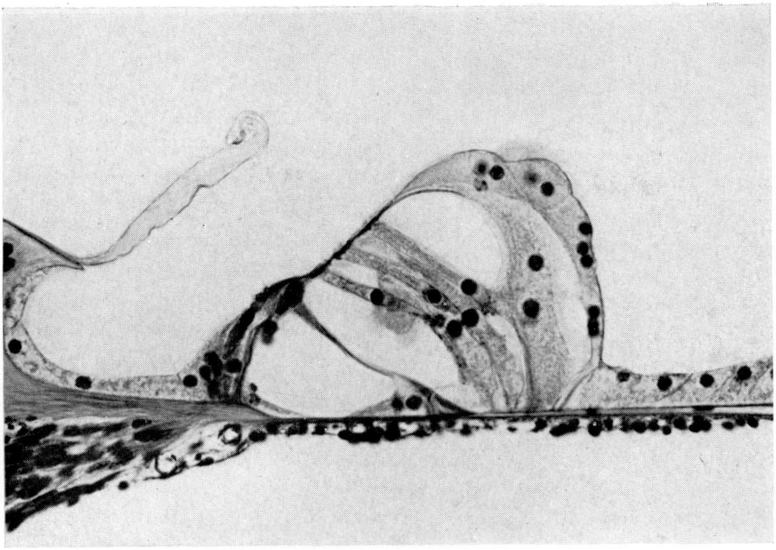

FIG. 4. Normal organ of Corti from the guinea-pig cochlea. Third coil.

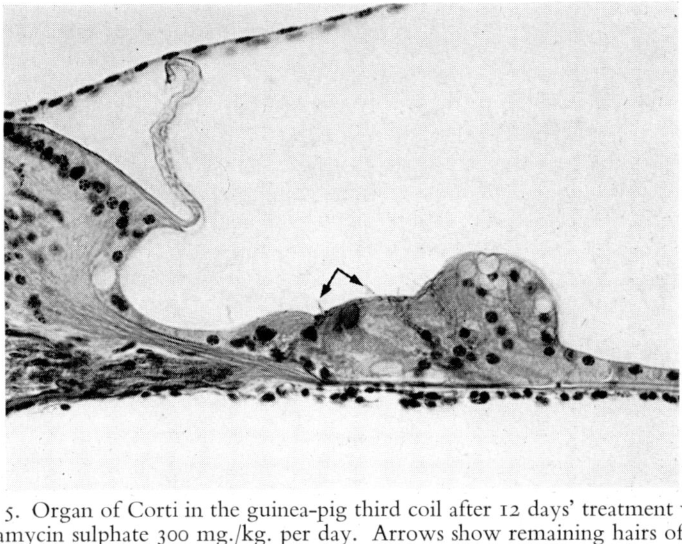

FIG. 5. Organ of Corti in the guinea-pig third coil after 12 days' treatment with kanamycin sulphate 300 mg./kg. per day. Arrows show remaining hairs of still intact inner hair cells and degenerated outer hair cells.

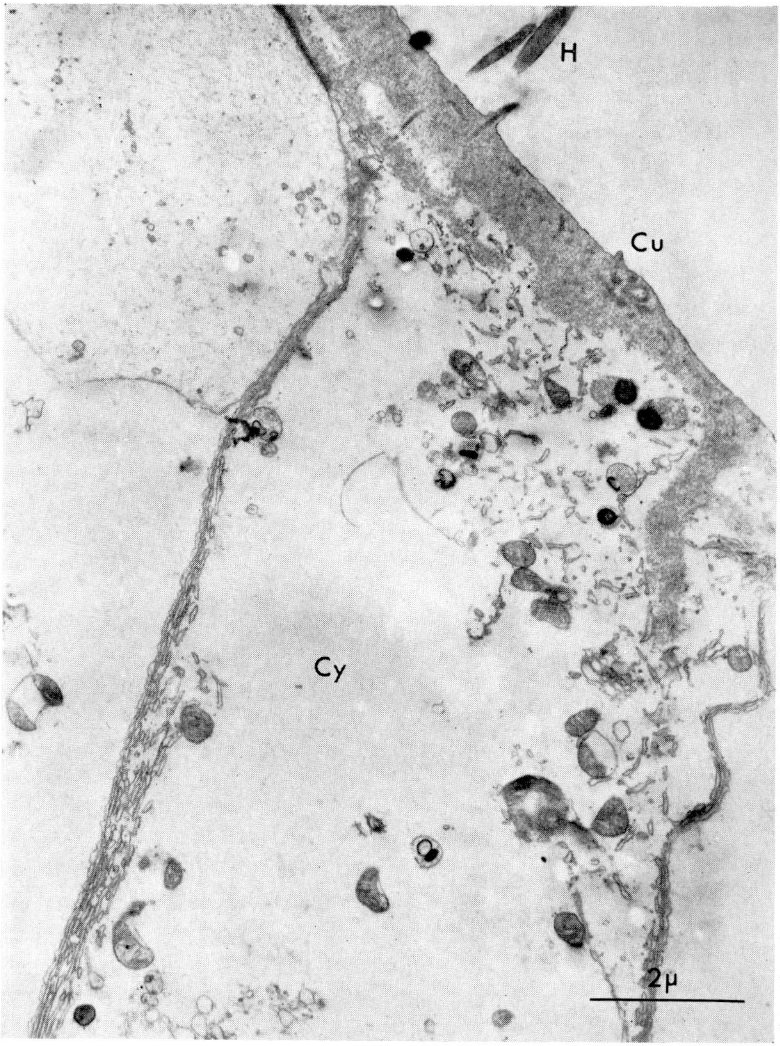

FIG. 6. Top of outer hair cell from guinea-pig cochlea during kanamycin intoxication showing disappearance of cytoplasmic matrix and ribosomes. The cytoplasm (cy) appears empty and watery. Hairs (H) and cuticle (Cu) still intact.

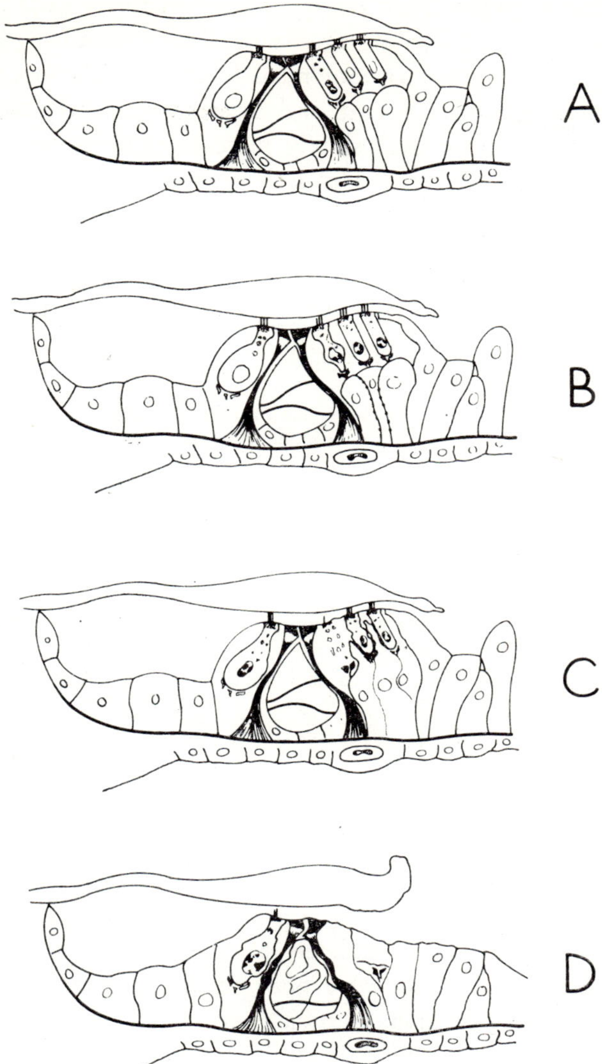

FIG. 7. Schematic drawing illustrating stages of degeneration of the organ of Corti during kanamycin intoxication, A–D.

biotics can be given in low dosages for a rather long time without ototoxic action. High dosages will always produce ototoxic effects. When owing to poor renal function, the concentration in the blood remains constant, or decreases very slowly, the endolymph concentration will slowly increase and the sensory cells will have no time to recover from the ototoxic action. Irreparable damage will then occur even when the antibiotic is given in very low dosage. That an ototoxic effect can appear in some patients even after very low doses of an antibiotic was pointed out by Cawthorne and Ranger (1958). This is illustrated by a number of cases selected from our clinic (Table 2).

Table 2—*Examples of dose and intoxication in a few representative cases of ototoxic reactions*

Case No.	*Age*	*Antibiotic*	*Total dose*	*Days of administration*	*Renal function*	*Vestibular damage*	*Hearing disorders*
1	34	Kanamycin	6 g	21	very poor	none	deafness tinnitus
2	41	Streptomycin Kanamycin	unknown 13+6 g	unknown	normal	none	deafness
3	54	Streptomycin Neomycin	unknown 2, 5 g	unknown 5	normal	none	deafness
4	61	Streptomycin Kanamycin	4 g 3 g	8 6	anuria	total	none
5	68	Neomycin	7 g	14	very poor	none	deafness tinnitus

Especially interesting are case 1, to which I will return, and case 4, the woman who was given 4 grams of streptomycin during a period of anuria and completely lost her equilibrium function. These two patients had very poor renal function, but ototoxicity has also occurred in cases with normal renal function.

Severe antibiotic intoxication is illustrated by case 1. A 34-year-old woman, with a *Proteus* infection after a kidney operation, was given a total dose of 6·5 g. of kanamycin during a period of 42 days. Owing to her poor renal function and the tendency to

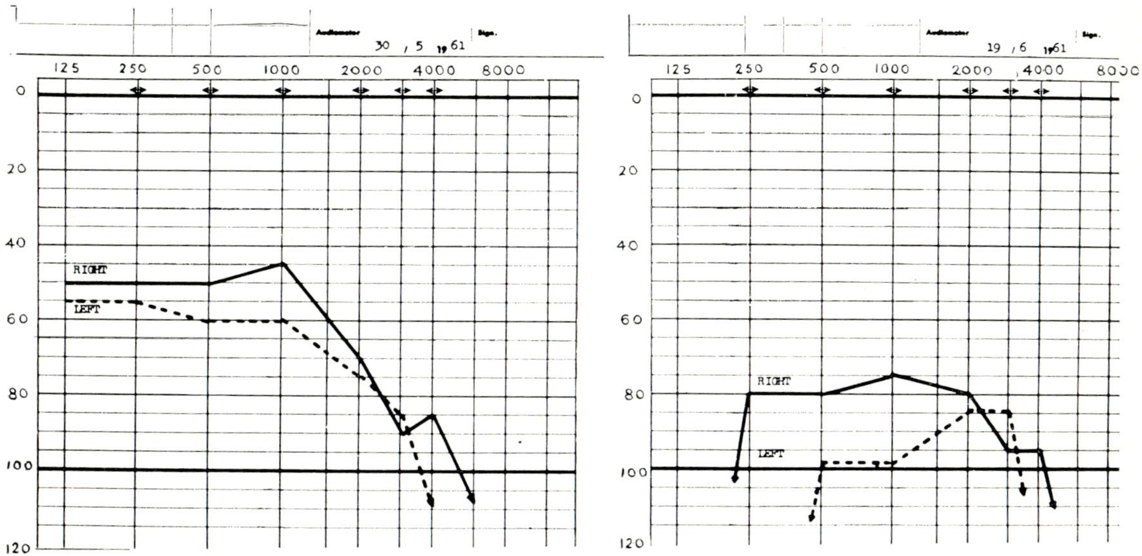

FIG. 8. Audiogram taken from case 1 on the 3rd and on the 23rd day after cessation of kanamycin treatment, demonstrating the rapid decay in hearing.

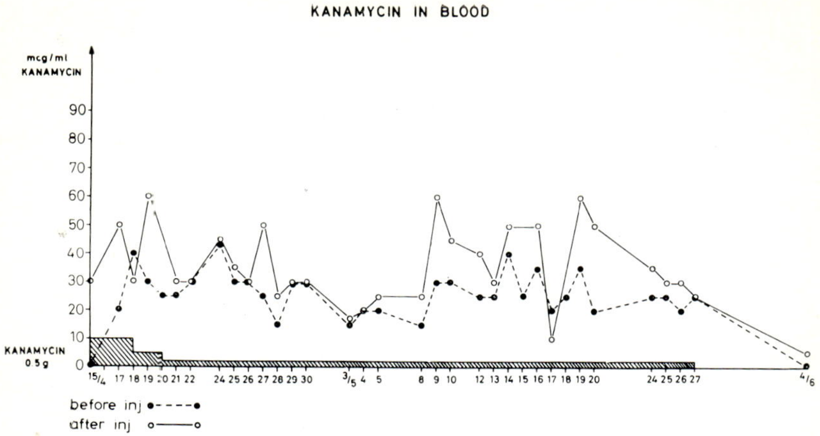

FIG. 9. Variations in level of the kanamycin concentration in the blood in case 1. The creatinine clearance was 12 ml./min.

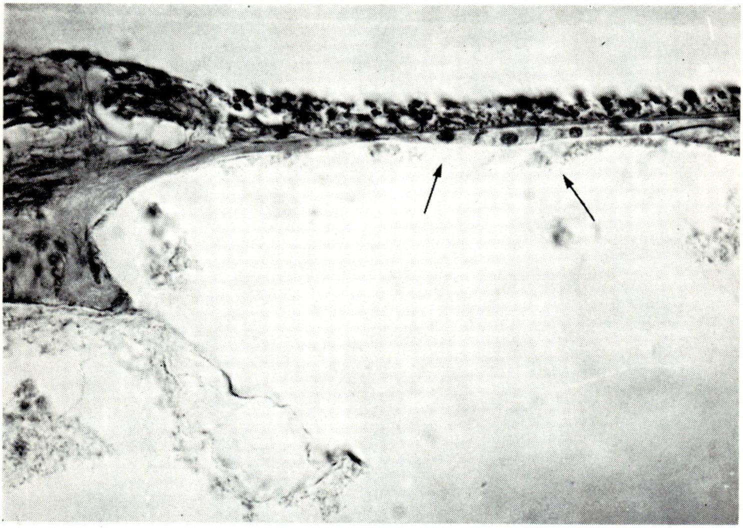

FIG. 10. Section from the basal coil of the organ of Corti of case 1 two months after kanamycin intoxication. Arrows demonstrate remaining Boecher cells. All other supporting cells and hair cells have degenerated.

accumulate kanamycin in the blood, the daily dosage was reduced from 0·5 g. during the first few days to 0·125 g. subsequently (Fig. 9). After 42 days tinnitus developed, and an audiogram showed that her hearing was severely reduced (Fig. 8). Kanamycin was stopped, but the disturbances in hearing progressed, and after another week there was no demonstrable hearing. The patient died 2 months later, and the temporal bones showed severe degeneration of the hair cells in the whole organ of Corti (Fig. 10).

Kanamycin has recently been discussed as the antibiotic of choice for treatment of infections with Gram-negative bacteria in children because of the other toxic actions of chloramphenicol and the tetracyclines. Even if the number of cases of hearing disorders is small when kanamycin is given in low dosage for a few days to persons with normal renal function, the disastrous effect of damage to the inner ear in children must be borne in mind before a child is given kanamycin.

Before an ototoxic antibiotic is used, the possibility of using other antibiotics should be excluded. Ototoxic drugs should be given only on vital indications, when no cure can be achieved with other treatment. When ototoxic antibiotics are given, the patient should be referred to a hospital with a bacteriological department capable of following the blood concentration daily. Preferably a test dose should be given, and the disappearance of the antibiotic from the blood during 24 hours should be studied. When a considerable delay in the excretion of the antibiotic through the kidney is observed it should be realized that the drug cannot be given in a therapeutic dose without damage to the labyrinth.

REFERENCES

Berg, K. (1951). *Acta oto-laryng. Suppl.*, **97,** 1.

Carr, D. T., Brown, H. A. and Pfuetze, K. H. (1950). *J. Amer. med. Ass.*, **144,** 65.

Cawthorne, T. E. and Ranger, D. (1957). *Brit. med. J.*, **i,** 1444.

Covell, W. P. (1936). *Arch. Otolaryng.*, **23,** 633.

Daly, J. F. and Cohen, N. L. (1965). *Ann. Otol.*, **74**, 521.
Duvall, A. J. and Wersäll, J. (1964). *Acta oto-laryng.*, **57**, 581.
Finegold, S. M., Winfield, M. E., Nishizawa, A., Kantor, E. A., Kvinge, V. E., and Hewitt, W. L. (1958–1959). *Antibiot. Ann.*, **6**, 606.
Geraci, J. E., Heilman, F. R., Nichols, D. R. and Wellman, W. E. (1958). *Proc. Mayo Clin.*, **33**, 172.
Hackney, R. L., King, E. Q., Marshall, E. E., Harden, K. A. and Payne, H. M. (1953). *Dis. Chest.*, **24**, 591.
Hawkins, J. E. and Lurie, M. H. (1952). *Ann. Otol.*, **61**, 789.
Hawkins, J. E. (1959). The ototoxicity of kanamycin. *Ann. otol.*, **68**, 698.
Hinohara, T. (1961). *Otolaryngology* (Tokyo), **4**, Suppl. 1, 49.
Hindshaw, H. C. and Feldman, W. H. (1945). *Proc. Mayo Clin.*, **20**, 313.
Koide, Y., Hato, A. and Reiko, H. (1966). *Acta oto-laryng.*, **61**, 332.
Lundquist, P. G. and Wersäll, J. (1966) *Z. f. Zellforsch.* **72**, 543.
McCabe, P. A. and Dey, F. L. (1965). *Ann. Otol.*, **74**, 312.
Patterson, W. C. and Gulick, W. L. (1963). *Ann. Otol.*, **72**, 50.
Rüedi, L., Furrer, W., Luthy, F., Nager, G. and Tschirren, B. (1952). *Laryngoscope*, **62**, 333.
Shambaugh, G. F., Derlachi, D. L., Harrison, W. H., House, H., House, W., Hildgard, W., Schuknecht, H. and Shea, J. J. (1959). *J. Amer. med. Ass.*, **170**, 1657.
Umezawa, H. 1958). *Ann. N.Y. Acad. Sci.*, **76**, 20.
Wersäll, J. and Flock, Å. (1964). *Life Sciences*, **3**, 1151.
Wersäll, J. and Hawkins, J. E. (1963). *Acta oto-laryng.*, **54**, 1.

DISCUSSION

Philipszoon: Dr. Wersäll mentioned the possibility that streptomycin might act also on the central auditory and vestibular nuclei, but there is another piece of evidence that these drugs mainly act peripherally on the sensory epithelia. We studied patients with dead labyrinths after streptomycin intoxication and found that stimulation of the posterior cervical nerve roots in these patients still provoked neck-torsion nystagmus. Such nystagmus is evoked in a subject sitting in a rotatable chair while his head is fixed; the trunk is moved relative to the head. This type of nystagmus requires functioning vestibular nuclei. This supports Dr. Wersäll's hypothesis that these drugs mainly act peripherally.

Hinchcliffe: The literature on the earlier studies of streptomycin intoxication indicated that there are not only end-organ but also neuronal changes. Some of these, I understand, were artifacts and others are probably secondary to the primary end-organ change. Would Dr. Wersäll care to comment on the absence of a systematic programme for testing the ototoxic effects in chronic toxicity studies?—should one have a particular systematic programme, or is this not feasible because of the time involved and the difficulty of choosing the right animal? Perhaps we should go back to Hawkins' studies (Hawkins, J. E. and Lurie M. H. *Ann. Otol.*, 1952, **61,** 789; 1953, **62,** 1128) because they showed a differential effect of streptomycin and other ototoxic drugs on cochlear microphonics as against action potentials, and on inner hair cells versus external hair cells. Are these observations still valid?

Wersäll: Testing of ototoxic effects in animals will have to include physiological and histological tests, preferably both light and electron microscopy. The effect on hearing should be tested by behavioural as well as electrophysiological methods. Vestibular tests should include electronystagmographic studies of labyrinthine responses to controlled acceleration. Cats and dogs are fairly easily trained to respond to acoustic stimuli; guinea-pigs require a more complicated training but can also be trained. The histological studies are most easily performed on guinea-pigs but could also be done on cats. Vestibular testing is fairly easily performed on all these animals in a well equipped laboratory. Monkeys will have to be excluded from routine testing, I presume, because of the cost. When an animal is chosen for studies of ototoxic effects the variation in blood concentration after injection of the drug has to be studied as species vary considerably in the rate of secretion of the drug through the kidneys.

DRUGS AND THE AUDITORY PATHWAY

B. J. Key

Department of Experimental Neuropharmacology, University of Birmingham

In studying the pharmacology of the specific sensory pathways, one is struck by the apparent resistance of the auditory pathway to the effects of drugs administered to animals by the systemic route. Substances such as acetylcholine, adrenaline, noradrenaline, 5-hydroxytryptamine and atropine are without effect on evoked macro-responses. This lack of effect, however, may be due entirely to their inability to pass the blood-brain barrier after systemic administration, or alternatively to their rapid breakdown. Certainly, these substances have been shown to influence neural activity within the central nervous system after topical or iontophoretic application (Bradley and Wolstencroft, 1965; Curtis, 1965; Krnjević, 1965). I shall not however discuss this class of drugs, but rather those substances which when injected systemically produce, or appear to produce, significant changes in the amplitude of potentials evoked in cortical or subcortical regions of the auditory pathway. Of the drugs which have direct effects, the barbiturates are probably the most consistent and provide a basis for comparison with the effects of other drugs.

French and co-workers (1953), in investigating the neural basis of the anaesthetic state, demonstrated that barbiturates effectively blocked conduction in the central brain-stem at a stage of anaesthetic depression when transmission of impulses in the lateral lemniscus was unimpaired. Indeed, in cat *encéphale isolé* preparations small intravenous doses of pentobarbitone have little effect on auditory potentials. Figure 1 demonstrates this point.

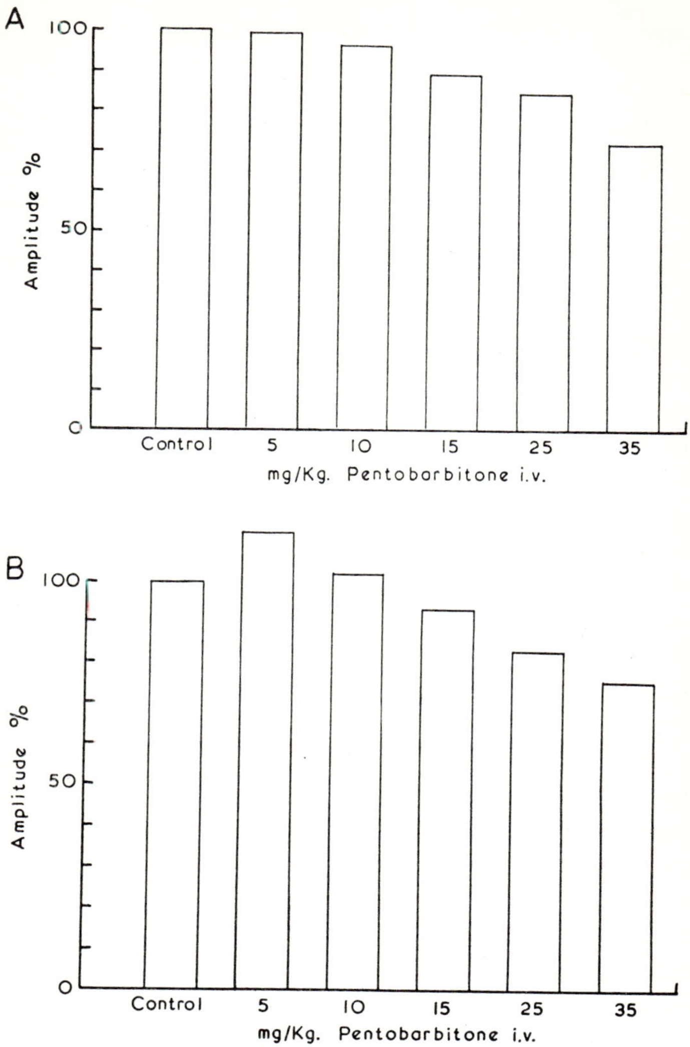

FIG. 1. The effect of incremental doses of pentobarbitone on the mean amplitude of evoked potentials recorded from the rostral portion of the lateral lemniscus in cat *encéphale isolé* preparations.

A. Typical experiment showing progressive decrease in amplitude.

B. Typical experiment showing initial increase in amplitude with small doses.

Here the mean amplitudes of potentials evoked in the rostral portion of the lateral lemniscus have been plotted as a percentage of control readings following incremental doses of pentobarbitone. Doses of 5 to 10 mg./kg. induced no significant changes in amplitude. There was in fact, in a minority of cases, as illustrated in Figure 1B, a slight increase in the mean amplitude at these dose levels.

The main features of the effect of pentobarbitone however, are firstly the progressive attenuation in the amplitude of the potentials when doses greater than 15 to 20 mg./kg. are used and secondly, a decrease in variability. Such changes are common to all sub-cortical recording positions in the auditory pathway but rather complicated at the cortex by the marked changes in background activity accompanying administration of this drug.

With the advent of psychotomimetic and tranquillizing drugs attention was focused on the possibility that they might modify sensory information within the primary projection pathway. It has become obvious, however, over recent years that the specific sensory pathways are no longer to be regarded as simple relay systems. Neurones of the auditory system are subject to inhibitory and facilitatory influences, intrinsically from within the primary pathway as well as extrinsically from other brain structures (Hernández-Peón *et al.*, 1957; Killam and Killam, 1957; Whitfield and Allanson, 1956; Galambos, 1960; Stephens and Key, 1964). Moreover, the electrical activity may be modified at the periphery as well as subsequent synapses within the brain. For example, transmission of sound through the middle ear may be attenuated by at least 25 decibels by the activity of the intra-aural muscles (Galambos, 1960). Incoming auditory information may also be modulated at the periphery by the centrifugal inhibitory system of the olivo-cochlear bundle (Galambos 1956; Desmedt 1960). Centrally, from the level of the cochlear nuclei to the primary auditory cortex, a number of mechanisms appear to control the flow of information through the brain-stem and thalamus (Killam and Killam, 1957; Stephens and Key, 1964).

Such mechanisms could well account for the spontaneous variability in the amplitude of responses evoked in the auditory pathway and primary auditory cortex of unanaesthetized animal preparations. Indeed, Galambos (1960) has suggested that the fluctuation in amplitude may be connected with the significance attached to the stimulus by the animal. If this is so, then the variations in response may reflect the interaction between the animal and its environment. Thus drugs which alter this relationship between the animal and its environment, by changing responsiveness to sensory stimuli for example, may modify electrical activity within the sensory pathway, not necessarily by a direct effect, but also by an action elsewhere in the central nervous system.

Lysergide (LSD 25) is probably a good example of this class of drug. From behavioural evidence small doses of 5 to 30 μg./kg. intravenously or intraperitoneally, increase the responsiveness of cats to sensory stimuli, lower the threshold for arousal and increase generalization and distractability (Bradley and Elkes, 1957; Bradley and Key, 1958; Key, 1961a, 1964). Electrophysiological data however, in terms of potentials evoked within the auditory system, present only equivocal changes. For example, Rovetta (1956), using lysergide applied topically to the primary auditory cortex or injected intravenously in doses up to 40 μg./kg., found little change in potentials evoked by acoustic stimulation, but Brown (1961) found that as little as 1·5 μg./kg. attenuated evoked cortical activity. These results were in contrast to the earlier work of Purpura (1956), who observed an enhancement of primary cortical responses with doses as low as 2 μg./kg.

This ambiguity may be resolved by considering the type of preparation employed, and the experimental situation. Using cats carrying permanently implanted sub-cortical and cortical recording electrodes in situations where the amount of ambient sensory stimulation differs, we find that lysergide induces different effects. For example, in semi-soundproofed conditions click-evoked primary potentials recorded in the auditory cortex increase in amplitude after 10 μg./kg. of lysergide given intraperitoneally. This effect is shown in Figure 2A, where each point

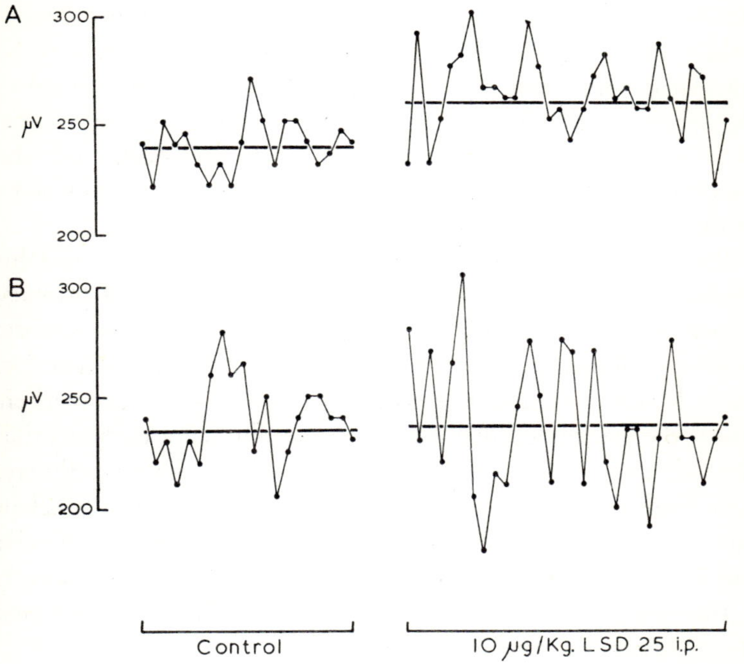

FIG. 2. The effect of lysergide (LSD 25) on the amplitude of consecutive primary responses recorded from the auditory cortex of an unrestrained chronic cat preparation.

A. Experiment carried out in semi-soundproofed conditions.
B. Experiment using the same animal in the open laboratory.
Black bar indicates the mean amplitude.

represents the amplitude of consecutive potentials in the sample and the black bar indicates the mean amplitude. In the open laboratory, illustrated by Figure 2B, where the level of extraneous stimulation had increased, the same dose of lysergide administered to the same cat now only increased the variability in the amplitude of the responses. Thus, in this situation, a decrease or increase in the mean amplitude could be merely a matter of sampling time.

These differential effects may also be observed by first altering the meaning or the significance of the test stimulus experimentally. By the use of appropriate training techniques it is possible to induce alterations in the attentive ability of cats which may be correlated with changes in the amplitude of potentials evoked in the specific auditory pathway. There is still some controversy as to how, why and even where these changes occur, but the concept that changes do occur and are related to the significance of the stimulus is gaining acceptance.

For example, repetitive presentation of an auditory stimulus results in the progressive decrease in the amplitude of primary responses evoked, not only at the cortex, but also in the specific pathway (Hernández-Peón, 1955; Galambos, Sheatz and Vernier, 1956; Marsh *et al.*, 1961). According to Dunlop and co-workers (1964) the percentage alteration in the amplitude of the potentials depends upon the recording site within the auditory pathway, very little change occurring at the level of the cochlear nucleus but more marked alterations appearing at the inferior collicular and medial geniculate levels. Probably more significant however, is the observation that the response level decreases in the first few minutes of the habituation procedure.

Conditioning the animal to pay attention to the acoustic signal, by pairing it with a noxious stimulus, induces an increase in the amplitude of auditory potentials recorded at sub-cortical and cortical placements (Jouvet and Hernández-Peón, 1957; Galambos *et al.*, 1956; John and Killam, 1959). In contrast, simultaneous presentation of two different stimuli, thereby producing interaction and distraction, results in attenuation of the auditory potentials (Hernández-Peón, 1959; Marsh *et al.*, 1961). According to Starr (1964) such attenuation in the lower levels of the auditory pathway is a passive reflection of middle ear muscle activity, while the changes in the cortical potentials depend, in addition, upon central mechanisms.

If lysergide is tested in animals previously conditioned or habituated different results are obtained (Stephens and Key, 1965). In these experiments using unrestrained cat preparations, recordings were taken simultaneously from the auditory cortex, indicated in Fig. 3 by the continuous line, and the lateral lemniscus, indicated by the broken line. Again the points represent the amplitude of consecutive primary potentials and the black bar the mean amplitude. In a conditioned animal (Fig. 3A), where the amplitude of the potentials has increased above control levels, 10 μg./kg. lysergide, given intraperitoneally, produced no striking effect on the amplitude of all potentials. Instead there was a wider fluctuation, which resulted in some cases in a significant decrease in the mean amplitude.

On the other hand, if we take an animal which has been previously habituated to the acoustic signal, thereby inducing a gradual decrease in the amplitude of the responses (Fig. 3B), we see again, after the administration of lysergide an increased fluctuation in the level of the response. In this case, in contrast to the effect shown in Fig. 3A, the result is a slight increase in the mean amplitude. The mean amplitude, however does not usually return to control levels.

Such changes could well be indirect effects due to the increased distractability which occurs with this drug (Key, 1964), for they do not occur in pentobarbitone-anaesthetized preparations. Thus they illustrate quite clearly the relationship between the effect of the drug and the level of significance of the stimuli. It is interesting to note that the changes observed after lysergide were not progressive; additional injections up to 30 μg./kg. induced no further change.

Differential effects on evoked potentials within the auditory pathway are not confined to substances which produce alerting or increased responsiveness. Chlorpromazine has been shown to

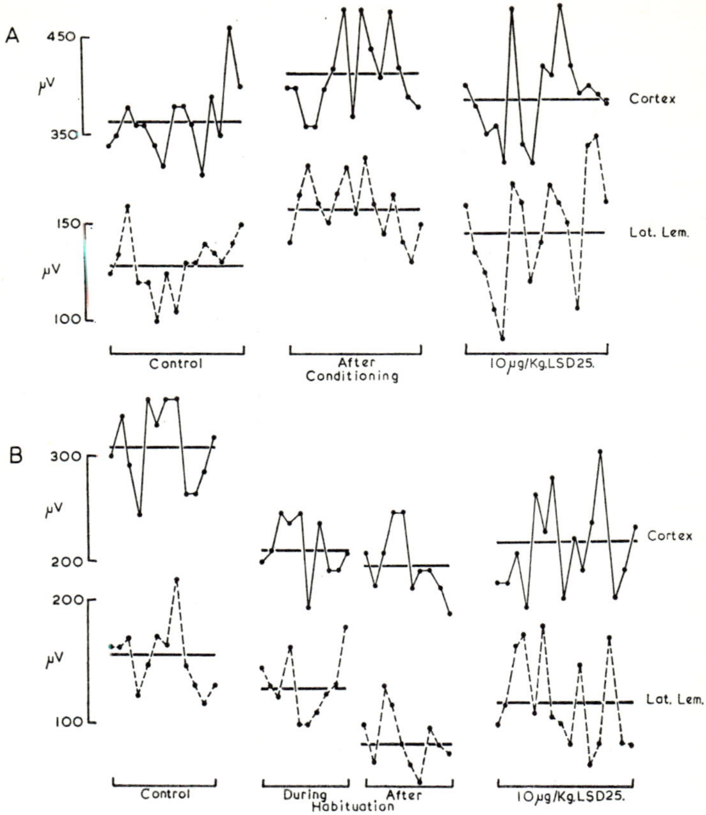

FIG. 3. The effect of lysergide (LSD 25) in unrestrained chronic cat preparations in relation to

A. Conditioning, B. Habituation.

•——• Consecutive primary potentials recorded from the auditory cortex.

•----• Responses recorded simultaneously from the lateral lemniscus.

Black bar indicates the mean amplitude.

FIG. 4. The effect of chlorpromazine on the amplitude of consecutive primary responses recorded from the medial geniculate body.

A. A cat conditioned to the auditory signal.

B. A naïve animal. C. A cat habituated to the auditory signal.

Black bar indicates the mean amplitude.

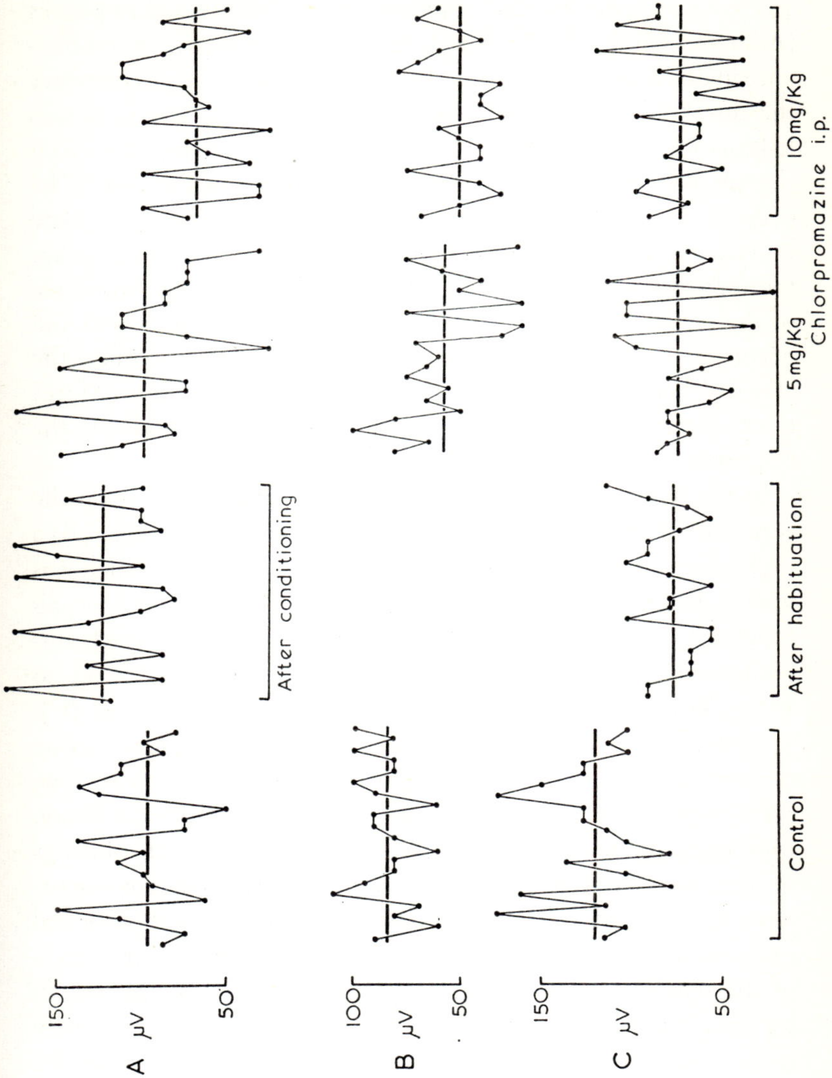
A μV
150
50
B μV
100
50
C μV
150
50
Control
After conditioning
After habituation
5 mg/Kg
10mg/Kg
Chlorpromazine i.p.

block conditioned avoidance behaviour (Cook and Weidley, 1957), or increase the rate of extinction of conditioned responses (Ader and Clink, 1957). This drug also induces a state of indifference in cats to auditory stimuli (Bradley and Hance, 1957), increases the threshold for arousal (Bradley and Key, 1958) and facilitates habituation (Key, 1961b). The effect of chlorpromazine on evoked potentials in relation to conditioning is shown in Fig. 4A. The evoked responses were recorded from the medial geniculate body in unanaesthetized cat preparations. After 5 or 10 mg./kg. intraperitoneally of this drug there was a decrease in the amplitude of the primary potential. This effect was usually quite rapid and occurred within the first minute or so of the trial. Unlike the effect of barbiturates the change was not related to dose. Moreover, there was still some variability in the amplitude of the responses.

In the naïve animal, there was either no change following the administration of chlorpromazine or, as in the case of Fig. 4B, a slight decrease in the mean amplitude of the potentials, which was usually less marked than in the conditioned animal. In animals previously habituated to the auditory signal by continued, unreinforced presentation, chlorpromazine, again in doses up to 10 mg./kg. had very little effect on the evoked responses (Fig. 4C).

These results make it unlikely that drugs such as chlorpromazine or lysergide, substances which influence auditory responsiveness, exert their effects by a direct action on the auditory pathway. Moreover, the results indicate that in assessing the effects of drugs on responses evoked in a system exhibiting spontaneous fluctuation in response level, it is necessary to consider the environmental situation just as much as the type of preparation or the parameters of the sensory stimulus involved. They also emphasize that in certain circumstances consideration of mean amplitudes, especially from limited samples, may yield misleading or inconclusive results.

To conclude, in assessing the effects of drugs in relation to changes in perception it may be profitable to study the controlling influences on the specific pathways rather than to consider direct effects.

REFERENCES

Ader, R. and Clink, D. W. (1957). *J. Pharmacol. exp. Therap.*, **121**, 144.
Bradley, P. B. and Elkes, J. (1957). *Brain*, **80**, 77.
Bradley, P. B. and Hance, A. J. (1957). *Electroenceph. clin. Neurophysiol.*, **9**, 191.
Bradley, P. B. and Key, B. J. (1958). *Electroenceph. clin. Neurophysiol.*, **10**, 97.
Bradley, P. B. and Wolstencroft, J. H. (1965). *Brit. med. Bull.*, **21**, 15.
Brown, B. B. (1961). *Fed. Proc.*, **20**, 320.
Cook, L., and Weidley, E. (1957). *Ann. N.Y. Acad. Sci.*, **66**, 740.
Curtis, D. R. (1965). *Brit. med. Bull.*, **21**, 5.
Desmedt, J. E. (1960). *In* Neural mechanisms of the auditory and vestibular systems, (Rasmussen, G. L. and Windle, W. F.), p. 152. Springfield: Thomas.
Dunlop, C. W., McLachlan, E. M., Webster, W. R. and Day, R. H. (1964). *Nature (Lond.)*, **203**, 874.
French, J. D., Verzeano, M. and Magoun, H. W. (1953). *A.M.A. Arch. Neurol. Psychiat.*, **69**, 519.
Galambos, R. (1956). *J. Neurophysiol.*, **19**, 424.
Galambos, R. (1960). *In* Neural mechanisms of the auditory and vestibular systems, (ed. Rasmussen, G. L. and Windle, W. F.), p. 137. Springfield: Thomas.
Galambos, R., Sheatz, G. and Vernier, V. G. (1956). *Science*, **123**, 376.
Hernández-Peón, R. (1955). *Acta neurol. lat-amer.*, **1**, 256.
Hernández-Peón, R., Jouvet, M. and Scherrer, H. (1957). *Acta neurol. lat-amer.*, **3**, 144.
Hernández-Peón, R. (1959). *Acta neurol. lat-amer.*, **5**, 279.
John, E. R. and Killam, K. F. (1959). *J. Pharmacol. exp. Ther.*, **125**, 252.
Jouvet, M. and Hernández-Peón, R. (1957). *Electroenceph. clin. Neurophysiol.* Suppl. No. 6, p. 39.
Key, B. J. (1961a). *Psychopharmacologia (Berl.)*, **2**, 352.
Key, B. J. (1961b). *Nature (Lond.)*, **109**, 275.
Key, B. J. (1964). *Psychopharmacologia (Berl.)*, **6**, 39.
Killam, E. K. and Killam, K. F. (1957). *In* Reticular formation of the brain (ed. Jasper, H. H., Proctor, L. D., Knighton, R. S., Noshay, W. C. and Costello, R.T.), p. 111. Boston: Little, Brown and Co.
Krnjević, K. (1965). *Brit. med. Bull.*, **21**, 10.
Marsh, J. T., McCarthy, D. A., Sheatz, G. and Galambos, R. (1961). *Electroenceph. clin. Neurophysiol.*, **13**, 224.
Purpura, D. P. (1956). *A.M.A. Arch. Neurol. Psychiat.*, **75**, 122.
Rovetta, P. (1956). *Electroenceph. clin. Neurophysiol.*, **8**, 15.

Starr, A. (1964). *Exper. Neurol.*, **10**, 191.
Stephens, R. J. and Key, B. J. (1964). *Electroenceph. clin. Neurophysiol.*, **16**, 623.
Stephens, R. J. and Key, B. J. (1965). *In* Neuro-psychoparmacology, (ed. Bente, D. and Bradley, P. B.), vol. 4, p. 306. Amsterdam: Elsevier.
Whitfield, I. C. and Allanson, J. T. (1956). *J. Physiol.*, **134**, 2P.

DISCUSSION

Salomon: In the cat pentobarbitone 5 mg./kg. abolished spontaneous activity recorded electromyographically in the stapedius muscle. The spontaneous activity is responsible for a change in sound transmission amounting to 6 db maximum. The increase in activity you found in the recorded activity after this dose of pentobarbitone may be due to this effect.

Key: An alternative explanation for the slight increase in the amplitude of evoked potentials after pentobarbitone is that in the acute preparations the electrodes have to be orientated to the desired position. The acoustic stimuli are presented during this procedure, so that even before the recording has begun the animal has already heard them a number of times. It may be therefore, that the animal has become partly habituated to the acoustic stimulus before the start of the experiment. Now it has been shown that barbiturates overcome habituation, in which case the amplitude of the evoked response will increase slightly before any general depressant effect is seen. (Hernández-Peón, R. Central mechanisms controlling conduction along central sensory pathways. *Acta neurol. lat-amer.*, 1955, **1**, 256–264).

Blane: Dr. Key referred to the increased level of evoked potentials in auditory nerve centres of the cat after conditioning to a sound signal. This level was reduced to the control level or lower by chlorpromazine. Is it possible to deduce from this anything about the animal's actual hearing and consequent behaviour? Animals conditioned to respond to a sound signal are widely used in the pharmacological evaluation of drugs—for example conditioned-avoidance behaviour of the rat using a Cook and Weidley, or Skinner apparatus. In assessing the results from such tests I doubt if the possibility is commonly considered that the animal is hearing the signal less and less well as the dose of drug is increased. This possibility is probably remote but ought to be borne in mind.

Key: Certainly, such an effect should be considered, for chlorpromazine does produce a progressive increase in the threshold for sensory-induced arousal. (Bradley, P. B. and Key, B. J. A comparative study of the effects of drugs on the arousal system of the brain. *Brit. J. Pharmacol.*, 1959, **14**, 340–349.) However, in assessing the effect on hearing, the use of evoked potentials has certain disadvantages, in that even with stimuli of constant intensity they tend to show spontaneous changes which may be related to the degree of attention rather than auditory acuity. Moreover, the changes which occur after chlorpromazine has been given still fall within the limits of this normal variation.

Admittedly, the use of evoked potentials could be misleading, for one does not really know what the potential represents. It may well be that one is not dealing with the same neurone population after the administration of the drug. Thus it would be difficult to say what part of hearing is changed when alterations in these evoked potentials occur.

Grossman: I wonder if the primary effect of lysergide (LSD) (greater fluctuations of response magnitude) could be explained as a fluctuation in the animal's attentiveness to the stimulation itself. An increased response may be given when the animal is paying attention to the experimenter and the response may be decreased while the animal is responding to something other than that part of the environment which is controlled. That might account for the differential effects which have been recorded in soundproof and non-soundproof environmental conditions.

Key: Yes, that is how I interpret the effect of lysergide. Behavioural tests show that this drug increases distractability, although I am not aware of any published reports that it definitely affects attentive ability in cats or in man. (Key, B. J. The effect of LSD-25 on the interaction between conditioned and non-conditioned stimuli in a simple avoidance situation. *Psychopharmacologia*, 1964, **6**, 319–326.). The attentiveness of the animals appears to fluctuate quite a lot under the effect of lysergide, so that they pay attention to one stimulus on some occasions but not on others. Perhaps the animals are paying attention all the time, but paying attention to different stimuli, which, previously classified as irrelevant, have become more significant under the effect of the drug.

This effect, of course, would only be shown with doses up to 30 μg./kg. i.p. Higher doses appear to decrease responsiveness to sensory stimuli.

King: It can be shown in a conditioned-avoidance situation under chlorpromazine that the animal still hears the signal stimulus. One can train the animal not only in shock-avoidance, but also in food-approach to another signal. We have done this and shown an attenuation of shock-avoidance behaviour when the food-approach responses are not affected at all—several people have done this (e.g. Ray, O. S. *Psychopharmacologia*, 1963, **4**, 326). The animal can certainly hear the stimulus, but in the case of the shock-avoidance it doesn't choose to respond.

THE PHARMACOLOGICAL BEHAVIOUR OF THE COCHLEAR NUCLEUS

I. C. WHITFIELD

Neurocommunications Research Unit, University of Birmingham

THAT few, if any, neurally active substances reach the neurones of the cochlear nucleus by the systemic route is suggested by the complete lack of any reference in the literature to synthetic or naturally occurring drugs which disrupt the basic hearing mechanism. There are of course substances, such as salicylates, and antibiotics (streptomycin, kanamycin) which damage the receptor mechanism, but streptomycin has no histological effect on brainstem nuclei (McGee and Olszewski, 1962). Similarly the hallucinogens, which by definition produce structured distortions of sensory processes, can be discounted as acting at this level (cf. Whitfield and Allanson, 1958).

Up to 10 years ago, little or no work seems to have been done on the pharmacology of the auditory pathway beyond the receptor sites. In 1957, Allanson and Whitfield, in an endeavour to elucidate the mechanism of afferent inhibition (Galambos, 1944) in the cochlear nucleus, investigated the effect of strychnine on the neurones of this nucleus. They found that neither systemic nor topical application of this substance had any influence on the course of the inhibition. Subsequently Whitfield and Allanson (1958) tried a great number of known neurally active substances by these routes, again with no influence whatever on the activity of the nucleus as recorded from single units in its efferent pathway.

It seemed likely that the substances were not reaching the receptor sites by the systemic route, and so recently we have begun to re-investigate the problem using local application of the drugs. For this purpose we have employed the micro-tap of Comis, Evans, and Whitfield (1964) which enables drug application to single neurones, and current stimulation of cell bodies, to be separately and independently controlled.

Use of this method confirmed the earlier result that strychnine has no influence on the afferent inhibitory process and that picrotoxin is likewise without effect. However, local application of certain compounds does influence the neuronal activity. Glutamate strongly excites all neurones on which it has been tested, whereas γ-amino-butyric acid completely inhibits all neurones. There is reason to think that the effects of these substances are non-specific (Curtis, Phillis and Watkins, 1959) and that they do not represent the mimicking of physiologically present transmitters.

More interesting have been the results with acetylcholine and noradrenaline. These substances have no action when administered systemically (Whitfield and Allanson, 1958), but have a pronounced effect when locally applied.

Acetylcholine produces excitation in about 80% of units in the antero-ventral cochlear nucleus (Comis and Whitfield, 1966). It has a similar effect on neurones in the dorsal nucleus. Inhibition has not been observed. *Per contra*, both adrenaline and noradrenaline produce inhibition of activity in about the same proportion of cells. Excitation has not been observed with these drugs. The excitatory and inhibitory effects referred to can be observed not only as influences on the background activity of the neurone, but also on the discharges produced by peripheral sound stimuli.

The acetylcholine system has been investigated in some detail. The presence of true cholinesterase in both the dorsal and ventral cochlear nuclei has been established (Fig. 1) by the use of Lewis's (Lewis and Shute, 1959) modification of the Koelle technique. It seems unlikely that acetylcholine represents the *afferent* excitatory transmitter since the neurones of the auditory nerve do not appear to be cholinergic (Rossi, 1961), and section of the auditory nerve

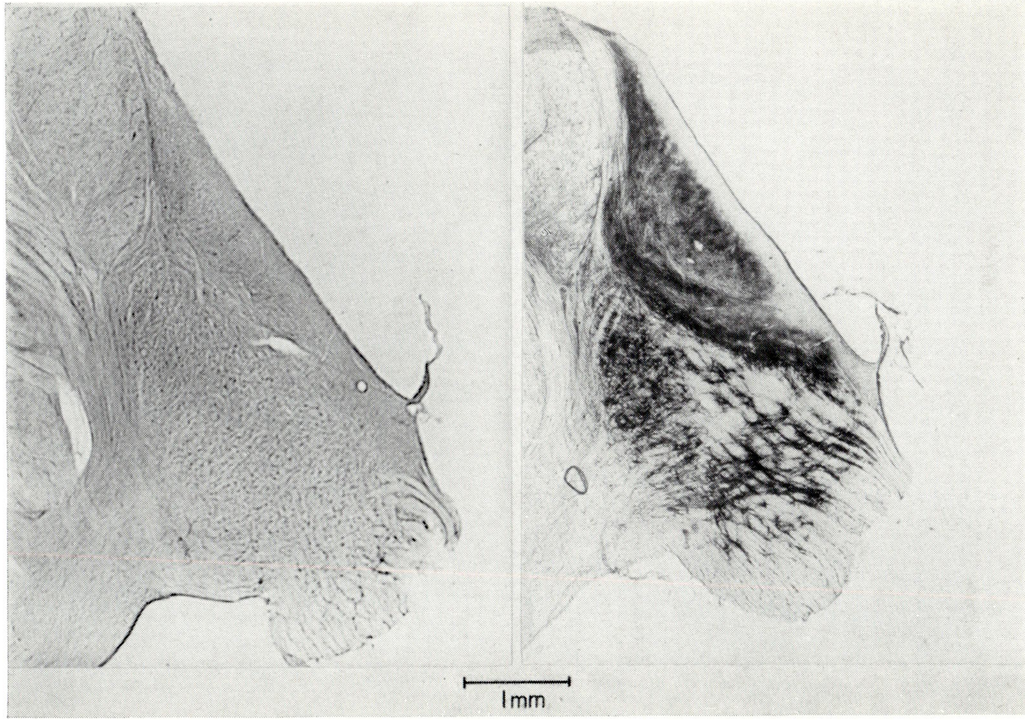

FIG. 1. Transverse section through the dorsal and ventral cochlear nuclei of the cat. Right: stained for true cholinesterase by Lewis's method. Left: Ditto, after, treatment with eserine.

facing page 168

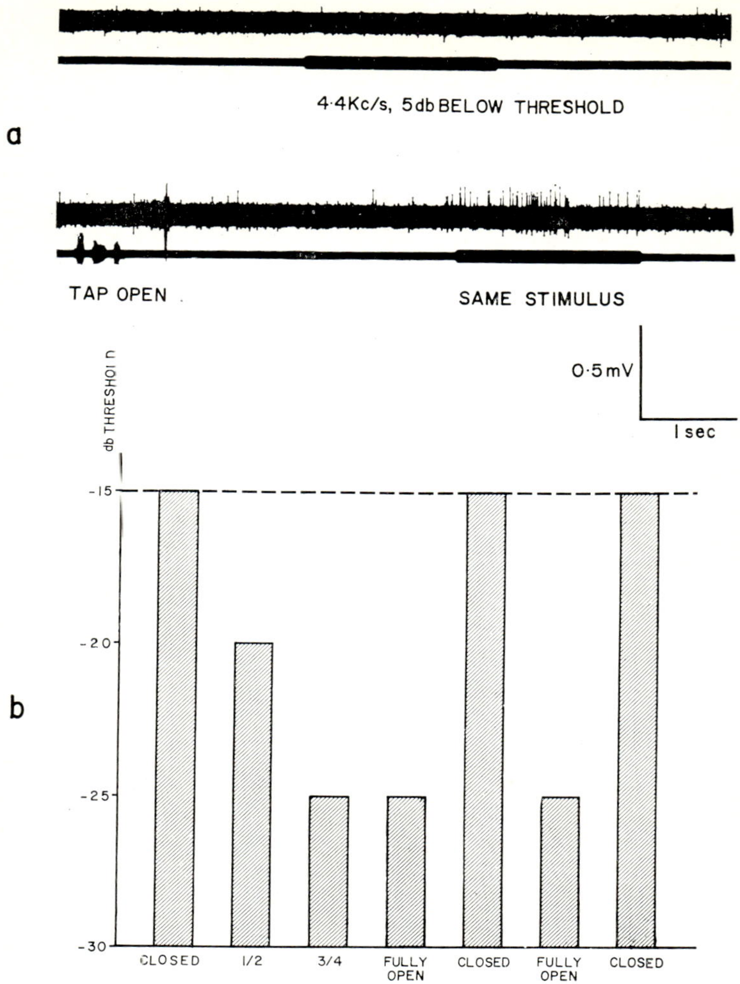

FIG. 2. (a) Upper trace: Unit in antero-ventral cochlear nucleus responsive to a tone of 4·4 kc/s, stimulated with this tone at an intensity 5 db. below threshold, and therefore not responding; Lower trace: same unit in the presence of acetylcholine (tap open). The unit now responds to the previously sub-threshold stimulus.

(*b*) The effect of acetylcholine on the threshold of response of a neurone in the antero-ventral cochlear nucleus to sound stimuli. When the tap is closed, the normal threshold is -15 db. Opening the tap and applying acetylcholine locally to the neurone lowers progressively the threshold to sound as the rate of application is increased. "Tap fully open" represents a rate of about 5×10^{-12} moles/sec. The vertical bars are for immediately successive records (from Whitfield and Comis, 1967).

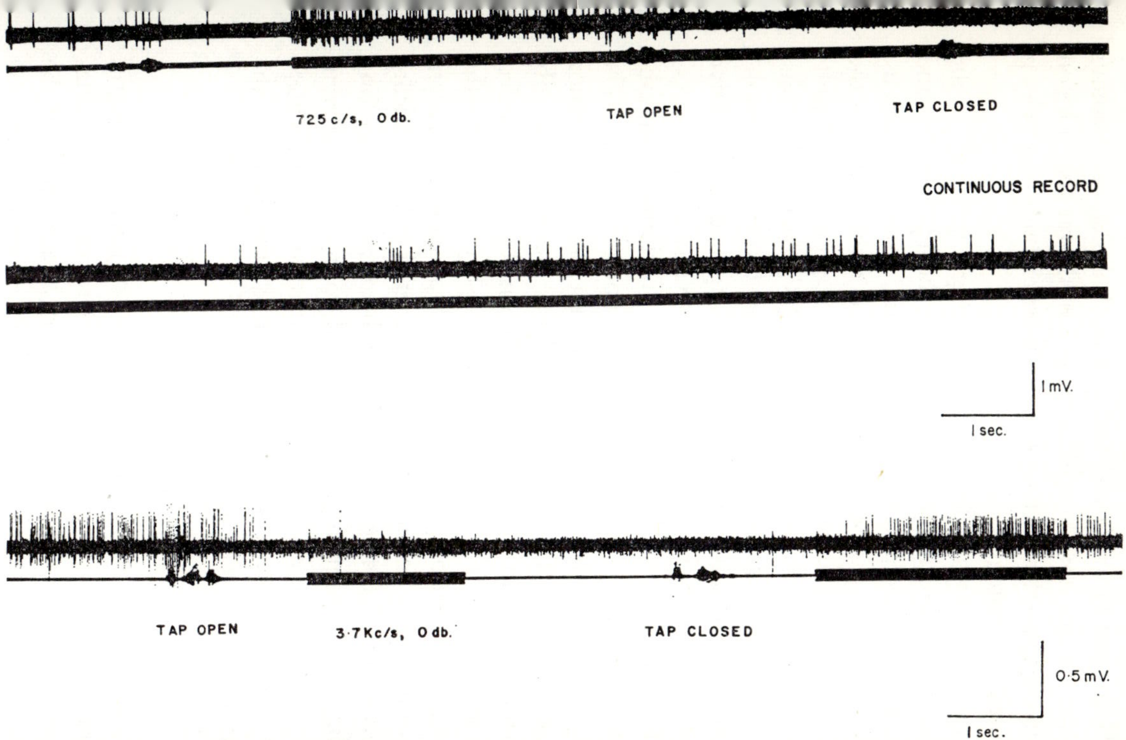

FIG. 3. The effect of blocking agents on the response of neurones in the antero-ventral cochlear nucleus to a sound stimulus. *Above:* response of a neurone to a continuous tone of 725 c/s. At 'tap open' atropine was applied directly to the neurone, causing a failure of the response. After the tap is closed the response gradually recovers. The upper and middle traces form a continuous record. *Below:* the effect of dihydro-β-erythroidine in blocking both 'spontaneous' activity and activity in response to a tonal stimulus. Different unit from that illustrated above (from Whitfield and Comis, 1967).

does not result in loss of staining from the nucleus. On the other hand, Shute and Lewis (1965) found that cholinesterase staining was reduced in the dorsal cochlear nucleus of the rat after a lesion placed in the brain stem, which suggests these endings may belong to a centrifugal system.

Rasmussen (1960) has described a centrifugal pathway in the cat with cells of origin in the lateral nucleus of the superior olive and terminating in the ipsilateral antero-ventral cochlear nucleus. Stimulation of this pathway produces effects on neurones in the anteroventral cochlear nucleus similar to those produced by application of acetylcholine to the same neurones (Whitfield and Comis, 1967). The most interesting of these effects are those on the threshold to sound stimulation. If acetylcholine is applied to a sensitive neurone in a quantity insufficient to cause it to discharge, it nevertheless lowers the threshold sufficiently for a previously subthreshold sound stimulus now to produce a response (Fig. 2a). The lowering of the threshold is dependent on the rate of application of the acetylcholine (Fig. 2b), and may be as much as 10–15 db. Presumably the centrifugal pathway is normally partly active, because application of atropine or dihydro-β-erythroidine to the cochlear nucleus neurone raises the threshold to sound stimulation, so that quite intense sound stimuli are prevented from producing a discharge (Fig. 3). It seems probable that these drugs are blocking the endings of the centrifugal pathway and not the direct afferent excitation, because they also prevent stimulation of the cochlear nucleus neurones normally brought about by stimulation of the superior olivary site (Fig. 4).

Discussion

The cochlear nucleus has four main classes of fibres entering it. The afferent fibres coming from the peripheral receptor mechanism may produce excitation or inhibition at a neurone in the nucleus. Likewise, there are centrifugal fibres coming from the brain stem and terminating in the nucleus; these, too, may

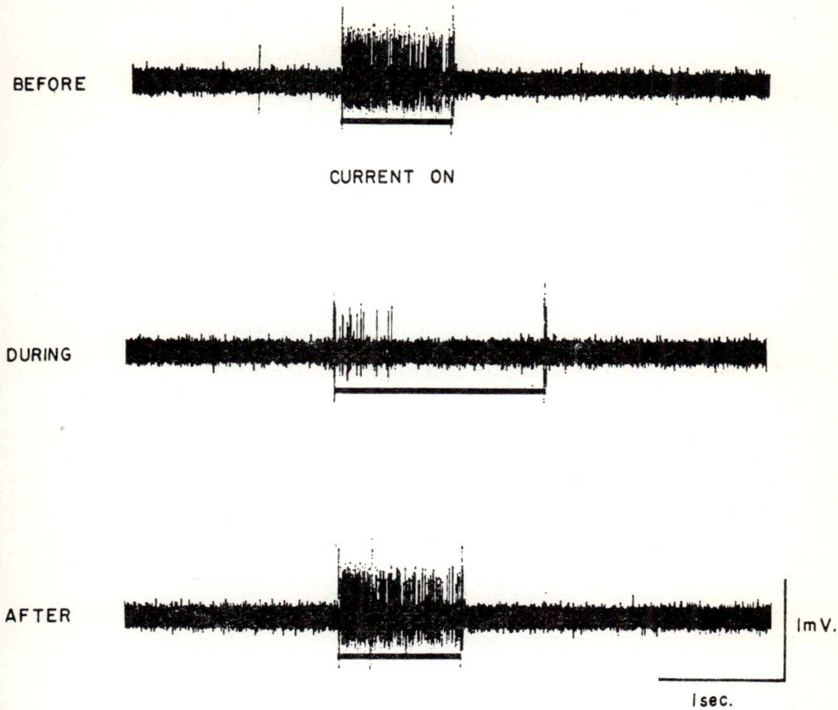

FIG. 4. Effect of atropine on the activity induced in a neurone of the antero-ventral cochlear nucleus by direct current stimulation of the superior olive. (a) before, (b) during, (c) 2 minutes after, local application of atropine (5×10^{-12} mole/sec.) to the neurone. Horizontal bar indicates current stimulation, 6×10^{-5}, amp. +ve.

produce excitation or inhibition. It is possible to stimulate each of these four classes of fibres separately or in combination, so that the system forms a powerful tool, in conjunction with local drug application, for the study of the pharmacology of central synaptic transmission.

The nature of the afferent excitatory and inhibitory transmitters has not yet been elucidated. Although glutamate and γ-amino-butyric acid respectively excite and inhibit all neurones in the nucleus, there is no reason at present to regard them as transmitters. Strychnine, which interferes with post-synaptic inhibition at motor neurones (Bradley, Easton and Eccles, 1953), has no influence whatever on the afferent inhibition in the cochlear nucleus. Picrotoxin, which is said to block presynaptic inhibition (Eccles, Schmidt and Willis, 1963), likewise has no influence on the inhibition (Comis, unpublished observation).

On the other hand, the possibility of identifying the transmitters for the centrifugal pathways is much more hopeful. Acetylcholine mimics the effect of stimulation of the lateral-olivary/cochlear nucleus pathway, and the effects of stimulation of this pathway are blocked by cholinergic blocking agents. Furthermore cholinesterase is abundantly present in the cochlear nucleus and there is evidence that this is linked with the centrifugal pathways, rather than with the afferent pathways. The status of adrenaline or noradrenaline as the centrifugal inhibitory transmitter is much less sound. According to Fuxe (1965) the cochlear nucleus of the rat contains some, though very little, noradrenaline. No data are at present available for the cat and no suitable adrenergic blocking agent has yet been found which would enable us to test whether the inhibitory effects of centrifugal fibre stimulation can be blocked by such substances.

Acknowledgement

Work here reported which was carried out in our laboratories was supported by the Royal Society and by the U.S. Air Force Office of Scientific Research under Grant A.F. EOAR 63-115 through the European Office of Aerospace Research (OAR) United States Air Force.

Summary

1. The neurones of the cochlear nucleus are unaffected by systemic application of a great range of neurally active substances.

2. The afferent inhibitory response is unaffected even by locally applied strychnine or picrotoxin.

3. Local application of acetylcholine excites, and of adrenaline or noradrenaline inhibits, the majority of neurones in the

anteroventral cochlear nucleus. The reverse effects have not been seen.

4. Cholinesterase is present in the cochlear nuclei and is probably related to centrifugal pathways.

5. Locally applied acetylcholine lowers the threshold of neurones in the antero-ventral cochlear nucleus to peripheral sound stimuli by up to 15 db. A similar result is obtained by direct-current stimulation of the lateral nucleus of the superior olive. Both these effects are blocked by atropine or dihydro-β-erythroidine.

REFERENCES

Allanson, J. T. and Whitfield, I. C. (1957). The effect of strychnine on inhibition in a sensory pathway. *J. Physiol.*, **134,** 12–13.

Bradley, K., Easton, D. M. and Eccles, J. C. (1953). An investigation of primary or direct inhibition. *J. Physiol.*, **122,** 474–488.

Comis, S. D., Evans, E. F. and Whitfield, I. C. (1964). A micro-tap for controlling the application of drugs to single neurones. *J. Physiol.*, **173,** 4–6P.

Comis, S. D. and Whitfield, I. C. (1966). The effect of acetylcholine on neurones of the cochlear nucleus. *J. Physiol.*, **183,** 22–23P.

Curtis, D. R., Phillis, J. W. and Watkins, J. C. (1959). The depression of spinal neurones by γ-amino-η-butyric acid and β-alanine. *J. Physiol.*, **146,** 185–203.

Eccles, J. C., Schmidt, R. F. and Willis, W. D. (1963). Pharmacological studies on pre-synaptic inhibition. *J. Physiol.*, **168,** 500–530.

Fuxe, K. (1965). Distribution of monoamine nerve terminals in the central nervous system. *Acta. physiol. scand.*, **64,** Suppl. 247, 39–85.

Galambos, R. (1944). Inhibition of activity in single auditory nerve fibres by acoustic stimulation. *J. Neurophysiol.*, **7,** 287–303.

Lewis, P. R. and Shute, C. C. D. (1959). Selective staining of visceral efferents in the rat brain stem by a modified Koelle technique. *Nature, Lond.*, **183,** 1743–4 (and personal communication).

McGee, T. M. and Olszewski, J. (1962). Streptomycin sulphate and dihydrostreptomycin toxicity. Behavioral and histopathologic studies. *Arch. Otolaryng.*, **75,** 295–311.

Rasmussen, G. L. (1960). Efferent fibres of the cochlear nerve and cochlear nucleus. *In* Neural Mechanisms of the Auditory and Vestibular Systems (Ed. Rasmussen, G. L. and Windle, W. F.), Chap. 8. Springfield: Thomas.

Rossi, G. (1961). L'acétylcholinesterase au cours du development de l'oreille interne du cobaye. *Acta oto-laryng.* Suppl. 170, 1–91.

Shute, C. C. D. and Lewis, P. R. (1965). Cholinesterase-containing pathways of the hind brain: afferent cerebellar and centrifugal cochlear fibres. *Nature, Lond.*, **205**, 242–246.

Whitfield, I. C. and Allanson, J. T. (1958). A study of the effect of some neurally active drugs on inhibition in the auditory pathway. *Arch. ital. Biol.*, **96**, 29–37.

Whitfield, I. C. and Comis, S. D. (1967). A reciprocal gating mechanism in the auditory pathway. *In* Cybernetic Problems in Bionics (Ed. Oestreicher, H. L. and Moore, D. R.), New York: Gordon & Breach.

DRUGS INHIBITING MOTION SICKNESS

SOME ELECTRONYSTAGMOGRAPHIC STUDIES OF THE EFFECT OF DRUGS UPON THE LABYRINTH

A. J. Philipszoon

Amsterdam

Motion sickness is a clinical syndrome consisting of dizziness, nausea, vomiting and a general feeling of malaise which may arise when people are in conveyances constantly subject to many accelerations, for example on ships, in aeroplanes, trains, and cars. The ancient Egyptians experienced it when riding on camels (Ferreri, 1957).

Changes in speed can be perceived by the vestibular organ, the eyes and the proprioceptive system. It is generally assumed that sea-sickness is caused by overexcitation of the labyrinth (Quix, 1923; De Wit, 1953, 1958). Other unpleasant stimuli, such as an overfilled stomach or being in a confined space may have a contributory effect in causing sea-sickness, and psychical factors also play an important part in determining its severity.

We may, however, be reasonably certain that overstimulation of the vestibular organ is a necessary link in the genesis of motion sickness. Rather strong evidence for this view is the fact that people without inner ears do not become sea-sick. In 1896 James found that deaf-mutes were refractory to sea-sickness. Sjöberg (1931) could not produce experimental sea-sickness in dogs whose labyrinths had been removed.

De Wit showed that people who are particularly prone to sea-sickness have a steep cupulogram, which indicates a hypersensitive labyrinth, compared with persons who are little troubled by sea-sickness. He also drew attention to the fact that people with vestibular affections get sea-sick sooner than healthy people. A sensitive labyrinth as shown by cupulometry also appears to predispose to air-sickness (Krijger, 1954).

Nieuwenhuijsen (1958) found a correlation between the number of motions of a ship per unit time and the percentage of sea-sick persons on board. According to Quix (1923) excitation of the otoliths is more important in the genesis of sea-sickness than excitation of the semicircular canals. McNally and Stuart (1942) reviewed the literature on the physiology of the labyrinth in relation to motion sickness, and concluded that linear accelerations are most important as a cause of motion sickness.

Since the vestibular organ is essential for sea-sickness, methods were sought to investigate the effect of drugs on vestibular reactions. Until recently it was difficult to record vestibular reactions objectively, but now eye movements provoked by vestibular stimulation can be adequately recorded by electronystagmography. This is based upon the fact that the retina is charged negatively as against the cornea: hence the eye is to be considered as a dipole, the electrical axis of which coincides with the optical axis. Any movement of the eye gives a change of the field power in the region near the eye. The nystagmograph records the eye movements by these changes in field power (Fig. 1).

A great advance in the drug treatment of motion sickness occurred in 1947 when Gay and Carliner treated a pregnant woman who suffered from urticaria with the antihistamine dimenhydrinate (diphenhydramine chlorotheophyllinate, Dramamine). This woman also happened to suffer from severe car-sickness. Not only did the patient recover from her urticaria, but also no longer experienced car-sickness when she used the drug. Extensive investigation of the effect of antihistamines against motion sickness followed. Some of the many publications on the subject are listed in the references at the end of this paper.

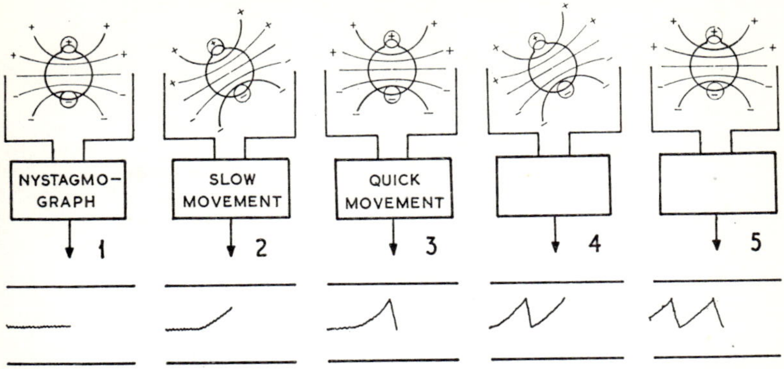

FIG. 1. Diagram showing principle of electronystagmography. The eye movements are recorded via changes in the field-potential.

We have studied the effect of drugs upon eye movements provoked by angular and linear acceleration and also the effect of drugs upon positional nystagmus after labyrinthectomy and alcohol intoxication. A method was also developed to study the effect of drugs upon the corneo-retinal potential difference, since an influence upon this potential difference could change the nystagmogram even when the eye movements are not affected.

Effect of drugs upon eye movements provoked by angular acceleration

To study the effect of drugs upon eye movements provoked by stimulation of the semicircular canals we devised a rotating table which could be used to provoke a constant rotatory nystagmus in rabbits. Since in rabbits a small rotatory stimulus already provokes distinct nystagmus, rotation through a small angle was sufficient. The rabbit was strapped to a board, and its head fixed in a clamp. It was then put on the rotating platform, a table with a circular top supported by ball bearings about its axis. The table could be rotated through an angle of 30° by a simple weight and pulley arrangement (Fig. 2). In order to check whether the table indeed turned at the same speed over the same angle in every rotation, the axis of the pulley was connected with the axis of a linear potenti-

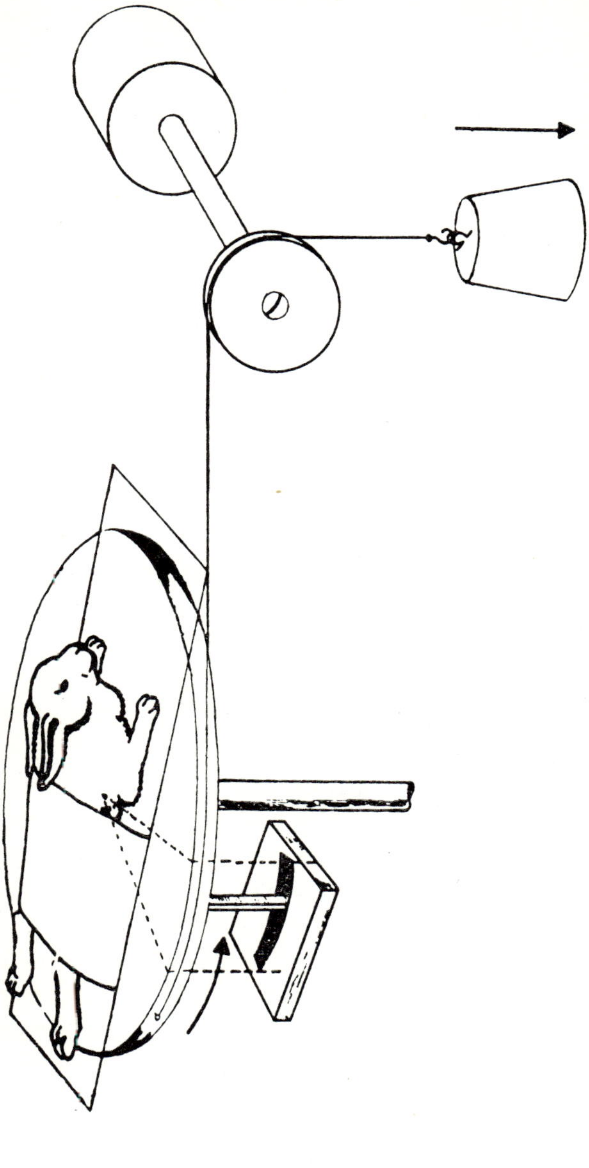

Fig. 2. Diagram of rotating table for rabbits.

ometer. The position of the pulley could be directly recorded via a second channel of the recording apparatus by means of the potentiometer, which was part of a Wheatstone bridge. Subcutaneous needles fixed to the skin with collodion were used as electrodes. The two recording electrodes were fixed in front of and behind the eye; the earth electrode was fixed to the head in the midline.

In order to exclude possible effects of light on the corneo-retinal potential difference and to exclude optokinetic stimuli the rabbit was put in the dark by screening it with cardboard and a lightproof photographic cloth. Experiments were not begun until the rabbit had been in the dark for half an hour because after that time the potential difference of the eye is quite constant.

We investigated the effects of the antihistamine cinnarizine, of of chlorpromazine, of hyoscine and of pentobarbitone (Fig. 3). The drugs were injected intraperitoneally. Normal saline solution never influenced the nystagmus.

Cinnarizine clearly suppressed the nystagmus, while the rabbit was still alert. After the test it behaved normally. Chlorpromazine also influenced the nystagmus, but only the quick phase. The slow phases accumulated, so that a deviation of the eye to one side was apparent on the nystagmogram. The eye did not return to its original position. On the record the curve returns slowly to its original position, but this is an artefact due to the response characteristics of the amplifying system.

Hyoscine, a drug which is clinically effective in motion sickness, did not suppress the nystagmus, and indeed increased its amplitude. This finding suggests that the effect of hyoscine in motion sickness cannot be due to suppression of vestibular excitability. Gutner, Gould and Batterman (1951) also found this influence of hyoscine.

Pentobarbitone suppressed the nystagmus in a dose which simultaneously produced complete anaesthesia.

To study the influence of cinnarizine on angular acceleration in man we used cupulometry (Van Egmond, Groen, and Jongkees,

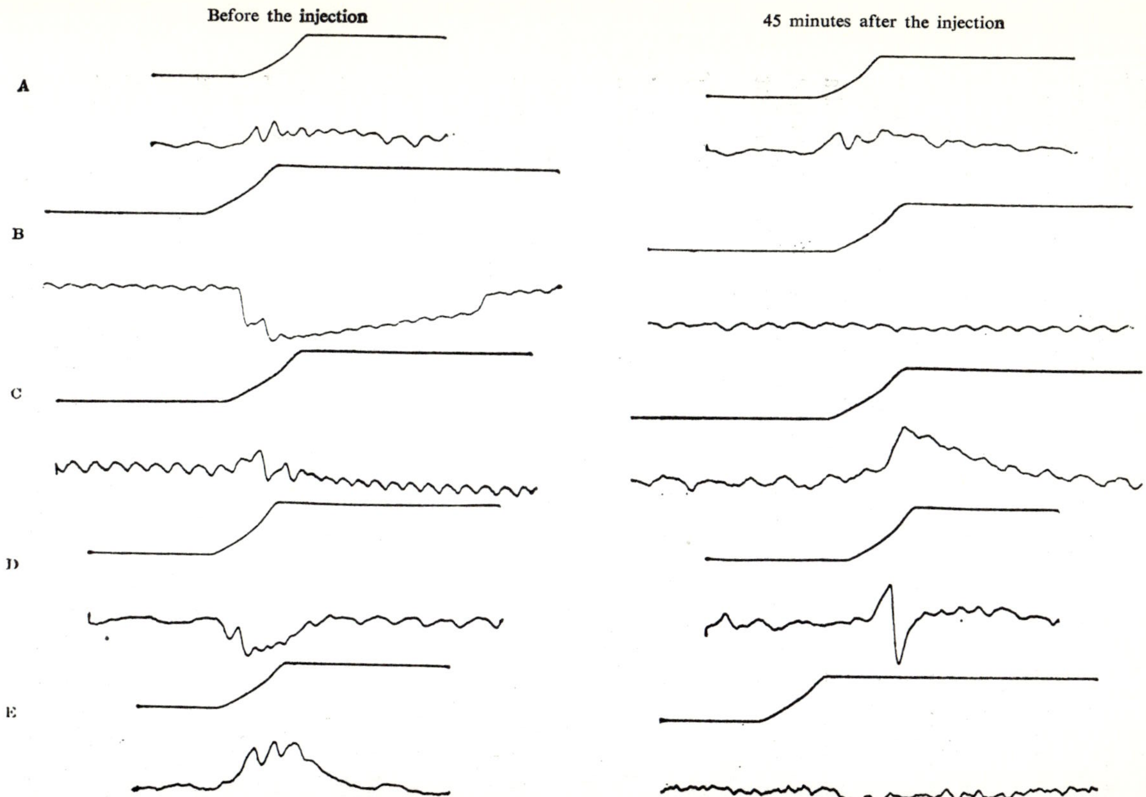

FIG. 3. Rotation tests in rabbits. The upper line represents the movement of the table. The lower line represents the eye movement. A normal saline solution 10 ml.; B. cinnarizine 40 mg./kg.; C. chlorpromazine 8 mg./kg.; D. hyoscine 500 mg./kg.; E. pentobarbitone 20 mg./kg.

1948, 1949, 1952), a rotation test using small innocuous stimuli of physiological intensity. The duration of the post-rotatory nystagmus and of the after-sensation is measured. The subject sits in a rotating chair with the head bent forward 30°. The horizontal semicircular canals are then situated in the plane of rotation, so that only the horizontal canals are stimulated. The subject is gradually set in rotation until a constant velocity is reached. After

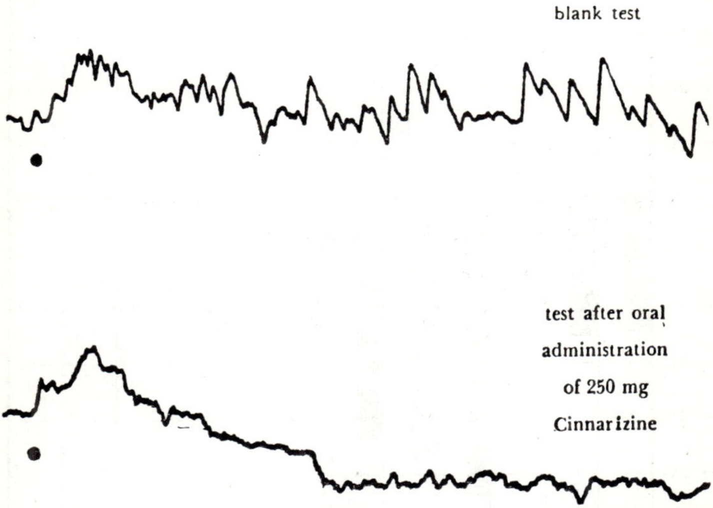

FIG. 4. Suppression of post-rotatory nystagmus in a human subject after cinnarizine.

a period of rotation at constant velocity the chair is stopped within one second. It is thus possible to administer precisely measured stimuli to the cupula. Our subjects were rotated both to the left and to the right with velocities of 20°/sec, 36°/sec and 60°/sec; the speed was checked with a stopwatch. The subject was screened off with black curtains, and the nystagmus was recorded with eyes closed.

The effect of cinnarizine (25 mg.) was compared with that of a placebo in a double-blind procedure. Cupulograms were made before and 3 hours after administration of the treatment. The durations in seconds of the post-rotatory nystagmus in the six rotation tests (20°/sec., 36°/sec. and 60°/sec. to the left and to the right) performed for each cupulogram were added together.

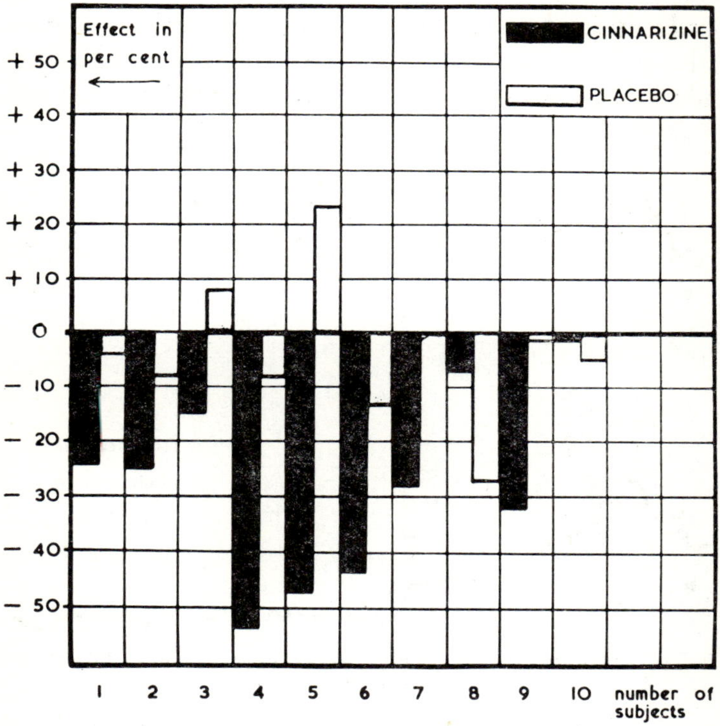

FIG. 5. Effects of cinnarizine on post-rotatory nystagmus in 10 subjects. The difference between the total duration of the nystagmus in the test, after the subject had taken cinnarizine or the placebo, and the total duration of the blank test before, is expressed as a percentage of the total duration of the blank test (see text).

The same was done for the durations of the after-sensation. Thus we obtained for each cupulogram a value both for the post-rotatory nystagmus and for the post-rotatory sensation. In order to be able to express the effect of the drug or of the placebo as a number, we expressed the difference between the values for nystagmus and sensation obtained in the blank test and in the test after the administration of drug or placebo as a percentage of the value found in the blank test. Cinnarizine significantly reduced post-rotatory nystagmus (Figs. 4 and 5) and the after-sensation (Fig. 6).

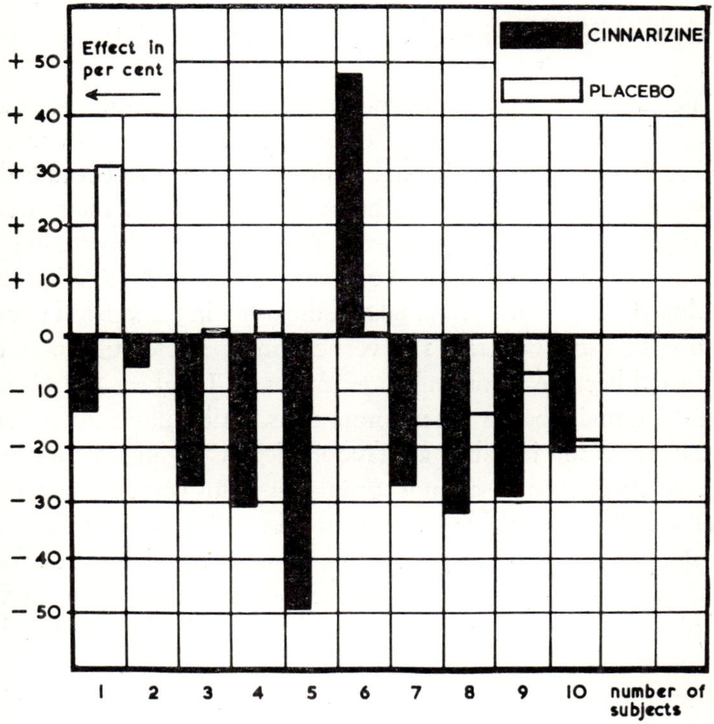

FIG. 6. Effects of cinnarizine on post-rotatory sensation in 10 subjects. The difference between the total duration of the sensation in the test, after the subject had taken cinnarizine or the placebo, and the total duration of the blank test before, is expressed as a percentage of the total duration of the blank test (see text).

Effects of drugs on eye movements provoked by linear acceleration

Since overstimulation of the otoliths is important in the production of motion sickness, we also investigated the effect of drugs upon reflexes caused by linear acceleration. The parallel swing appeared to be a suitable instrument for the purpose. Jongkees and Groen (1946) described compensatory eye movements in rabbits that were swung on a parallel swing. They observed these eye movements with the unaided eye. We developed a method of recording the eye movements with the aid of the nystagmograph (Philipszoon, 1959; Jongkees and Philipszoon, 1960).

The parallel swing is a stretcher hung from four cables of equal length fastened to its corners. It can be swung in two directions. The surface remains horizontal while it is swinging because the cables are joined to the ceiling perpendicularly above their points of attachment to the stretcher. The manner of swinging is shown in Figs. 7 and 8. Two kinds of linear acceleration are produced, one in the horizontal and the other in the vertical plane, both with a sine pattern. The vertical linear acceleration may be neglected because according to estimates by Jongkees and Groen (1946) it remains below the minimum perceptible if the dimensions of the swing and its cables are favourable. As no angular acceleration arises the cupulae are not stimulated. This was demonstrated after selective otolith destruction in rabbits by the technique of Versteegh (1927), when no eye movements could be provoked on the parallel swing, whereas on the torsion swing which applies angular accelerations eye movements could still be provoked by stimulating the cupulae (Fig. 10) (Philipszoon, 1962c).

For rabbits we made a parallel swing that could be swung sideways. The swing moved to and fro in 22 seconds. The initial amplitude was 22 cm., the cable length 112 cm.

Initially we swung the rabbit along its longitudinal axis and tried to record compensatory eye movements by placing the electrodes in front of (rostrally) and behind (caudally) the eye, but even with a very great excursion no eye movements could be recorded. This particular motion probably causes only rotatory eye movements, the eye rotating its optical axis, which coincides

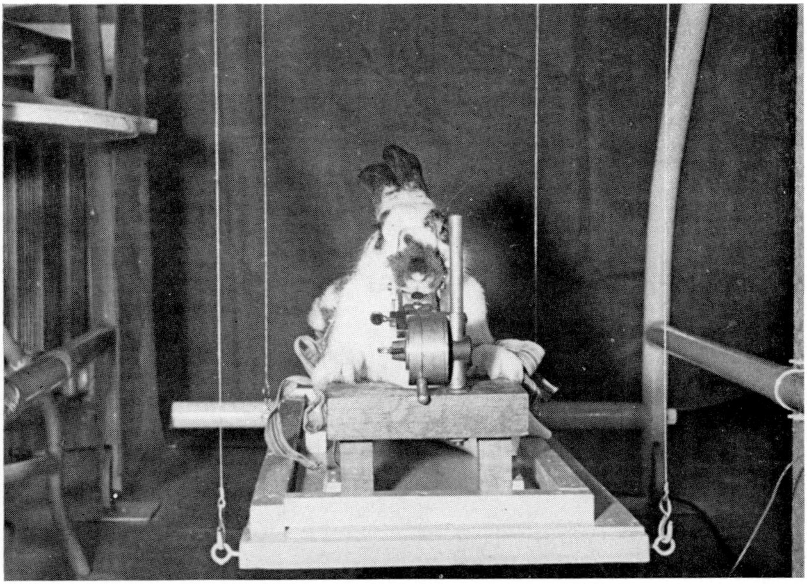

Fig. 7. Rabbit on parallel swing.

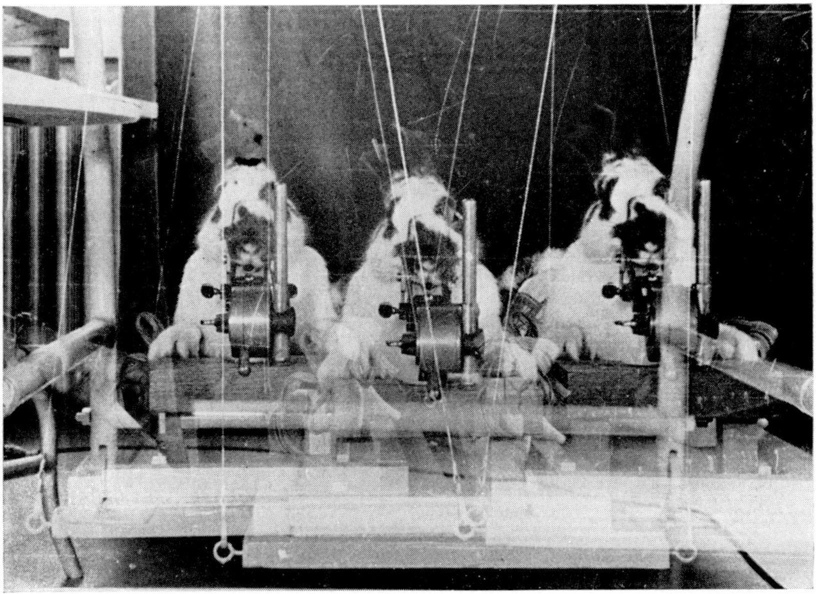

Fig. 8. Movement of parallel swing: three super-imposed photographs.

facing page 184

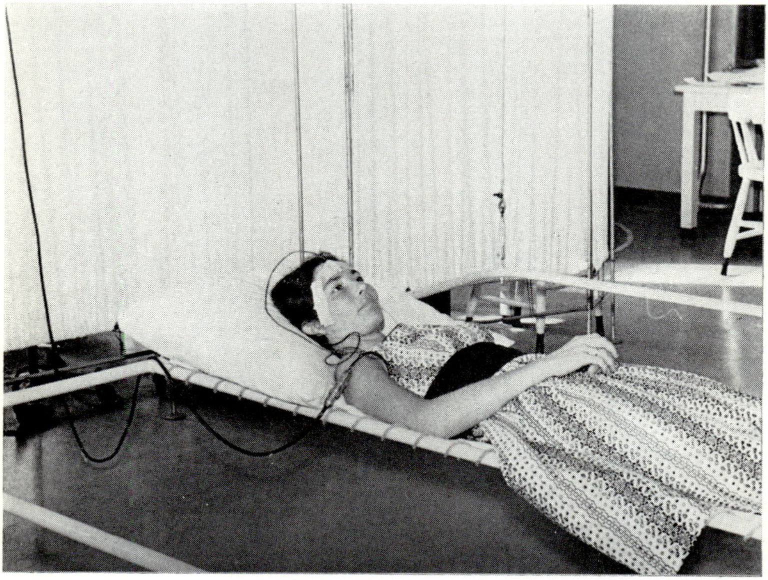

FIG. 9. Human subject on parallel swing.

with the electrical axis. The field potential therefore does not record eye movements. However, compensatory eye movements could be recorded when we swung the rabbit sideways. The

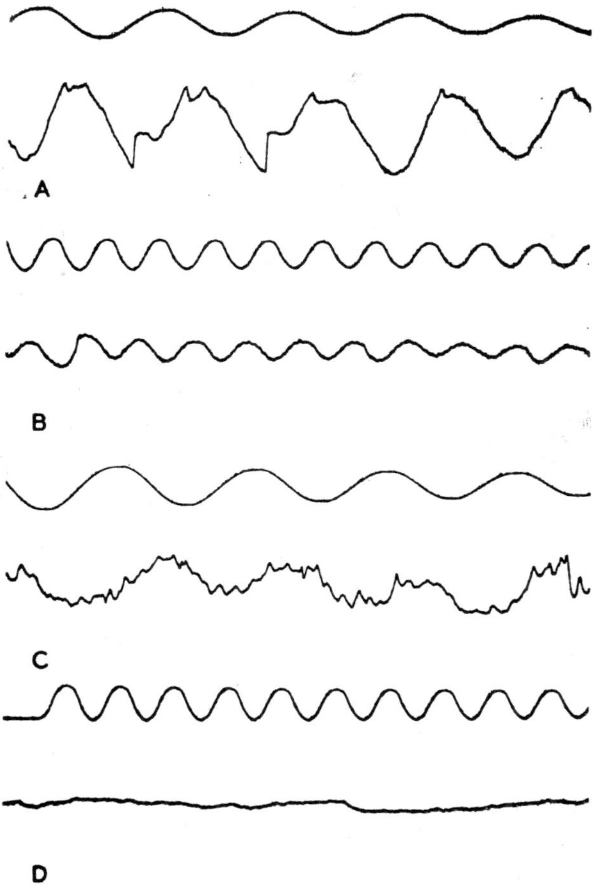

FIG. 10. Selective otolith destruction. The upper line records the movements of the swing, the lower one the eye movements. A. Torsion swing (angular acceleration) before operation. B. Parallel swing (linear acceleration) before operation. C. Torsion swing after operation: there is still a response. D. Parallel swing after operation: no response.

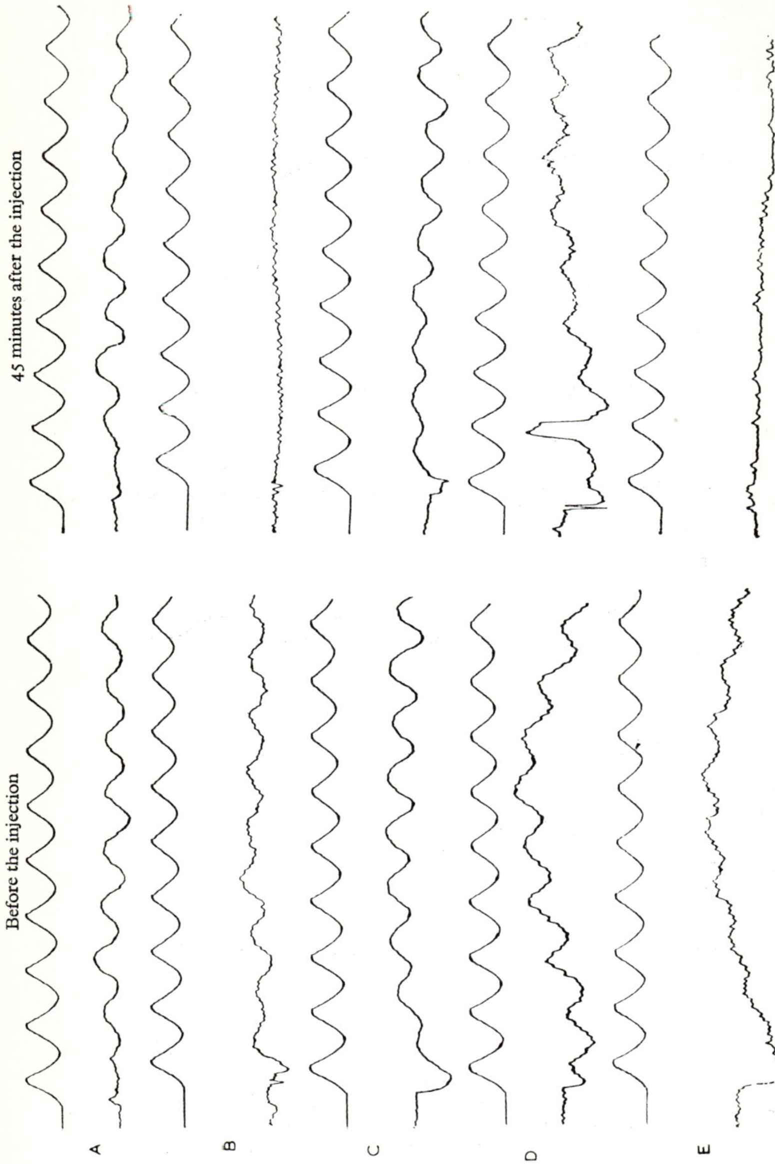

FIG. 11. Parallel swing tests in rabbits. The upper line represents the movement of the swing, the lower line represents the eye movement. A. normal saline solution 10 ml.; B. cinnarizine 40 mg./kg.; C. chlorpromazine: 8 mg./kg.; D. hyoscine 5 mg./kg.; E. pentobarbitone 40 mg./kg.

electrodes were placed above and below the eye in these experiments.

As in the rotation tests the rabbit was fixed on a board, its head held in a clamp, and the experiments were carried out in the dark. The mechanical movement of the swing was recorded by means of a potentiometer whose axle was placed end to end with the turning point of one of the four cables and connected with it.

We investigated the same drugs as in the rotation test. Cinnarizine clearly suppressed the eye movements on the swing. Neither chlorpromazine nor hyoscine affected the eye movements (Fig. 11). Pentobarbitone suppressed the eye movements only when complete anaesthesia had been reached, just as in the rotation tests.

We also constructed a parallel swing for human subjects (Fig. 9). Cinnarizine prevented the eye movements here too (Fig. 12).

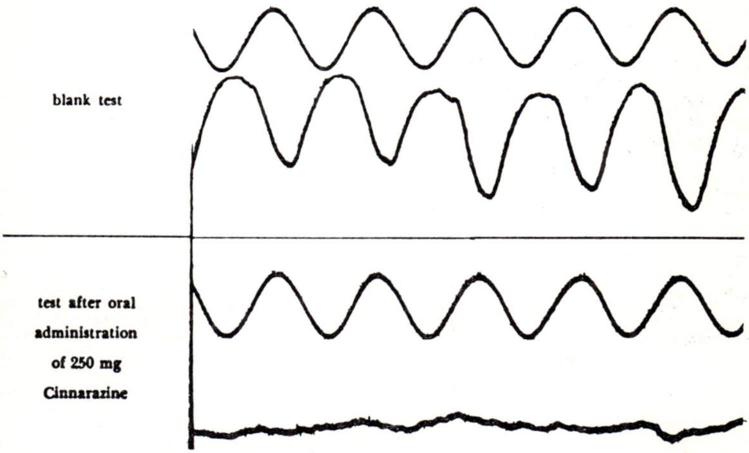

FIG. 12. Suppression of compensatory eye movements on parallel swing in a human subject after cinnarizine.

Positional nystagmus

We have also studied the effect of cinnarizine on positional nystagmus after unilateral and bilateral labyrinthectomy, and

7*

upon nystagmus provoked by ethyl alcohol (Bos, 1962; Bos and Philipszoon, 1963). The nystagmus was studied in the prone position, on the right side, on the left side, supine, and with the head upwards.

The movements of both eyes were recorded simultaneously.

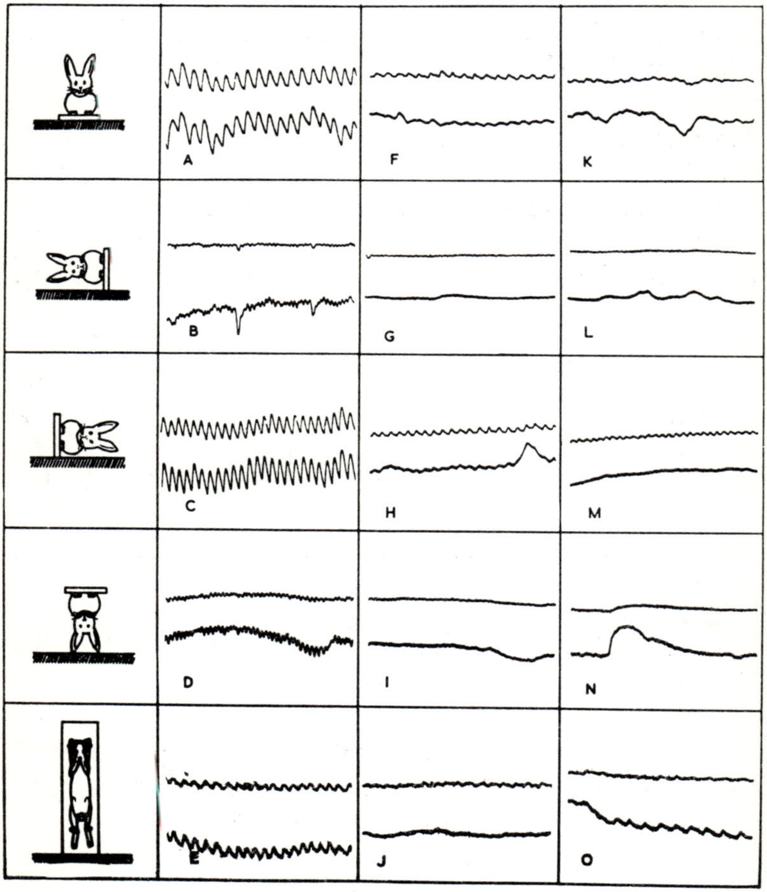

FIG. 13. The effect of cinnarizine upon positional nystagmus after one-sided labyrinthectomy. *Upper tracing:* right eye. *Lower tracing:* left eye. A–E: before injection. F–J: 20 minutes after injection of cinnarizine. K–O: 40 minutes after injection.

Cinnarizine clearly influenced the positional nystagmus after unilateral and bilateral labyrinthectomy (Figs. 13 and 14), but did not influence alcohol nystagmus (Fig. 15). The labyrinthectomies were performed by the method of De Kleijn and Versteegh (1935); 96% ethanol was diluted and administered by stomach tube.

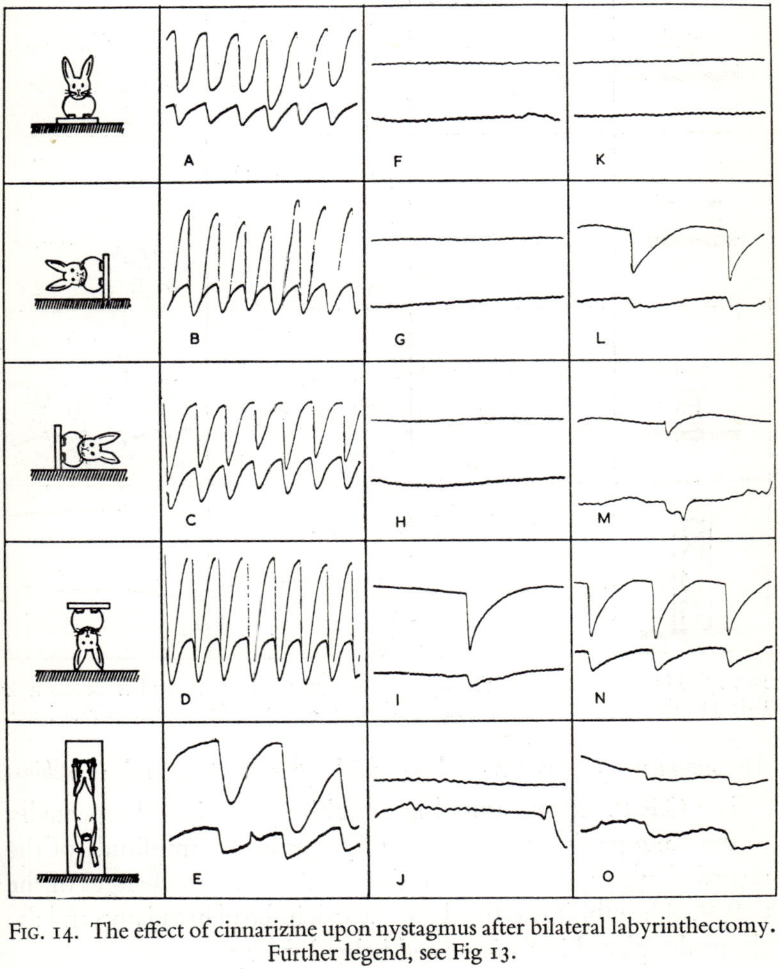

FIG. 14. The effect of cinnarizine upon nystagmus after bilateral labyrinthectomy. Further legend, see Fig 13.

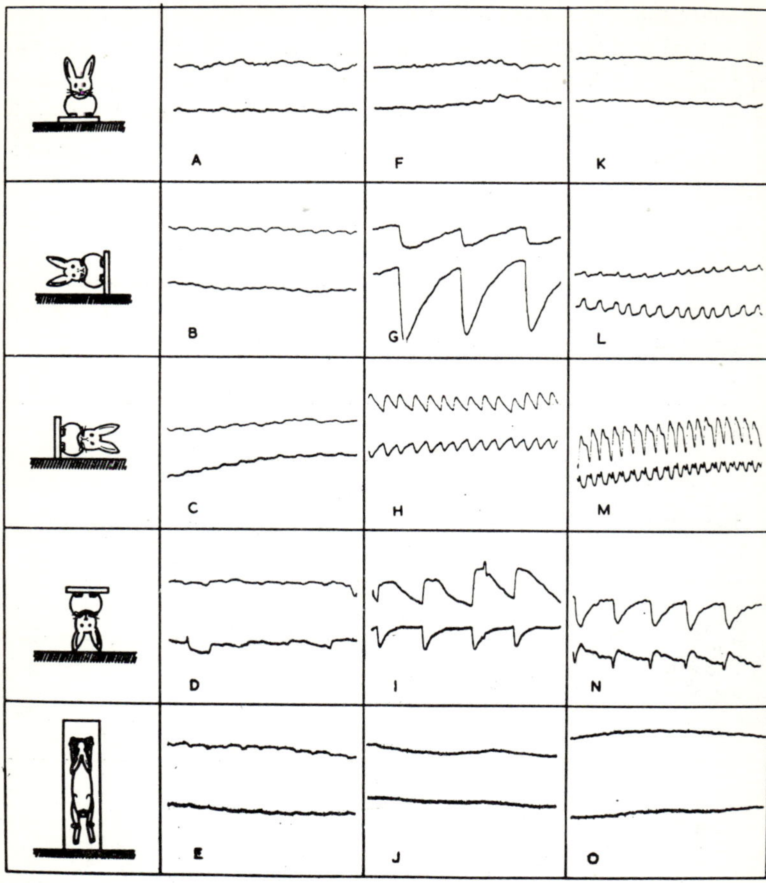

FIG. 15. The effect of cinnarizine upon alcohol nystagmus. A–E: before alcohol. F–J: 30 minutes after alcohol consumption. K–O: 30 minutes after cinnarizine.

Measurement of corneo-retinal potential difference (C.R.P.) in rabbits

The C.R.P. was measured in a rabbit eye subjected repeatedly to the same passive movement. Changes in the amplitude of the recorded eye movement could thus be due only to changes of the C.R.P. The rabbit was fixed on a board, its head in a clamp and the electrodes placed in front of and behind the eye.

After corneal anaesthesia with 0·5% amethocaine, a thread was sutured to the cornea. One end was led via a small pulley to an electro-magnetic relay, and the other end fastened to a small counterweight via another pulley (Fig. 16). When the relay was actuated the eye was drawn forward; when it was released the counterweight pulled the eye back to its original position. The movement of the relay was recorded on the paper and checked by fixing to the lever of the relay a thread connected via a pulley

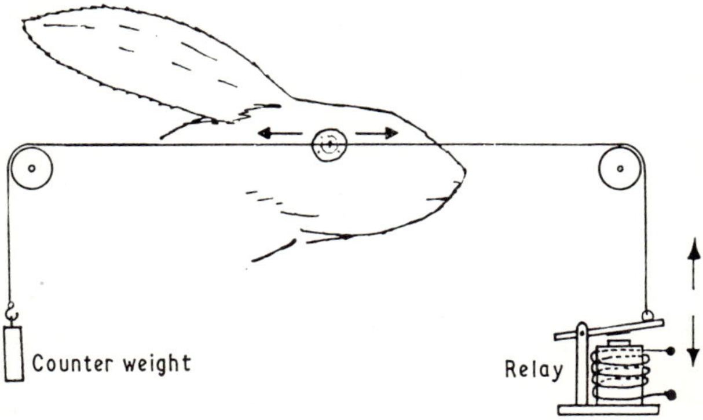

FIG. 16. Diagram showing method of measuring the corneo-retinal potential difference.

to another counterweight. The rotation of the latter pulley wheel was recorded on the second channel of the recording system. The position of the axle of the pulley was linearly converted into a voltage. During the first half hour in the dark, and especially during the first 15 minutes, the C.R.P. clearly decreased, but only very slight spontaneous changes in the C.R.P. occurred after a rabbit had been in the dark for half an hour or more. We therefore began the vestibular tests half an hour after having put the rabbits in the dark.

Fig. 17 shows that cinnarizine, chlorpromazine, hyoscine and pentobarbitone do not affect the C.R.P. and also demonstrates that sodium iodate ($NaIO_3$) decreases and sodium azide (NaN_3)

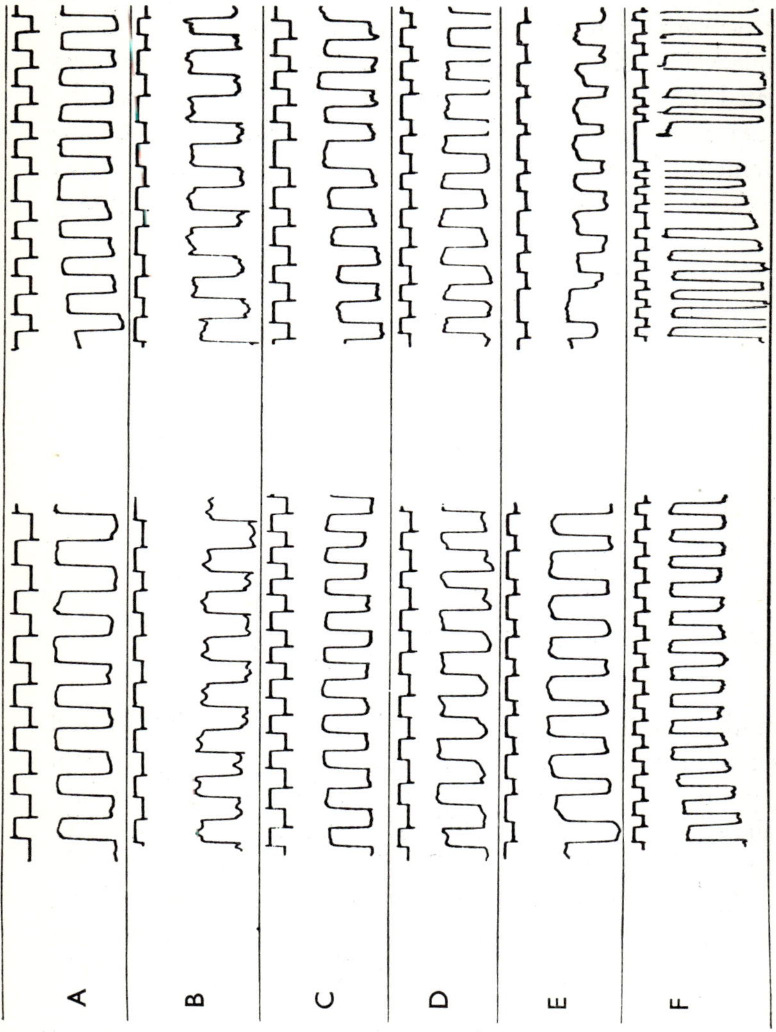

FIG. 17. Effects of some drugs upon the corneo-retinal potential difference. The upper line records the movements of the relay, the lower line the movements of the eye. A. Cinnarizine. B. Chlorpromazine. C. Hyoscine. D. Pentobarbitone. E. Sodium iodate. F. Sodium azide.

increases the C.R.P., as described by Noell (1952) and Heck and Papst (1957).

Summary

Over-stimulation of the labyrinth is an essential feature of motion sickness. The effects of drugs upon the vestibular have been investigated by electronystagmography. The semicircular canals in rabbits were stimulated on a rotating table. The antihistaminic drug cinnarizine clearly suppressed the nystagmus; chlorpromazine only suppressed the quick nystagmus phase; hyoscine intensified the nystagmus, indicating that its effect in motion sickness cannot be due to inhibition of the labyrinth; pentobarbitone only influenced the nystagmus in doses inducing complete anaesthesia. Cupulometry in man clearly demonstrated suppression of post-rotatory nystagmus and sensation. The drugs were also tested in rabbits subjected to linear acceleration to stimulate the otoliths. Cinnarizine suppressed the compensatory eye movements; chlorpromazine and hyoscine did not affect them, and pentobarbitone only suppressed them when the rabbit was fully anaesthetized. In human subjects cinnarizine also diminished similar compensatory eye movements.

Cinnarizine clearly suppressed positional nystagmus in rabbits after unilateral and bilateral labyrinthectomy, but not alcohol nystagmus.

None of the drugs influenced the corneo-retinal potential difference.

REFERENCES

(**denotes reports on antihistamines in motion sickness not cited in the text.*)

*Arner, O., Diamant, H. and Goldberg, L. (1954). Effects and side-effects of motion sickness preparations. *Acta otolaryng.* (*Stockh.*), *suppl.* **116,** 19.

*Aschan, G., Bergstedt, M. and Goldberg, L. (1957). The effect of some antihistaminic drugs on positional alcohol nystagmus. *Acta otolaryng.* (*Stockh.*), *suppl.* **140,** 79.

*Bartalena, G. (1955). Azione degli antistaminici di sintesi sugli effetti della stimolazione vestibolare. *Boll. Mal. Orecch.*, **73,** 500.
*Beaumont, F. K. (1949). Antihistamine drugs and sea-sickness. *Brit. med. J.*, **ii,** 1473.
*Bergström, O. and Koch, H. (1956). The effect of chlorpromazine on the vestibular function. *Acta otolaryng.* (*Stockh.*), **46,** 484.
Bos, J. H. (1962). On vestibular nystagmus without causative endolymph displacement. Amsterdam. Thesis.
Bos, J. H. and Philipszoon, A. J. (1963). Some forms of nystagmus provoked by stimuli other than accelerations. *Pract. Oto-rhino-laryng.* (*Basel*), **25,** 108.
*Carbonara, L. and Salonna, F. (1956). Effetti del Largactil sulla funzionalità vestibulare. *Boll. Mal. Orecch.*, **74,** 47.
*Chinn, H. I., Noell, W. K. and Smith, P. K. (1950). Prophylaxis of motion sickness. *Arch. intern. Med.*, **86,** 810.
*Cojazzi, L. and Pivotti, G. (1952). Richerche sperimentali sull'azione della Dramamina. *Valsalva*, **28,** 348.
Egmond, A. A. J. van, Groen, J. J. and Jongkees, L. B. W. (1948). The turning test with small regulable stimuli: Cupulometry. *J. Laryng.*, **62,** 63.
Egmond, A. A. J. van, Groen, J. J. and Jongkees, L. B. W. (1949). The mechanics of the semi-circular canal. *J. Physiol.*, **110,** 1.
Egmond, A. A. J. van, Groen, J. J. and Jongkees, L. B. W. (1952). The function of the vestibular organ. *Pract. Oto-rhino-laryng.* (*Basel*), **14,** suppl. 2.
*Felistati, D. (1956). La chloropromazina (Prozin) in otorinolaringoiatria. *Arch. Ital. Otol.*, **67,** 709.
*Fermin, H., Deinse, J. B. van, and Hammelburg, E. (1950). The effect of dimenhydrinate upon the labyrinth. *Acta otolaryng.* (*Stockh.*), **38,** 543.
Ferreri, G. (1957). Le mal des transports (cinétose). Cours internat. sur l'appareil vestibulaire. Paris: Presses universitaires de France.
Gay, L. N. and Carliner, P. E. (1947). The prevention and treatment of motion sickness. *Bull. Johns Hopk. Hosp.*, **84,** 470.
*Gay, L. N. and Carliner, P. E., (1949). The prevention and treatment of motion sickness. *Science*, **109,** 359.
*Glaser, E. M. and Hervey, G. R. (1951). The prevention of sea-sickness with hyoscine, Benadryl and Phenergan. *Lancet*, **ii,** 749.
*Glaser, E. M. and McCance, R. A. (1959). Effect of drugs on motion sickness produced by short exposures to artificial waves. *Lancet*, **i,** 853.
Guns, P., Gillain, A. and Doyen, E. (1953). Antihistaminiques et le mal du mouvement. *Ann. Otolaryng.* (*Paris*), **70,** 496.
Gutner, L. B., Gould, W. J. and Batterman, R. C. (1951). Action of dimenhydrinate (Dramamine) and other drugs on vestibular function. *Arch. Otolaryng.* (*Chic.*), **53,** 308.
*Gutner, L. B., Gould, W. J. and Cravocaner, A J. (1954). Effects of cyclizine hydrochloride and chlorcyclizine hydrochloride upon vestibular function. *Arch. Otolaryng.* (*Chic.*), **59,** 503.

*Gutner, L. B., Gould, W. J. and Swift Hanley, J. (1955). Effect of meclizine hydrochloride (Bonamine) upon vestibular function. *Arch. Otolaryng. (Chic.)*, **62**, 497.

Heck, J. and Papst, W. (1957). Ueber den Ursprung des corneo-retinalen Ruhepotentials, Elektroretinographie. Hamburger Symposium 1956, *Bibl. ophthal. (Basel)*, **48**, 96.

James, W. (1896). Minor sea-sickness, its cause and relief. *N.Y. med. J.*, 552.

Jongkees, L. B. W. and Groen, J. J. (1946). The nature of the vestibular stimulus. *J. Laryng.*, **61**, 529.

Jongkees, L. B. W. and Philipszoon, A. J. (1960). Some nystagmographical methods for the investigation of the effect of drugs upon the labyrinth. *Acta Physiol. Pharmacol. Neerlandica*, **22**, 220.

*Jongkees, L. B. W. and Philipszoon, A. J. (1964). Electronystagmography in the study of clinical problems, physiology and pharmacology of the vestibular system. *Acta otolaryng. (Stockh.), suppl.* **189**.

Kleijn, A. de and Versteegh, C. (1935). Näheres über die Auslösungsstelle der Labyrinthreflexe in peripheren Labyrinth. *Acta otolaryng. (Stockh.)*, **22**, 327.

*Krejci, F. and Bornschein, H. (1952). Die Wirkung von Dimenhydrinat auf vestibuläre Reaktionen und Hörfunktion. *Arch. Ohr.-Nas. und Kehlk.-Heilk.*, **162**, 152.

*Krejci, F. and Bornschein, H. (1955). Zur Frage einer Beeinflussung des Spontannystagmus durch Dimenhydrinat. *Pract. Oto-rhino-laryng. (Basel)*, **17**, 337.

Krijger, M. W. W. (1954). The significance of the labyrinth in aviation. Utrecht Thesis.

McNally, W. J. and Stuart, E. A. (1942). The physiology of the labyrinth reviewed in relation to seasickness and other forms of motion sickness. *War Med. (Chicago)*, **2**, 683.

Nieuwenhuijsen, J. H. (1958). Experimental investigations on sea-sickness. Utrecht, Thesis.

Noell, W. K. (1952). Azide-sensitive potential difference across the eye-bulb. *Am. J. Physiol.*, **170**, 217.

*Oosterveld, W. J. (1963). Effects on central nystagmus, Amsterdam, Thesis.

*Oosterveld, W. J. (1965). De werkzaamheid van twee middelen tegen zeeziekte, beoordeeld naar hun effect op de vestibulaire oogbewegingen. *Ned. Tijdschr. v. Geneesk.*, **109**, 844.

*Palmer, J. M. (1950). Dramamine and sea-sickness. *Brit. med. J.*, **ii**, 948.

*Pfaltz, C. R. and Pfaltz, R. (1963). Zur Prüfung der Wirksamkeit vestibulär angreifender Pharmaka. *H.N.O. Wegweiser*, **II**, 165.

Philipszoon, A. J. (1959). The effect of some drugs upon the labyrinth. Amsterdam, Thesis.

*Philipszoon, A. J. (1961). De invloed van cinnarizine bij duizeligheid; een electronystagmografisch onderzoek bij 55 patiënten. *Ned. Tijdschr. v. Geneesk.*, **105**, 657.

*Philipszoon, A. J. (1962a). Some experiments on the function of the vestibular organ. *Pract. Oto-rhino-laryngol.* (*Basel*), **24,** 344.

*Philipszoon, A. J. (1962b). The influence of cinnarizine on the labyrinth and on vertigo. *Clin. Pharmacol. Therap.*, **3,** 184.

Philipszoon, A. J. (1962c). On the proper stimuli for otoliths and semi-circular canals. *Acta Physiol. Pharmacol. Neerlandica*, **11,** 317.

*Pichler, H. (1953). Klinische Erfahrungen mit Dimenhydrinat bei Labyrinthreizsymptomen und Morbus Ménière. *Mschr. Ohrenheilk.*, **87,** 24.

Quix, F. H. (1923). Le mal de mer. Paris, Monogr. O.R.L. Internat. 8.

*Richards, A. B., Hughes, F. W. and Forney, R. B. (1963). Evaluation of anti-motion sickness drugs by component measurements of nystagmus in guinea pigs. *Current. Therap. Res.*, **5,** 587.

*Riskaer, N. and Permin, P. (1954). Susceptibility of the vestibular apparatus to antihistamines and D.F.P. *Acta otolaryng.* (*Stockh.*), **44,** 89.

*Salerno, G. (1955). L'azione del largactil sui disturbi vestibulari. *Ann. Laring.* (*Torino*), **54,** 1.

Sjöberg, A. A. (1931). Experimentelle Studien über den Auslösungsmechanismus der Seekrankheit. *Acta otolaryng.* (*Stockh.*), *suppl.* 14.

Versteegh, C. (1927), Ergebnisse partieller Labyrinth Exstirpation beim Kaninchen. *Acta otolaryng.* (*Stockh.*), **11,** 393.

Winston, J., Rubin, A., Lewis, J. and Rehberger, J.M. (1950). The effects of dramamine upon cochlear function and the vestibular responses to turning in normal subjects. *Ann. Otol.* (*St. Louis*), **59,** 622.

Wit, G. de (1953). Sea-sickness (motion sickness). A labyrinthological study. *Acta otolaryng.* (*Stockh.*), *suppl.* **108.**

Wit, G. de (1958). Zeeziekte, een vorm van overprikkelingssyndroom. *Ned. Tijdschr. v.Geneesk.*, **102,** 2227.

DISCUSSION

Hösli: In your experiments testing the action of drugs upon the labyrinth of rabbits you studied the nystagmus during acceleration over a very short period of time. I would like to ask you if during this short period of acceleration there was enough time to investigate the drug action on the component of the nystagmus due to acceleration without interference from the opposite nystagmic effect of deceleration?

Philipszoon: We never saw an effect of deceleration, just a few beats of perrotatory nystagmus and that was sufficient for the investigation. We first investigated 20 animals and gave them normal saline solution which did not abolish the nystagmus.

Norris: I would like to clarify a small but potentially misleading point.

You showed (Fig. 3) that pentobarbitone eradicated the vestibular nystagmus, though you said that the animal was completely anaesthetized. Did you not use sub-anaesthetic doses of barbiturates? If so, did you not then confirm the finding that a barbiturate has no effect on the vestibular nystagmus at doses which abolish the optokinetic nystagmus? (Rashbass, C. and Russell, G. F. M. Action of amylobarbitone sodium on the vestibulo-ocular reflex. *Brain*, 1961, **84**, 329–335).

Philipszoon: Yes, we tried a series of doses on a logarithmic scale, but when the eye movement disappeared there was anaesthesia.

CENTRALLY ACTING DRUGS AND AUDITORY FLUTTER

G. M. Besser

Departments of Medicine and Pharmacology, The Medical College of St. Bartholomew's Hospital, London

Intermittent sound signals are perceived as being continuous when the interruption rate is greater than a critical threshold for the subject. This was demonstrated by Miller (Miller, 1948; Miller and Taylor, 1948) and confirmed by Symmes, Chapman and Halstead (1955). In most respects the physiological characteristics of this threshold (the auditory flutter fusion threshold or AFF) are similar to those of the visual critical flicker fusion threshold (CFF). The outstanding difference is the greater sensitivity of the auditory pathways to intermittency, since flutter can be detected at frequencies much higher than those at which visual flicker disappears. Fig. 1 represents flicker and flutter stimuli diagrammatically. If a visual stimulus with a mark: space (or on:off) ratio of 1:1 is used then a mean CFF of about 35–40 interruptions per second (i/sec.) will be recorded. However if an auditory stimulus is used with a similar mark: space ratio then fusion will not occur until frequencies greater than 1000 i/sec. are reached. If the ratio is 9:1 (that is 9 parts of noise to 1 of quiet) then the mean AFF will be of the order of 35–45 i/sec. Studies on animals and man have indicated that fusion of auditory signals depends on central rather than peripheral mechanisms (Chapman, Symmes and Halstead, 1955; Chartrian, Peterson and Lazarte, 1960; Goldstein, Kiang and Brown, 1959; Symmes and Wegener, 1963; Peak, Goldstein and Kiang, 1962).

Since flicker fusion is remarkably sensitive to the actions of psychotropic drugs, it is surprising that so little work has been reported on the effects of these compounds on flutter fusion. The only previous report is that of Eysenck and Easterbrooke (1960) who studied the actions of sodium amylobarbitone, dexamphetamine and meprobamate but could not detect any alterations in the flutter fusion process.

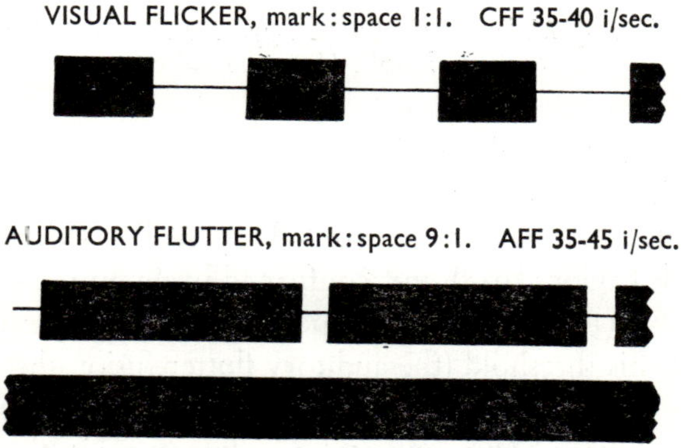

FIG. 1. Diagrams of (a) visual flicker stimulus with a mark: space ratio of 1 : 1 and (b) auditory flutter stimulus with a ratio of 9 : 1. A continuous sound stimulus is also shown. The values for the mean critical flicker-fusion threshold (CFF) and auditory flutter-fusion threshold (AFF) were similar when these signals were used. In AFF determinations a signal containing alternating 1-second periods of interrupted and continuous sound was used.

With Miss Duncan and Professor Quilliam, I have looked again at the psychopharmacology of auditory flutter fusion using a more sensitive technique (Besser, Duncan and Quilliam, 1966; Besser, 1967a; Besser and Duncan 1967). A random noise signal which could be interrupted at rates varying continuously between 1·5 and 275 i/sec. was used, each interruption cycle having a mark: space ratio of 9 : 1. The interruptions were switched on and off every 1 second so that the final signal, presented binaurally to the subject, consisted of alternating 1-second periods of interrupted or continuous noise (Fig. 1). The starting flutter rate was 100 i/sec., well above fusion, and the signal was re-presented in a descending sequence of flutter rates, initially in steps of 10 i/sec. but finally in steps of 1 i/sec. when the point about 10 i/sec. above the subject's threshold was reached. This had been previously

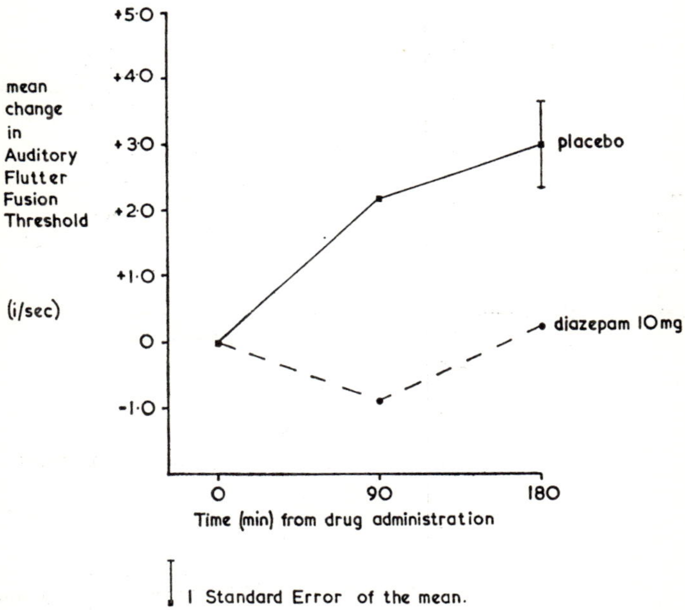

FIG. 2. The mean changes in AFF following placebo or diazepam (10 mg.) treatment over 180 minutes in 6 subjects. The pre-treatment mean threshold for the placebo was 38·93 i/sec. and for diazepam 40·67 i/sec.

approximately determined. The critical threshold for fusion was taken to be the highest interruption rate at which flutter could be distinctly heard and below which it was consistently reported.

Drug studies were double-blind and placebo-controlled and treatments were taken at 7-day intervals. Results were subjected to analysis of variance for factorial designs (Snedecor, 1956).

When studied over a 3-hour period, oral doses of central depressants such as amylobarbitone (100 mg.), diazepam (10 mg.) and chlorpromazine (25 and 50 mg.) significantly depressed the AFF, whereas racemic amphetamine (10 and 15 mg.) raised it. Each drug study involved 6 subjects.

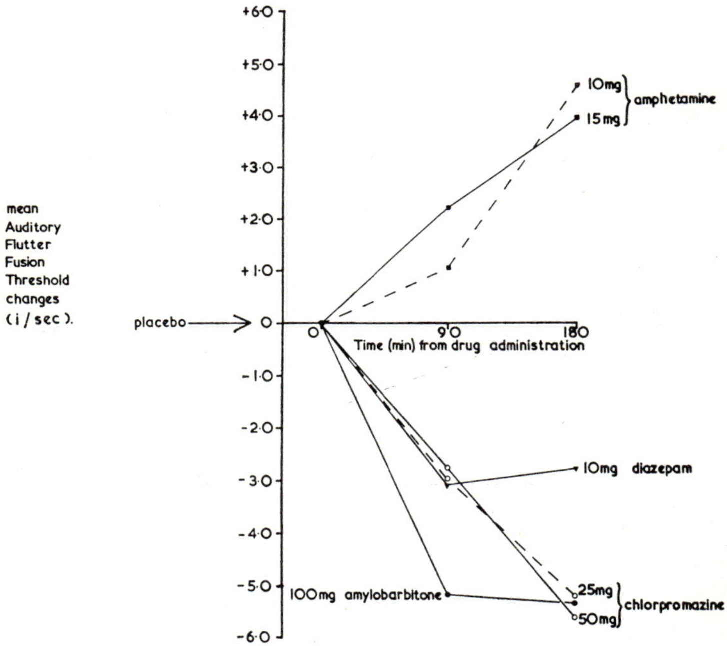

FIG. 3. Effects of amylobarbitone, diazepam, chlorpromazine and amphetamine on AFF over 180 minutes. The placebo values are represented by the zero baseline. Means from 6 subjects are given.

Figure 2 shows the changes in the threshold following a placebo and a 10 mg. dose of diazepam. The pre-treatment mean threshold on the placebo was 38·93 i/sec. and on the active drug 40·67 i/sec. The mean threshold rose after placebo over the 3 hours, as is usual when studies are started in the morning (Besser, 1967b). However, on diazepam the threshold was 3·07 i/sec. less than on placebo 90 minutes after administration, and 2·75 i/sec. less at 180 minutes. The depression was significant at the 0·1% level.

Figure 3 shows a comparison of the active treatment effects of the drugs producing significant changes in AFF. Here the values on the placebo are represented by the zero baseline. The depressions of threshold due to diazepam and amylobarbitone are equally great 90 minutes after administration as at 180 minutes. With chlorpromazine, however, the drug effect is greater at 180 minutes than at 90 minutes, suggesting a different time course of action. The maximum change in threshold is about 5 i/sec. We might have missed changes of this order if we had altered the frequency of signal interruption in steps of 10 i/sec. over the whole range of stimulus frequency as did Eysenck and Easterbrooke (1960).

The time courses of action of the 3 central depressant drugs have been investigated further, recording, in 12 subjects each, the AFF and CFF concurrently over 8 hours (Fig. 4). The mark : space ratio for the CFF determinations was 1 : 1. Following amylobarbitone (100 mg.) and diazepam (10 mg.) the depression of the threshold was first seen at 30 minutes and was maximal at 2 hours. The amylobarbitone-induced effect wore off gradually over the 8 hours but the effect due to diazepam appeared to pass off more quickly in 6 hours. The depression due to chlorpromazine (50 mg.) was also evident by 30 minutes but was not maximal until 4 hours. The depression of flutter and flicker fusion thresholds were similar on all the drugs but greater in magnitude for flutter.

This technique differentiated between the actions of the aliphatic phenothiazine, chlorpromazine, which depressed the flutter fusion threshold in these doses, and the piperazine derivative, perphenazine, which had no effect in the therapeutically equivalent dose of 2 or 4 mg. A mixture of racemic amphetamine (15 mg.) and amylobarbitone (100 mg.) also had no effect on the threshold, indicating that the stimulant effect of amphetamine was offset

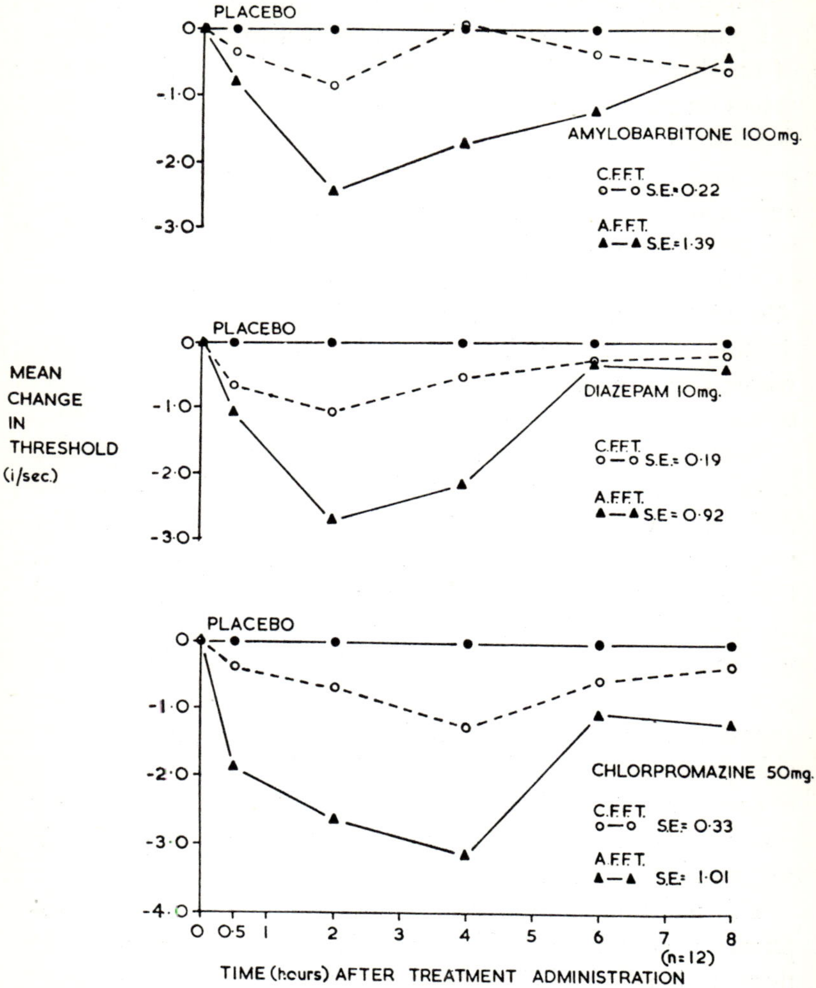

FIG. 4. Effects of amylobarbitone, diazepam and chlorpromazine over 8 hours, on CFF and AFF measured concurrently, in 12 subjects. The placebo values are represented by the zero baseline.

by the depressant effect of the barbiturate. In this respect the changes on the drug mixture resembled those found by Dickens, Lader and Steinberg (1965) when testing psycho-motor function, rather than mood. Meprobamate (400 and 800 mg.) had no effect on flutter fusion.

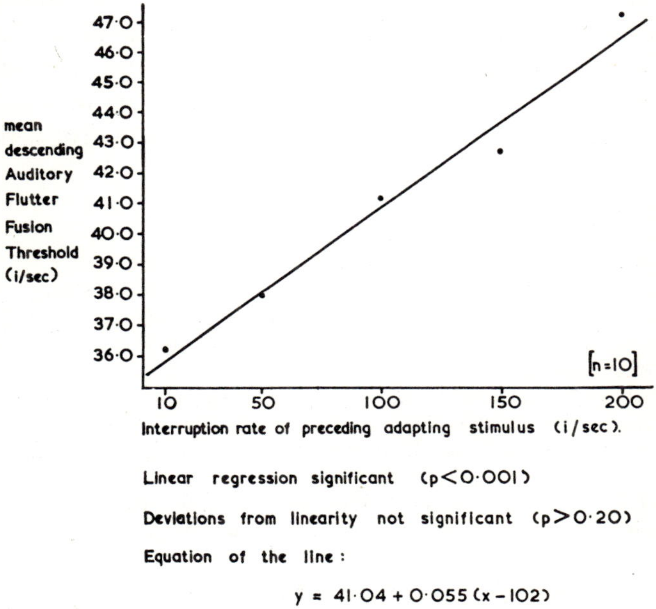

FIG. 5. Relationship between the interruption rate of adapting stimuli and the subsequently determined AFF. The adapting stimuli were presented for 60 seconds immediately before each threshold was determined. Means from 10 subjects are shown.

When interrupted stimuli were presented to subjects for 60 seconds immediately before measuring their threshold, the level of the threshold was directly and linearly related to the frequency of the preceding stimulus (Fig. 5) (Besser, 1967b). This shift in response is an example of perceptual adaptation, and occurs even if the preceding adapting stimulus frequency is above the critical threshold for fusion. Amphetamine, chlorpromazine and amylobarbitone, while altering the absolute level of the threshold, did not affect the shift in threshold due to the adapting stimuli.

The perceptual processes involved in auditory flutter fusion are thus highly sensitive to the effects of centrally acting drugs in moderate, therapeutic doses. In general the changes were similar to those seen in visual flicker fusion but of greater magnitude. The effects of preceding adapting stimuli on the flutter fusion thresholds were unaffected by the drugs. Measurement of the drug-induced depression of AFF provides a convenient and sensitive technique for following the time course of drug action.

REFERENCES

Besser, G. M. (1967a). *Brit. J. Pharmacol.*, **30,** 329–340.
Besser, G. M. (1967b). *Nature, Lond.*, **214,** 17–19.
Besser, G. M. and Duncan C. (1967). *Brit. J. Pharmacol.*, **30,** 341–348.
Besser, G. M., Duncan, C. and Quilliam, J. P. (1966). *Nature, Lond.*, **211,** 751.
Chapman, L. F., Symmes, D. and Halstead, W. C. (1955). *J. comp. physiol. Psychol.*, **48,** 421–425.
Chartrian, G. E., Petersen, M. C. and Lezarte, J. A. (1960). *Electroenceph. clin. Neurophysiol.*, **12,** 479–489.
Dickens, D. W., Lader, M. H. and Steinberg, H. (1965). *Brit. J. Pharmacol.*, **24,** 14–23.
Eysenck, H. J. and Easterbrooke, J. A. (1960). *J. ment. Sci,.* **106,** 855–857.
Goldstein, M. H., Jr., Kiang, N. Y-S. and Brown, R. M. (1959). *J. acoust. Soc. Amer.*, **31,** 356–364.
Miller, G. A. (1948). *J. acoust. Soc. Amer.*, **20,** 160–170.
Miller, G. A. and Taylor, W. G. (1948). *J. acoust. Soc. Amer.*, **20,** 171–182.
Peak, W. T., Goldstein, M. H. Jr. and Kiang, N. Y-S. (1962). *J. acoust. Soc. Amer.*, **34,** 562–570.
Snedecor, G. W. (1956). Statistical Methods, 5th Edition. Iowa: Iowa State Univ. Press.
Symmes, D., Chapman, L. F. and Halstead, W. C. (1955). *J. acoust. Soc. Amer.*, **27,** 470–473.
Symmes, D. and Wegener, J. G. (1963). *Fed. Proc.*, **22,** 678.

DISCUSSION

Whitfield: What did the stimuli actually look like when monitored with a microphone? Did the supra-threshold stimuli not contain an audible frequency?

Besser: When signals were used with supra-threshold interruption rates there was no detectable qualitative difference between the interrupted and continuous portions of the signal. Further, frequency analysis of the chopped random noise signal failed to demonstrate any predominant frequency, so that chopping did not alter the frequency spectrum of the signal. This confirmed the earlier findings of I. Pollack (*J. acoust. soc. Amer.*, 1951, **20,** 646).

Steinberg: The fact that both doses of amphetamine had the same effect suggests that a physiological limit of discrimination may have been reached.

Besser: The effects of the two doses of amphetamine (10 and 15 mg.) and the two doses of chlorpromazine (25 and 50 mg.) appeared to be equal and probably represented the maximum ceiling effects obtainable. Small doses of amylobarbitone (e.g. 50 mg.) did not cause any significant depression of flutter fusion threshold, unlike the large dose. I suspect that the absence of a differential dose response with smaller doses is due to the submergence of small alterations in the thresholds within the natural variation of the threshold on test repetition.

Session IV

Vision

Chairmen: Sir Stewart Duke-Elder and E. S. Perkins

THE EFFECTS OF DRUGS ON COLOUR VISION

IRWIN M. SIEGEL* and GEOFFREY B. ARDEN

Institute of Ophthalmology, University of London

THE perception of colour is but one of many kinds of visual sensation by which stimuli in the outside world are made known to us and, like other information received by the eye, requires the functional and structural integrity of a great number of specialized sense cells, interconnecting nervous pathways, and association centres in the brain. Any portion of this pathway may be affected by drugs. The highly magnified inset in Fig. 1 shows the essential structures in the retina concerned with vision. The pigment epithelium provides for the metabolic requirements of adjacent and avascular layers. The outer portions of the rods and cones, which are in intimate contact with the pigment epithelium, contain the light-sensitive pigments which initiate visual excitation. The photoreceptors synapse with the bipolar and horizontal cells. The lateral spread of the synaptic fields is actually very much larger than shown in the diagram. The bipolars and amacrines make extremely complicated synaptic connections with the third order neurones—the ganglion cells. The axons of the ganglion cells exit as the optic nerve. The functional properties of the ganglion cells can be investigated in detail by studying their spike discharge pattern. Receptors and the second order bipolars respond with slowly changing electrical potentials which comprise the components of the electroretinogram.

However, before light from a source (S) reaches the retina and

* On leave from the Department of Ophthalmology, New York University Medical Center.

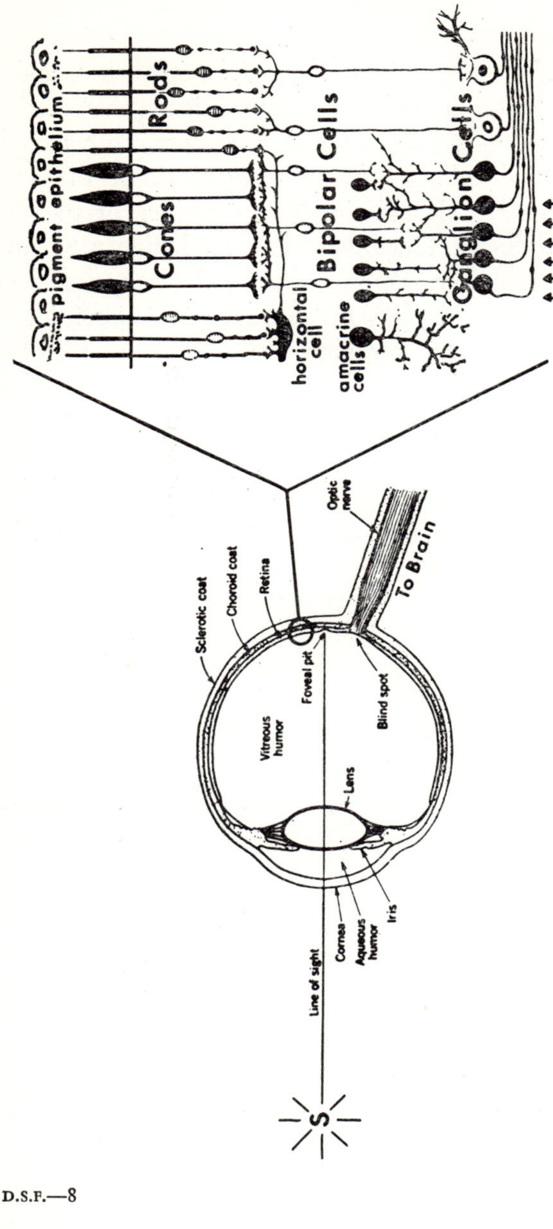

FIG. 1. Ocular anatomy concerned in colour detection. The path of light through the ocular media is shown and, in inset, the histology of the retina. Between the photoreceptors and bipolar cells, and the bipolar and ganglion cells lie complex synaptic layers, in which lateral connections predominate.

initiates visual excitation, it must first (as shown in the figure) pass through the cornea, crystalline lens and the transparent media. These fluids and tissues are not completely colourless, and the perception of colour is limited by their transmission characteristics. If these media undergo changes which cause them to behave like coloured filters, absorbing selectively portions of the visible spectrum, predictable changes in the appearance of the visual scene will be produced. Since the colour-mediating mechanisms are intact, most researchers do not consider these types of defects true changes in colour vision. However, they are of considerable toxicological importance. Ordinarily the brain can adequately compensate for alterations in the colour quality of an object. By changing the illuminating source from a tungsten to a fluorescent lamp, for example, colour identification is scarcely affected. However, colour photographs taken under these two lighting conditions would appear grossly dissimilar. This ability of the retina and brain to achieve 'colour constancy' fails if the relative proportions of the received wavelengths are altered by pre-retinal structures.

It is well known, for example, that the crystalline lens yellows as it ages (Said and Weale, 1959) and therefore decreases the amount of blue light which reaches the retina. The effect of this age change can be dramatically illustrated by contrasting the early pictures of J. M. W. Turner with ones painted in later life (Trevor-Roper, 1959). The latter have a predominantly orange cast to them, presumably because the blue and green wavelengths were absorbed by the lens before they reached the artist's retina, making the colours appear relatively warm in tone. Therefore, in mixing colours to match the subject, Turner did not feel the need to include blues. The opposite effect may be produced if the aged painter creates from memory. The intense blues used in Picasso's later studies may have been due to his attempt to match pigments to the more subdued blues he remembered. Drugs which produce changes in the ocular media and mimic aging would probably produce similar effects. The yellow vision occasionally noted in cases of picric acid poisoning or with intensive mepacrine therapy may be due to deposition of these substances or their coloured intermediates in the cornea or ocular media (Duke-Elder, 1954).

A frequently observed defect in colour vision produced by this type of mechanism is seen in the plastics industry. Workers exposed to several kinds of volatile heterocyclic amines develop 'blue-haze' vision (Mastromatteo, 1965; Mellerio and Weale, 1966). The amines are absorbed by the exposed cornea, which becomes oedematous and cloudy; enhanced light scatter through this tissue produces the visual defect. Routine clinical tests of colour vision may not be able to distinguish these effects from certain types of congenital colour anomalies.

Once inside the retina the light must proceed to the most posterior layer where two kinds of primary visual cells, the rods and cones are located. The rods contain the well-known photopigment, rhodopsin. They play no part in colour vision, being exclusively concerned with night vision, which is necessarily achromatic since the absorbed quantum, no matter what its wavelength, produces the same effect on the photopigment. Of course, the probability that the incident quantum will be absorbed depends on its wavelength; rhodopsin scarcely absorbs any red light. To perceive colour, however, it is necessary to possess at least two sorts of photopigment with different absorption bands so that the relative effect of a stimulus on the two pigments varies with its wavelength. Furthermore, since the receptors can only produce one type of signal it must follow that each photopigment is confined to a different class of receptor. Direct measurements on individual cones have shown that there are three types of pigment-containing cones with absorption bands centered in the red, green, and blue regions of the spectrum (Marks, Dobelle and MacNichol, 1964). The chemical constitution of these cone pigments is very similar to that of rhodopsin; all are conjugates of 11-*cis* Vitamin A aldehyde and a specific protein moiety (Wald, Brown and Gibbons, 1963). It is therefore most unlikely that a drug could attack the cone pigments and leave rhodopsin unharmed, or vice versa. It is certainly true that certain agents do specifically affect receptors, but not cones in particular.

The situation is quite different, however, if we consider not the pigments but their containers. The receptor cell is long (about one-third the thickness of the entire retina), complex in structure, and only a small part of it (the laminated outer portion) contains the photopigment. There is a mitochondria-rich section, located near the nucleus, and a synaptic zone in apposition to the bipolar cells. These synapses are quite different in rods and cones, and this is reflected in functional differences of the two systems. For example, (1) the rod system reaches its message-carrying capacity when the ambient illumination is quite low, while the cone system continues to transmit information even in very bright lights, (2) the rod system cannot follow a rapid series of stimuli (flicker), while the cone system can, (3) after exposure to a bright light, the rate of recovery of the rod system is much slower than that of the cone system. All these facts (derived from psychophysical and electrophysiological studies) point to the presence of much more powerful restorative processes in cones. It is not unreasonable therefore to suppose that cones require a more active metabolism (they are known to contain denser clusters of mitochondria than rods; Cohen, 1963), and hence a differential sensitivity towards metabolic inhibitors could affect colour vision preferentially.

Even greater differences between the two systems exist at the post-receptoral level. The particular properties of the rod system (e.g. high sensitivity, wide areal summation) are achieved by lateral retinal interconnections. The cone system also depends on these connections for its special roles in visual acuity and colour vision but in these processes the interplay results in a differencing mechanism rather than a summative one. Obviously, neurotoxic drugs, synaptic inhibitors, etc. can have markedly different effects on the two systems.

However, in considering any selective effects of drugs on colour vision, one must take account of the gross topographical segregation of cones in the fovea. The human retina is composed predominantly of rods; of the 130 million photoreceptors only about 6% or 7 million are cones. The portion of the retina we

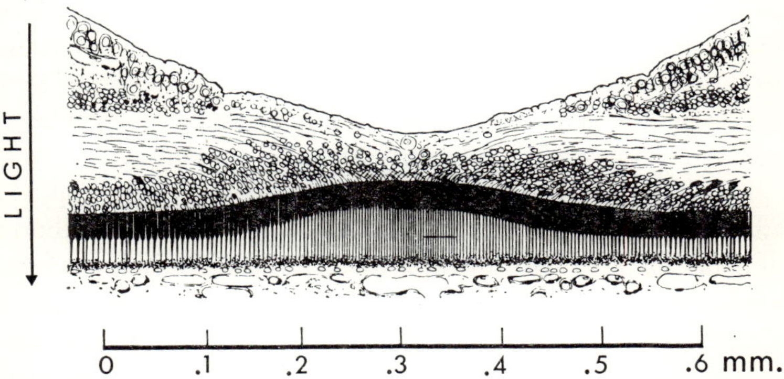

FIG. 2. Structure of the human fovea. This drawing shows the small pit which contains only cone receptors. At the margin of the drawing a few thin rods may be seen. In the fovea itself, the other retinal layers are displaced. In spite of the close packing of the cones in this region only a few per cent of the total number of colour vision receptors are located here (after Polyak, 1941).

use for direct fixation, the fovea centralis, is devoid of rods and contains only cones (see Fig. 2), but this unique portion of the retina is very tiny (0·07 mm.^{2}) and contains only a few per cent of the total number of retinal cones. In point of fact, very few animals possess a fovea (Duke-Elder, 1958) and many which lack this structure seem to have perfectly good acuity. The common feature about sharp-sighted animals is that a small specialized retinal area projects to a very large area of the visual cortex, and signals from other regions of the retina have less cortical representation (Poljak, 1933). Therefore when we speak of colour vision we are usually considering only our cortical projection, i.e. foveal vision, even though 98% of our colour receptors are *not* in the fovea. From the psychophysicist's point of view this may appear a reasonable attitude, but it is not acceptable to the neuropharmacologist. If a drug truly acts on the colour mediating mechanism it will exert its effect throughout the retina. It is possible that there may be some structural characteristics peculiar to the fovea which make it more liable to the action of drug toxicity (e.g. morphology and blood supply), but these factors may be allowed for. More importantly, the reverse is true of the peripheral retina. Damage to the fovea inevitably leads to complaints of acuity and loss of colour vision, whereas damage of large numbers of peripheral cones may not produce subjective colour disturbances.

It is clear, therefore, that the investigation of any drug reputed to affect colour vision must include an evaluation of the contribution of cones from all parts of the retina, thus distinguishing a foveal dysfunction from a diffuse dysfunction limited to one class of receptors and their connections. Judged on these criteria few drugs can be said to affect colour vision selectively. Chloroquine-induced retinopathy was first described in a patient who complained of night blindness (Hobbs, Sorsby and Freedman, 1959). Superficial testing might have suggested that the drug damaged the rods only. In subsequent patients, however, primary complaints included changes in colour vision (Okun, Gouras, Bernstein and von Sallmann, 1963)! It soon became apparent that this drug is not selective to either the rods or the cones but causes generalized disturbances originating in the outer part of the retina (Arden and Fojas, 1962), The presenting symptoms depends on whether the drug attacks the rod-dominated periphery or the cone-filled fovea. Many other drugs act similarly, amongst them are the phenothiazine NP 207 (Burian and Fletcher, 1958), some other phenothiazines (Weekly, Potts, Reboton and May, 1960) and ethambutol (Carr and Henkind, 1962). Some affect mainly the outer layers of the retina, others the inner layers and optic nerve.

None of them produce a true selective effect on the cone system. Evidence of colour-vision loss induced by toxic agents is usually based on tests which measure only foveal function, or colour fields in which boundaries of colour recognition for the whole retina are plotted out. The first kind of test is inadequate because only a minute portion of the cone mechanism is measured; and colour fields, although intrinsically useful, are not usually determined with test objects of matched luminosity and saturation. The clinician generally uses coloured test objects only as a means of reducing the stimulus brightness; hence a grey stimulus equated in brightness to a red would elicit the same field defects. Therefore the so-called red-green field defects produced by excessive amounts of alcohol and tobacco (Harrington, 1956) probably do not derive from damage specific to the colour mechanisms but to the luminosity sense which receives contributions from both cones *and* rods. We might add that in such conditions the visual fields tested with white objects are usually also defective.

Do drugs exist which affect only colour vision? Any such drug must be shown to leave intact all other visual mechanisms. For example, the ability to dark-adapt and the extent of the field of vision must remain unimpaired. Further, the effect on colour vision must, if the drug acts on the retinal level, be similar to the familiar forms of 'colour blindness'. These may range from the mild red-green confusion (protan and deutan types) to *complete loss* of colour vision (achromatopsia). However, these defects are usually associated with disturbances in the receptoral layers of the retina, while, as indicated above, drugs might act post-receptorally; hence the similarity between drug-induced colour defects and their congenital counterparts need not be complete. Two drugs at least fulfil these requirements. We shall present the effects of these drugs in some detail since the techniques used represent the adaptation to drug investigation of basic psychophysics and electrophysiology.

Furaltadone (Altafur)

Patient A, a 34-year-old woman, was admitted to hospital for a Caesarian section. Five days after surgery she developed a systemic staphylococcal infection. Furaltadone (Altafur, 5-morpholinomethyl-3-(5-nitrofurfurylideneamino)-2-oxazolidin-one)* 500 mg. four times daily was given and response to the drug was prompt. Therapy was continued for 8 days, at the end of which time she was sent home. Blood cultures, however, were still positive for staphylococcus and the patient was maintained on the same dosage of Altafur for about another week. It is estimated that this patient received about 2 g. daily for about 2 weeks, during which time she experienced sciatica, speech difficulty, slight loss of visual acuity, an inability to discriminate light shades of colour, and a severe dazzle effect in moderately bright light. Only the visual side-effects persisted after Altafur was discontinued. The test results which we shall consider were obtained 5 years after her illness (Siegel and Smith, 1967); the subjective disturbances remained unchanged during this long interval.

Ophthalmoscopic examination showed the ocular media, retinal vasculature and general appearance of the retina to be normal. Tests of colour vision included the familiar Ishihara plates, Farnsworth D-15 panel and 100-Hue Test, and measurements on the Nagel anomaloscope. The results indicated an equivocal red-green confusion which manifested itself only when the chroma of the stimuli were relatively desaturated. Visual acuity loss was not very great (only a few Snellen lines, 6/12), and the patient was not particularly disturbed by this loss, but found the presence of glare very troublesome: objects appeared as against 'dazzling white snowbanks'. Tests of acuity and colour vision established, therefore, that her foveal cones, though not entirely normal were still functioning quite well. The status of

* Altafur was withdrawn from the market in 1961 by its manufacturers, Eaton Laboratories, following a decision of the U.S. Food and Drug Administration.

the majority of retinal cones located outside the foveal region was determined by measuring the visual fields with a variety of stimuli. Fields were normal when tested with white targets (outer contour, Fig. 3A), but this might merely mean that the peripheral *rods* were normal. When coloured objects were used, patient A could not recognize any of the colours until they were brought

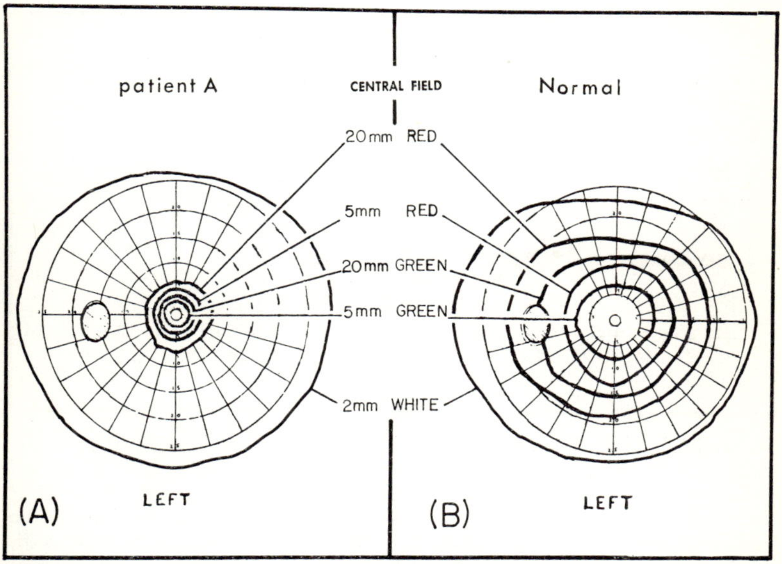

FIG. 3. Charts illustrating central visual fields in a case of drug-induced colour blindness and in a normal subject. Test objects used are indicated and were viewed at a distance of one metre. Patient A has normal-sized fields when tested with white objects but recognizes colours only in the perifoveal region.

to within a few degrees of the fovea (Fig. 3A), although they could be seen as far out as the white ones. Using very large coloured targets did not appreciably enlarge these fields, emphasizing that colour loss was severe, and involved very large areas of the retina.

If the eye is exposed to a bright light and then placed in darkness, the sensitivity increases with time. Thresholds can be determined during this dark-adaptation process by adjusting the intensity of the light so that the subject can 'just see' it. When the test light stimulates a retinal area that contains both rods and cones, say 10° away from the fovea, it can be seen (Fig. 4A, dashed lines) that the dark-adaptation curve has two distinct portions. The initial rapid increase in sensitivity seen during the first 10 minutes reflects cone activity, because these receptors dark-adapt very

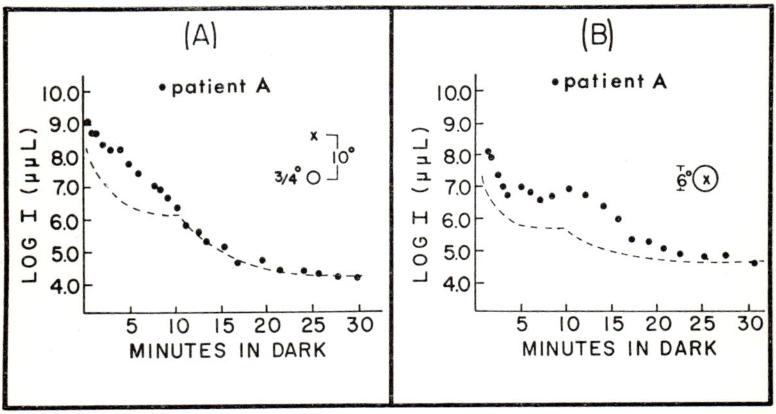

FIG. 4. Dark-adaptation curves in drug-induced colour blindness tested (A) in the peripheral retina and (B) in the parafoveal region. Location and size of stimuli indicated. Thresholds were determined following light adaptation to 8900 cd/m² for 7 minutes. Normal responses indicated by dashes. In the periphery, the patient has a monophasic curve, since cone function is absent. The rod threshold, reached after 25 minutes is quite normal. The parafoveal curve (B) demonstrates the presence of abnormal cone function.

rapidly. The later, slower increase is known to be associated with the very sensitive rods, because no colour sensation can be produced by any of these dim stimuli. After 15 minutes A's thresholds are exactly the same as that of the normal subject, tested under equivalent conditions; her rod thresholds are absolutely normal. However, early on in dark-adaptation patient A is about ten times less sensitive than the normal and thus produces a monophasic dark-adaptation curve. An identical function is obtained from patients with complete congenital colour blindness (achromatopsia)

(Goodman, Ripps and Siegel, 1963) and reinforces the view that in the retinal periphery only rod activity can be detected. We have already shown that some cone activity exists in the foveal and para-foveal areas of this subject's retina. If a large (6°) target is substituted for the smaller one and a dim red fixation light arranged so that the line of sight is centred on the stimulus (Fig. 4B) we can evaluate the contribution of any functional cones to the adaptation process. The data thus obtained show an unequivocal biphasic character, and cone activity, while admittedly less sensitive than normal, is revealed. Final rod thresholds were once again normal.

The results thus far presented show that A's peripheral cones cannot send signals to higher centres. The lesion might conceivably not be located in the retina, although the type of disturbance demonstrated by the quantitative tests makes this most unlikely. More specific localization can be obtained by the electroretinogram (ERG). This response represents the light-induced potential developed by the outer layers of the retina and has the virtue of being a completely objective record of certain crucial aspects of retinal function. Most important from the clinician's point of view, it is easily and quickly performed on adults and children alike. The one outstanding feature of the ERG, which makes it particularly useful in the present context, is that it reflects a massed response from the whole retina. By varying the intensity, wavelength, and temporal characteristics of the stimulus, we can distinguish rod from cone activity. Thus, a high-intensity stimulus, flashing on and off 30 times a second will evoke electrical activity from cones only (Dodt, 1951), since the rods cannot 'follow' a light flickering faster than 8 to 10 c.p.s. The normal ERG response to fast flicker can be seen in Fig. 5 (above the stimulus marker tracings) together with records from patient A and a congenital achromat. It must be noted that these records represent the activity from cones scattered throughout the retina, not only from those few per cent (important as they may be) which are closely packed in the foveal region. Indeed, persons who have, through accident or disease, lost the central area of their retinae produce ERGs that do not differ from those of the normal. The

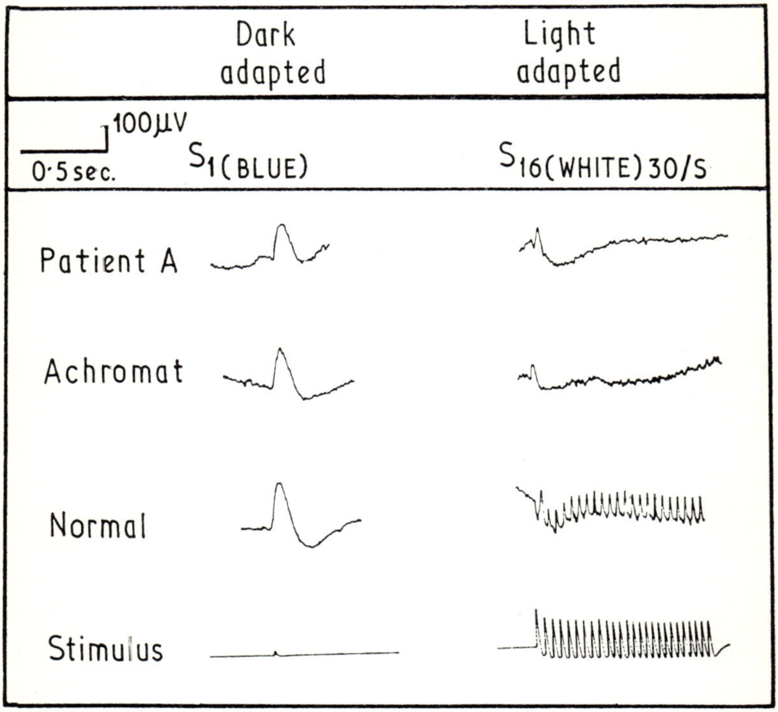

FIG. 5. Electroretinograms in drug-induced and congenital achromatopsia. A single weak blue stimulus delivered to the dark-adapted eye evokes a normal, positive going *b*-wave, showing that the response of the rod system in all the subjects is normal throughout the retina. The first of a train of stimuli delivered to the light-adapted eye evokes a small *b*-wave (derived from the rods). Subsequent flashes, which follow each other so quickly that the rod system cannot recover, evoke no measurable electrical activity; hence the rapid cone response, evident in the normal, is absent in patient A and the congenital achromat.

similarity between ERG records of patient A and the congenital achromat is striking. Both show rod responses (elicited by low intensity blue flashes in the dark-adapted eye) of normal amplitude.

This finding completes the evidence that the rod system is normal in A's retina. When the eye was light-adapted and exposed to the 30-second sequence of flashes the responses were greatly reduced. The single response produced by the onset of flicker in these latter records represents rod activity—which cannot recover fast enough to follow the successive flashes. We interpret the electrical silence during flicker stimulation as indicating a gross impairment to that portion of the cone system peripheral to the ganglion cells. Altafur, then, appears to have acted selectively on the cone system in this patient. One other drug has been investigated in sufficient detail also to be included in this category.

Troxidone

Troxidone (trimethadione, Tridione; 3,5,5-trimethyloxazolidine-2,4-dione) is an anticonvulsant that has been widely used for treating the petit mal forms of epilepsy. It was early noted that 50% or more of the treated adults reported a 'glare' effect amounting to photophobia while receiving the drug (Vail, 1946). Laboratory testing showed that complete loss of peripheral colour vision, reduction in visual acuity and a marked inability to discriminate a rapidly flickering light from a steady one, were induced when the subjects were light-adapted (Sloan and Gilger, 1947). Despite these visual disturbances, which were specific to cone activity and generalized to the entire retina, rod activity was shown to be perfectly normal. These effects could not be produced by exposing one eye to a bright field and simultaneously testing the contralateral eye, indicating that the level of involvement was pre-chiasmal and most likely retinal. What remains to be investigated is whether, like the furaltadone-induced defect, these patients would show a reduced electrical response to a bright flickering light localized to the photoreceptor-bipolar layers of the retina.

It would be of great interest to be able to designate with certainty the site and mode of action of these drugs. But the pharmacological action is undoubtedly as complicated as the physiological function on which it acts and the meagre knowledge we possess of these processes only allows us to speculate. The effect of furaltadone in patient A was irreversible, and this suggests its effects might have resulted from receptor cell death. However, though the effect of troxidone is similar, it is reversible and non-progressive. But if, on the other hand, the drugs produce their functional alterations by a common mechanism, it seems more reasonable to look for changes at a post-receptoral level, where interactions between activated retinal pathways occur. The final common path of impulses from rods and cones to higher centres is via the ganglion cells, and it is thought that the horizontal and amacrine cells impose very important neural modifications on this path. We also know that ganglion-cell discharges alter when the retinal illumination changes. In light-adaptation, the number of cones contributing to ganglion-cell activity (photopic receptive field) is large, and stimulating the peripheral portions of this field with light inhibits the response from the central area (Barlow, Fitzhugh and Kuffler, 1957). During dark-adaptation this lateral inhibition decreases. The groups of cells which inhibit and excite the ganglion cell have similar but not identical spectral sensitivities because each intermediate neurone will be connected to different numbers of red-, green- and blue-sensitive cones. Hence the response of the ganglion cell will change abruptly with small alterations in stimulus wavelength (Wagner, MacNichol and Wolbarsht, 1960) (see Fig. 6). This mechanism can explain how the three cone pigments produce messages which allow the organism to discriminate between the hundreds of different hues. A slight change in the inhibitory interactions of such a pooled pathway could grossly alter the relative balance of excitatory and inhibitory effects upon which the discrimination of colour might depend. The same experiments (Wagner, MacNichol and Wolbarsht, 1960) showed that ganglion-cell response can be changed qualitatively by altering the intensity of the monochromatic stimulus.

This could explain the finding that the peripheral colour vision in the troxidone patients changed greatly as ambient illumination was increased.

One attraction of this hypothesis is that if the rod system were similarly affected the unimodal luminosity response associated with this mechanism would not be affected in the same way.

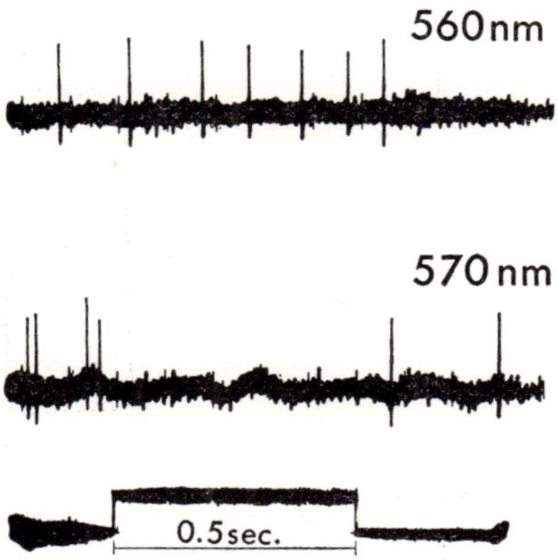

FIG. 6. Ganglion-cell discharges in the goldfish retina. A stimulus of 560 nm (yellowish-green) evokes a spike discharge in the cell. Shifting the wavelength to 570 nm (greenish-yellow) inhibits spontaneous activity. The duration of the stimulus is indicated by the step in the signal record (bottom trace) (after Wagner, McNichol and Wolbarsht, 1960).

However, a removal of inhibition might cause the dazzle which accompanies drug-induced achromatopsia. Finally, it is of interest to note that furaltadone and troxidone, though developed for treating very different conditions, are both derived from a 5-membered heterocyclic oxazole ring (Fig. 7). Further research on these drugs and other of their derivatives may help us to relate the remarkably similar defects these compounds produce to what appears to be a common feature in their structural configuration.

Troxidone, and to a less extent, furaltadone, would seem to have just those qualities which are of use to the vision physiologist studying retinal processes associated with colour vision. The effects appear wholly specific to the cone mechanism, leaving

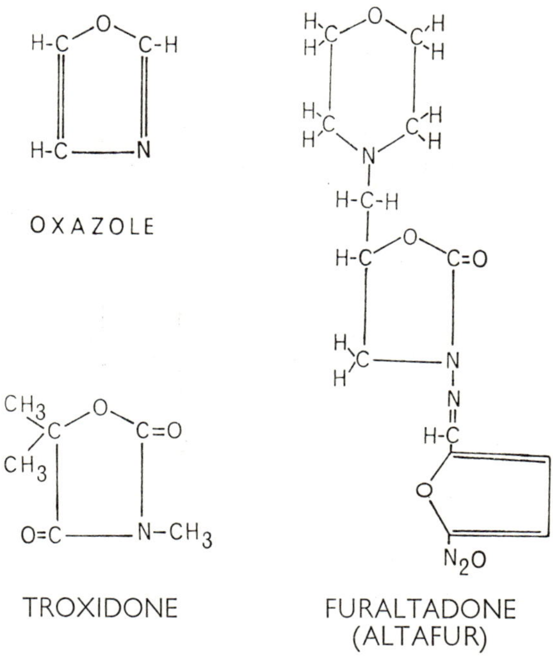

FIG. 7. Structural formulae of two drugs which cause specific damage to the cone system of the retina. Their relation to a 5-membered heterocyclic oxazole ring is shown.

rod sensitivity unimpaired, and with troxidone this disturbance has the unique distinction of being reversible.

Acknowledgement

This study was supported in part by a Research Fellowship Award from the U.S. Public Health Service (1 F11 NB 1470-01 VSN) to one of the authors (I.M.S.).

REFERENCES

Arden, G. B. and Fojas, M. R. (1962). Electrophysiological abnormalities in pigmentary degenerations of the retina. *Arch. Ophthal.*, **68**, 369.

Barlow, H. B., Fitzhugh, R. and Kuffler, S. W. (1957). Changes in organisation in receptive fields of cat's retina during dark adaptation. *J. Physiol.*, **137**, 338.

Burian, H. M. and Fletcher, M. C. (1958). Visual functions in patients with retinal pigmentary degeneration following the use of NP 207. *Arch. Ophthal.*, **60**, 612.

Carr, R. E. and Henkind, P. (1962). Ocular manifestations of ethambutol. *Arch. Ophthal.*, **67**, 566.

Cohen, A. I. (1963). Vertebrate retinal cells and their organisation. *Biol. Rev.*, **38**, 427.

Dodt, E. (1951). Elektroretinographische Untersuchungen zur Analyse des Flimmerphänomens im menschlichen Auge. *Ber. dtsch. ophthal. Ges.*, **57**, 242.

Duke-Elder, W. S. (1954). *Text Book of Ophthalmology*, vol. 6. London: Henry Kimpton.

Duke-Elder, W. S. (1958). *System of Ophthalmology*, vol. 1. London: Henry Kimpton.

Goodman, G., Ripps, H. and Siegel, I. M. (1963). Cone dysfunction syndromes. *Arch. Ophthal.*, **70**, 214.

Harrington, D. O. (1956). *The Visual Fields*. London: Henry Kimpton.

Hobbs, H. E., Sorsby, A. and Freedman, A. (1959). Retinopathy following chloroquine therapy. *Lancet*, **ii**, 478.

Marks, W. B., Dobelle, W. H. and MacNichol, E. F. (1964). Visual pigments of single primate cones. *Science*, **143**, 1181.

Mastromatteo, E. (1965). Heterocyclic amine exposure with urethane foams. *J. occup. Med.*, **7**, 507.

Mellerio, J. and Weale, R. A. (1966). Hazy vision in amine plant operatives. *Brit. J. ind. Med.*, **23**, 153–154.

Okun, E., Gouras, P., Bernstein, H. and von Sallmann, L. (1963). Chloroquine retinopathy. *Arch. Ophthal.*, **69**, 59.

Poljak, S. (1933). A contribution to the cerebral representation of the retina. *J. comp. Neurol.*, **57**, 541.

Polyak, S. (1941). *The Retina*. Chicago: Univ. of Chicago Press.

Said, F. S. and Weale, R. A. (1959). The variation with age of the spectral transmissivity of the living human crystalline lens. *Gerontologica*, **3**, 213.

Siegel, I. M. and Smith, B. F. (1967). Acquired cone dysfunction. *Arch. Ophthal.*, **77**, 8.

Sloan, L. L. and Gilger, A. P. (1947). Visual effects of Tridione. *Amer. J. Ophthal.*, **30**, 1387.

Trevor-Roper, P. D. (1959). The influence of eye diseases on pictorial art. *Proc. roy. Soc. Med.*, **52**, 721.

Vail, D. (1946). Tridione and the eye. *Amer. J. Ophthal.*, **29**, 606.

Wagner, H. G., MacNichol, E. F. Jr. and Wolbarsht, M. L. (1960). The response properties of single ganglion cells in the goldfish retina. *J. gen. Physiol.*, **43**, 45.

Wald, G., Brown, P. K., and Gibbons, I. R. (1963). The problem of visual excitation. *J. Opt. Soc. Amer.* **53**, 20.

Weekly, R., Potts, A., Rebotor J. and May, R. (1960). Pigmentary retinopathy in patients receiving high doses of a new phenothiazine. *Arch. Ophthal.*, **64**, 65.

DRUGS AND VISUAL THRESHOLDS

G. W. Granger and Hisako Ikeda

Department of Psychology, Institute of Psychiatry, and Department of Neurophysiology, Institute of Ophthalmology, University of London

Our aim in this paper is to show how visual threshold measurements, supplemented by electrophysiological techniques, can be used to throw light on the nature and site of drug action on the human visual system.

The old idea of the visual threshold was of a critical value of a light stimulus such that equal or stronger ones can be detected and weaker ones cannot. But observation has shown that there are stimuli which, if repeated many times at the same intensity, will sometimes be seen, sometimes not. It follows, therefore, that thresholds are definable only statistically, for instance as critical values of the stimulus variable at which the probability of detection equals 50% (but see (13)).

In the simplest case measurement consists in determining the least quantity of a test light that can be detected against a completely dark field to which the subject's eyes are fully adapted. The threshold thus obtained is known as an *absolute threshold*, in contrast to a *differential threshold* which is measured at background intensities other than zero. When the test stimulus and adapting field have the same spectral composition the quantity measured is usually known as an *intensity threshold* and it is with thresholds of this type that we have been concerned. We have studied a wide range of stimulus patterns of varying degrees of complexity, including the simplest case in which a single flash is applied against zero background. But here we shall consider only one type of pattern in which the luminance of the test light changes periodically, for it is at about this level of stimulus complexity that significant and interesting visual effects begin to appear from moderate doses of neurotropic drugs.

If a steady light is regularly interrupted at a low rate, an observer can readily detect this: the light appears to 'flicker'. Above a certain frequency, however, he cannot distinguish the intermittent stimulus from a steady light. The least frequency at which 'flicker' discrimination breaks down is known as the *flicker fusion frequency*, or, more usually, the *critical flicker frequency* (CFF), and this is what we have measured.

At this point it is important to emphasize an obvious but often neglected fact, namely, that the data from visual threshold experiments are *behavioural* in nature. Determining whether the subject can 'see' the stimulus or not is based on a *response*, verbal or otherwise, to a pattern of light stimuli falling on his retina. This response is the last of a complex chain of events in the sensory, central nervous and motor systems. Before one can conclude that variations in response following the administration of a drug are sensory in origin one must exclude a variety of non-sensory sources of variation, ranging from fluctuations in pupil size to changes in central decision processes and reaction time. This has hardly ever been done satisfactorily; in consequence, the significance of the vast majority of the 'visual' effects reported in the pharmacological literature remains in considerable doubt. In our own work we have tried to reduce extraneous sources of variation to a minimum and thereby secure more definitive sensory data.

We have studied a variety of drugs (including amphetamines, barbiturates, caffeine, adrenaline and meprobamate) but to illustrate our approach we propose dealing in some detail with only one of these, ethyl alcohol, for which we have electrophysiological as well as psychophysical data. Now it is known that alcohol dilates the pupil (11). This means that if pupil size is not controlled visual thresholds may appear to alter simply because more light reaches the retina. To control this variable we have used 'Maxwellian view' optics and made the beam diameter at the pupil plane smaller than the least diameter the pupil could assume when bright lights were shone into the eye. Our optical system also enabled us to control spectral distribution, angular size and other basic stimulus parameters, so that any drug effects we detected would at least be relatively free from the influence of extraneous sources of variation at the pre-retinal level.

It has been our general practice before testing the effects of a drug to first spend several experimental sessions with each subject to determine his usual threshold variability. In agreement with much previous vision research, we have found that once a subject has settled down to his task, and provided great care is taken to control the experimental conditions (retinal stimulus, state of adaptation of the eye, etc.), the CFF is remarkably stable and seldom varies more than $\pm$ 0·5 c/s from its initial value over a period of several hours. Having obtained extensive data on the reproducibility of the CFF under normal physiological conditions on different occasions, we then study the effects of the drug in a single experimental session, making repeated determinations of the threshold over a 2–3 hour period. Here we should mention that, contrary to some claims made by earlier workers, we have consistently failed to find any significant change in thresholds following the administration of placebos.

Our aim is to throw light on the mode and site of action of drugs on the visual system rather than to develop clinically useful tests. Therefore we have preferred to make detailed experimental studies of individual subjects, in the tradition of sensory physiology, rather than make more cursory statistical surveys of groups. In keeping with this approach, all the results presented in this paper represent individual data obtained on a single occasion But, as will be shown elsewhere in a fuller account of the experiments (3, 4) from which these illustrative data are taken, the main features of the drug effects we shall discuss appear to be reproducible between, as well as within, subjects.

Figure 1 shows some typical data for the time course of the effects of alcohol on the CFF. The drug was given in the form of absolute, 'Analar' reagent grade, ethyl alcohol, and was consumed over a period of 5–10 minutes about 2 hours after the subject had had a very light breakfast. Contrary to some earlier reports, we

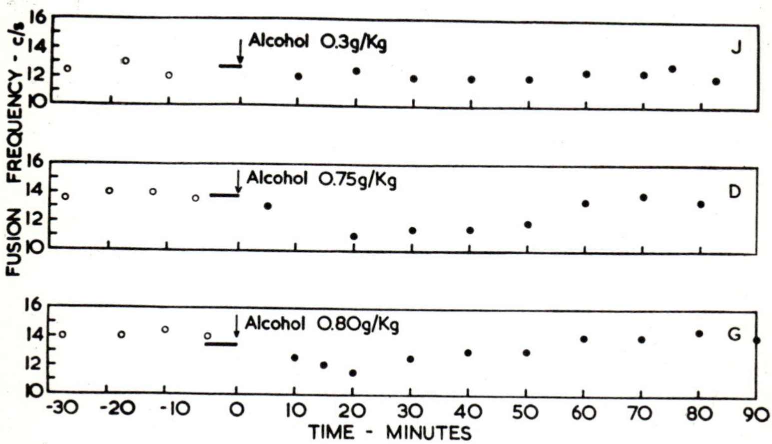

FIG. 1. Time course of the effect of ethyl alcohol on the foveal CFF: ○, control; ●, alcohol.

failed to observe any effect from the smallest dose we used (0·3 g./kg.): the measurements fall within the limits of normal variation. But, for a dose of 0·75 g./kg. there is a significant drop in the CFF. The data are for two different subjects: in both instances the CFF is depressed by about 2 c/s within 20 minutes of consuming the alcohol and shows a gradual return to normal values over the next hour.

The points in Fig. 1 represent mean values of the foveal CFF determined by a method of 'limits' in which, starting at a value above 'fusion', the frequency was gradually reduced until the subject first reported 'flicker' by pressing a response key. We have preferred to approach the threshold from 'fusion' to 'flicker' rather than from 'flicker' to 'fusion', for three reasons. First, because it provides better control of the adaptation of the eye. Secondly, because it makes the subject's task of fixation easier and hence reduces errors arising from eye movements. Thirdly,

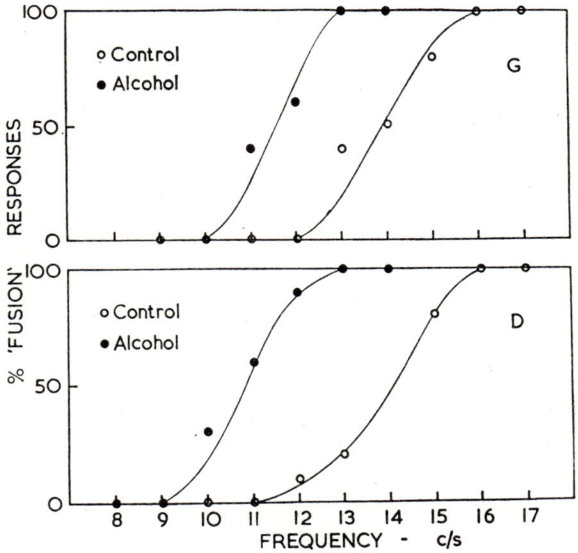

FIG. 2. Effect of ethyl alcohol on the relation between the percentage of 'fused' responses and frequency (in c/s). (10° test field, 150 trolands in retinal illumination; 0·5 sec. exposure; dark-adapted eye; central fixation.)

because it is known to be much less affected by the rate at which the frequency is changed (9).

Although this method of 'limits' is convenient for tracking the time course of a drug effect because it allows rapid determination of the threshold, it suffers from the obvious disadvantage that any increase in the subject's reaction time may cause a spurious decrease in the CFF. We decided, therefore, to check our result by a different method in which reaction time does not enter as a variable. In this second method the stimulus was exposed for a brief period at a fixed frequency and the subject simply had to report if the light was 'flickering' or 'fused' (3). This procedure was repeated at a number of different frequencies presented in a pre-determined random order. Typical data are shown for two subjects in Fig. 2, from which it will be seen that the S-shaped curves for per cent 'fused' responses as a function of frequency are shifted bodily along the frequency axis to lower frequencies. The extent of this shift varies a little between subjects but, for a given subject, is essentially the same as the drop found with the first method, for a comparable dose of alcohol.

This result not only enables us to exclude reaction time but the absence of any change in the range of 'uncertain seeing' makes it unlikely that the effects we have observed are due to a central action of the drug on decision processes. In keeping with this, we have found no change in the range of 'uncertain seeing' at the absolute threshold and no increase in the number of 'false positive' responses (i.e. reports of a 'sighting' when no stimulus is presented to the eye). But we cannot yet claim to have made any precise estimate of the drug's action on the subject's 'response criterion', within the framework of the decision theory of signal detection (13).

Having given grounds for rejecting explanations of the drug effect in terms of non-sensory variables we can say with some confidence that we are dealing with a *visual* effect and proceed with its analysis by psychophysical and electrophysiological methods.

Figure 3 shows the effect of a dose of 0·8 g./kg. ethyl alcohol on the relationship between foveal CFF and log stimulus intensity. The object of studying this function was to test the hypothesis, suggested by earlier work (2), that the visual effects of alcohol are analogous to placing a neutral density filter in front of the eyes, more light being needed to produce a given threshold response. If alcohol acts in this way it should cause a shift of the CFF/log intensity curve on the intensity axis to higher intensities, without change of shape. It is clear from Fig. 3 that a simple 'filter' hypothesis cannot account for our data. After alcohol the maximum CFF is lower and the curve as a whole is shifted downwards on the frequency axis, although our data do not cover a wide enough range of intensities to enable us to exclude a slight horizontal displacement as well. (It is interesting to note that barbiturates affect the CFF/log intensity relation in the same way (5) while adrenaline and respiratory alkalosis (6) cause an upward shift of the curve.)

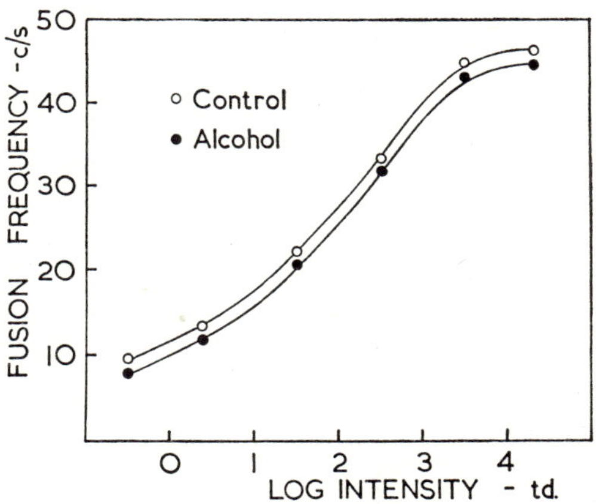

FIG. 3. Effect of 0·8 g./kg. ethyl alcohol on the foveal CFF log intensity relation.

These results suggest that, unlike anoxia and insulin hypoglycaemia which have a general 'filter' effect on all forms of intensity discrimination, through their depressant action on central nervous activity (2), alcohol may have a more specific action on neural organization within the visual system. The displacement of the curve along the vertical axis is of the kind that occurs when temporal or spatial parameters of the stimulus are varied and suggests that the drug may affect temporal or spatial summation or some other aspect of neural interaction. In the case of respiratory alkalosis we have in fact shown that the vertical shift of the

CFF/log intensity curve is associated with a change in spatial summation (6). But so far we have failed to find any obvious effects of alcohol on either spatial or temporal summation, in

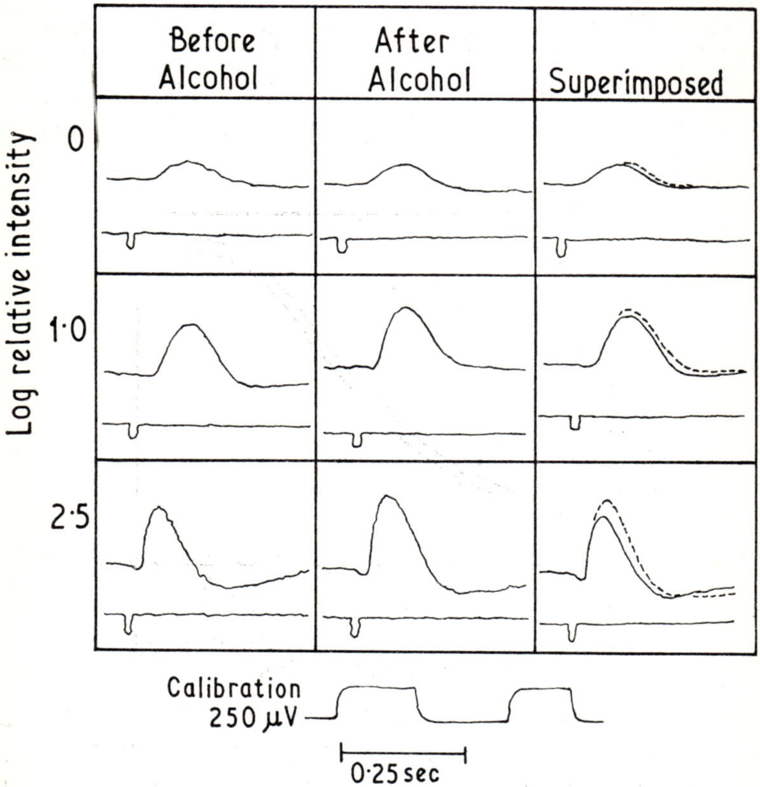

FIG. 4. Typical single flash ERGs recorded before (*left*) and after (*middle*) the administration of alcohol (0·75 g./kg.). On the right, the two traces are shown superimposed, with that taken after alcohol shown dotted. The highest intensity used was $1 \cdot 9 \times 10^5$ trolands in retinal illumination.

experiments with stimuli of different angular sizes and durations. From some preliminary measurements we have made with different light-dark ratios in the flicker cycle we suspect that the duration of the dark period between flashes may be a significant variable in the drug effect. This belief gains further support from observations we have made on the effect of alcohol on the electroretinogram (ERG) (7, 8) which, at the same time, enable us to say something about the site of the drug's action on the visual system.

Figure 4 shows a single flash ERG of the fully dark-adapted eye, before and after alcohol was administered. At the low intensity the typical rounded scotopic *b*-wave is recorded and alcohol has a negligible effect. But at the higher intensities it will be seen

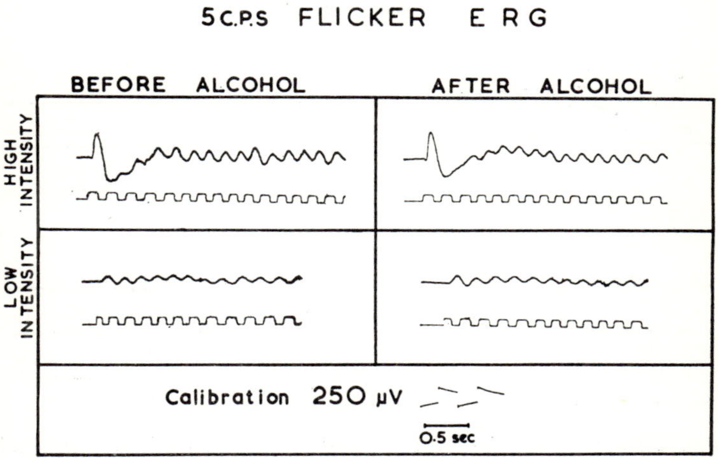

FIG. 5. Typical 5 c/s ERGs recorded before and after the administration of alcohol (0·75 g./kg.). The intensity used for the upper records was $1 \cdot 9 \times 10^4$, and that for the lower records 19 trolands in retinal illumination.

that alcohol lengthens the response and increases the amplitude of the *b*-wave. At first glance it might seem rather odd that the ERG amplitude should increase while the visual CFF decreases after alcohol. However, it will be evident from Fig. 5 that the lengthening of the response to a single flash by alcohol results in a different kind of effect when a flickering light is used.

When the eye is stimulated five times per second by a light of low intensity each ERG is small and no lengthening of the individual response occurs. At the high intensity the situation is different. Here, because of the lengthening of the response to the first flash, the ERG for the next response is suppressed completely by alcohol, while it is not under normal conditions. (Arden, Granit and Ponte (1) observed a similar effect from pentobarbitone, a finding of considerable interest in view of the similarity between the effects of alcohol and barbiturates on the visual CFF.)

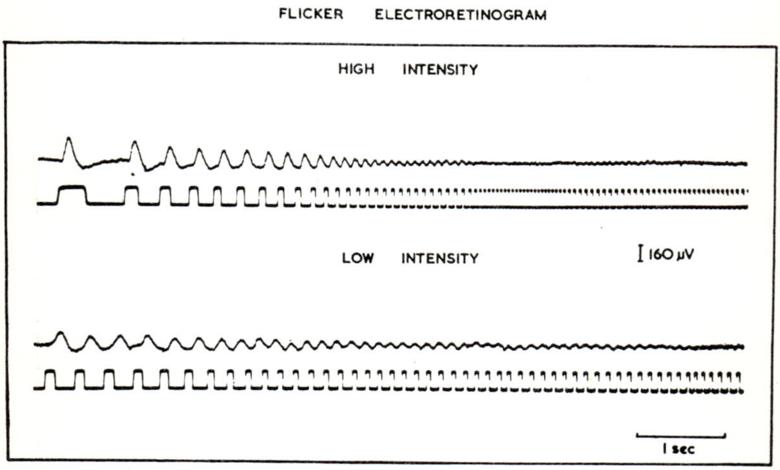

FIG. 6. Examples of the flicker ERG recorded when determining the ERG fusion frequency. The photocell traces (up = on) indicate the rate of flicker. The light intensity used for the upper record was $3 \cdot 9 \times 10^4$, and that for the lower records 39 trolands in retinal illumination.

The consequence of this suppression is, therefore, that the ERG fusion frequency is *reduced* by alcohol, as is the visual CFF.

Figure 6 shows an example of an ERG record from which one can determine the frequency at which the ERG ceases to follow the intermittent stimulus. And in Fig. 7 the ERG fusion frequency is plotted against log stimulus intensity. Following the administration of alcohol the ERG fusion frequency/log intensity curve is shifted downwards on the frequency axis, as was the corresponding curve for the visual CFF (Fig. 3).

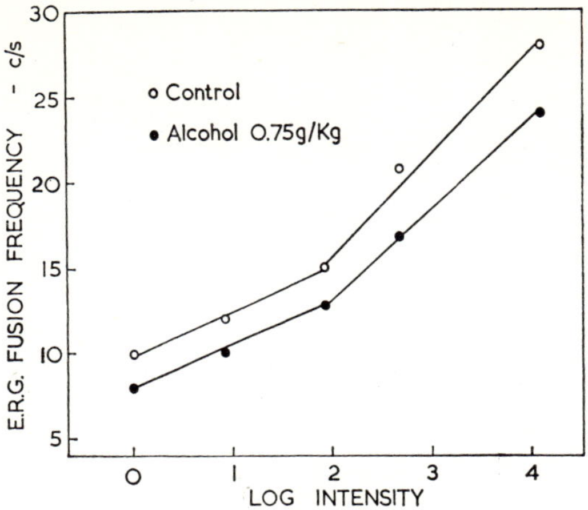

FIG. 7. Effect of alcohol on the relation between the ERG fusion frequency and the log intensity of the stimulus. The highest intensity used (4 log intensity in the abscissa) was $3 \cdot 9 \times 10^5$ trolands in retinal illumination.

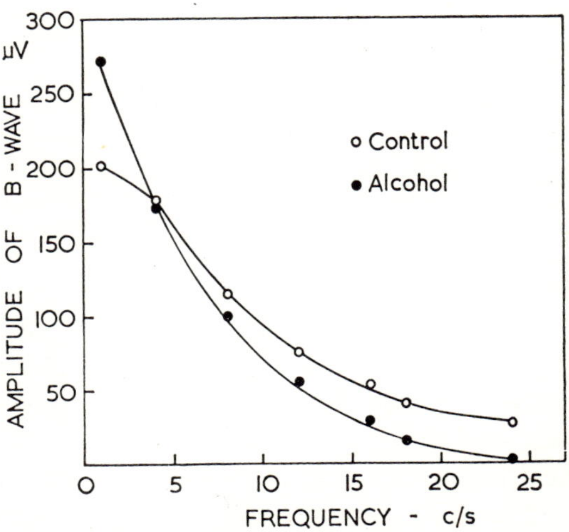

FIG. 8. Effect of alcohol on the relation between the *b*-wave amplitude and the rate of flicker (in c/sec.). Intensity of the stimulus was kept constant at $3 \cdot 9 \times 10^4$ trolands in retinal illumination.

What is happening here can be explained by Fig. 8 in which the amplitude of the flicker ERG is plotted against frequency. It will be seen that the control and alcohol curves cross. At the lower flicker rates the lengthening and increase of the individual responses after alcohol does not interfere with the response to the next flash because the dark interval is long enough for recovery to occur. But at the higher frequencies the size of the following response is suppressed.

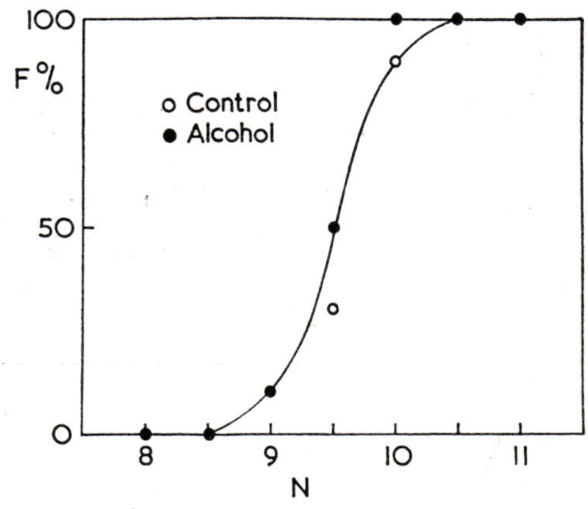

FIG. 9. Effect of ethyl alcohol (0·8 g./kg.) on the relation between the percentage of 'fused' responses and frequency (*N*), in c/s. Scotopic vision.

These electrophysiological observations show that alcohol affects the retina, somewhere between the photoreceptors and the bipolar cell layer (where the ERG originates), probably by prolonging the recovery time of a neural suppressive process elicited by each flash. And they suggest that the visual effects reflect the action of the drug on the retina, for two reasons. First, the downward shift of the ERG fusion frequency/log intensity curve is similar to the shift in the corresponding curve for visual CFF. Second, as we have shown elsewhere (8), the time course of the ERG and the visual changes is similar.

Despite an encouraging degree of correlation between the electrophysiological and psychophysical data it must not be forgotten that the ERG results showed that alcohol had a negligible effect at lower intensities when the relatively pure scotopic *b*-wave responses were evoked. This suggested to us that the scotopic CFF might prove more resistant to the action of alcohol than the photopic CFF which we had previously been measuring. To test this possibility we made some measurements of the CFF in the

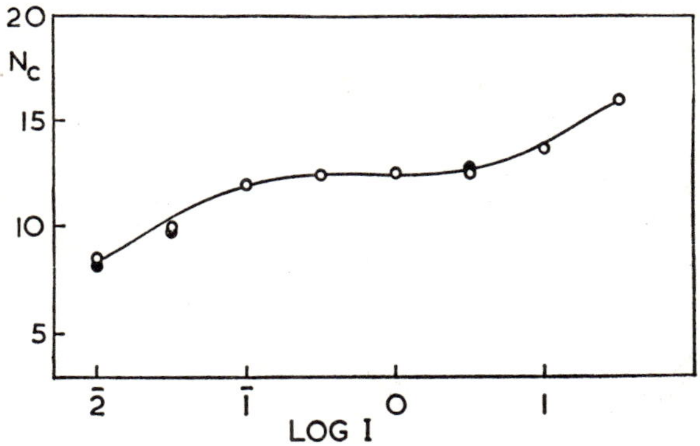

FIG. 10. Effect of ethyl alcohol (0·8 g./kg.) on the scotopic fusion frequency (N_c)/log intensity relation. (○, control; ●, alcohol).

parafoveal retina using 'blue' light of an intensity so low that its hue could not be detected by our dark-adapted subjects. Typical data for a single intensity level are shown in Fig. 9, which shows that alcohol in a dose large enough to depress the photopic CFF (Fig. 2) fails to produce a significant effect under scotopic conditions. Figure 10 shows an absence of drug effect at three different intensities over the scotopic range (3).

Evidence of a more compelling kind for supposing that the drug acts differently on 'cone' and 'rod' mechanisms comes from an experiment (4) in which use was made of the retinal direction effect. It is well known that under conditions of cone-mediated vision the luminous efficiency of a light ray entering the eye depends on its point of entry through the pupil (12), as shown in Fig. 11. It was interesting to find that the effect of alcohol on the parafoveal CFF could be made to disappear simply by adjusting the point of entry of the light beam from the centre to the edge of the pupil. The data for central entry, shown in the upper part of Fig. 12, were obtained with the test light set at an intensity just above the level at which the subject could clearly recognize its

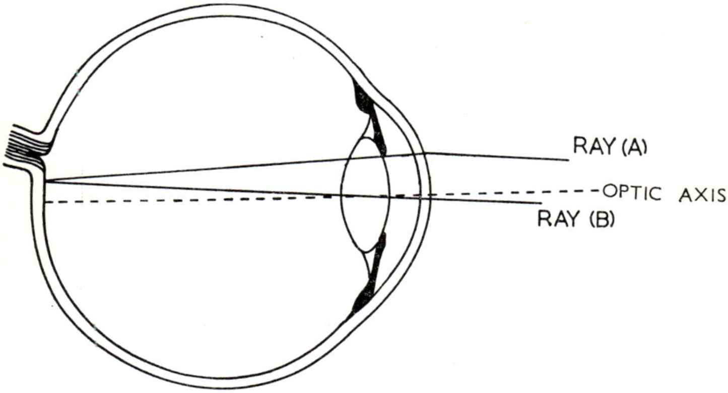

FIG. 11. Diagram illustrating the directional sensitivity of the retina. The marginal ray (A) is less effective as a stimulus for vision than ray (B) that reaches the same point on the retina by passing through the centre of the pupil.

colour ('orange'). On moving the point of entry of the test beam to the periphery of the pupil the light appeared colourless. The lower CFF and absence of drug effect with peripheral entry (lower part of Fig. 12) can be explained in terms of a shift from a response mediated by cones, which are directionally sensitive (i.e. to the angle at which the light strikes them) to one mediated by rods, which show hardly any directional effect.

We conclude from these results: (1) that the cone mechanism is more susceptible to alcohol than is the rod mechanism; (2) that the site of the drug's action is between the photoreceptors and the bipolar cell layer; and (3) that the duration of the dark interval between flashes and neural 'recovery time' are probably the significant variables underlying the drug effect.

These conclusions should be assumed to apply in the first instance to moderate doses of ethyl alcohol. Larger doses might

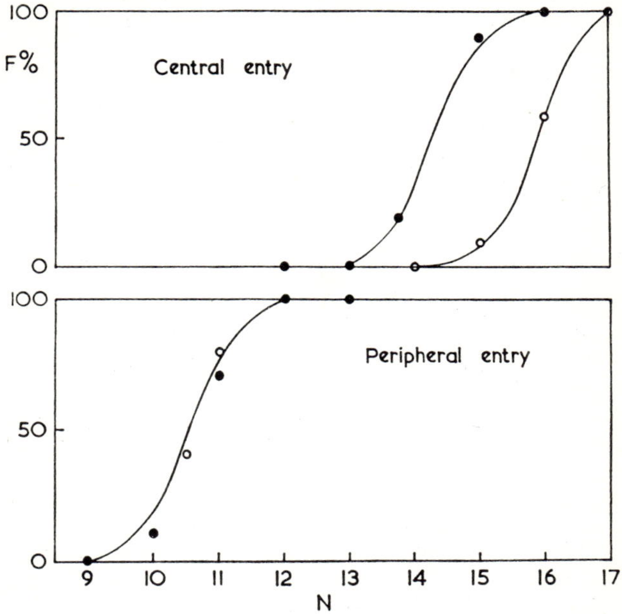

FIG. 12. Effect of ethyl alcohol (0·8 g./kg.) on the relation between the percentage of 'fused' responses (*F*%) and frequency (*N*), in c/s, under conditions of central and peripheral entry of the light beam through the pupil. (○, control; ● alcohol).

produce a different kind of effect on the cone mechanism and might also affect the rod mechanism. A 'filter' effect on both the 'rod' and 'cone' portions of the parafoveal dark-adaptation curve has in fact been observed in subjects who had consumed 'whisky equivalent to 180 cc. alcohol' (10).

Acknowledgements

We are grateful to the Medical Research Council for supporting the work reported in this paper.

REFERENCES

1. Arden, G. B., Granit, R. and Ponte, F. (1960). Phase of suppression following each retinal *b*-wave in flicker. *J. Neurophysiol.*, **23**, 305–314.
2. Granger, G. W. (1959). In Pfeiffer, C. C. and Smythies, J. R. (Eds.) *Int. Rev. Neurobiol., Vol. I.* New York: Academic Press.
3. Granger, G. W. Effect of ethyl alcohol on photopic and scotopic fusion frequencies. (To appear.)
4. Granger, G. W. Separation of the effects of ethyl alcohol on rod and cone fusion frequencies by means of the retinal direction effect. (To appear.)
5. Granger, G. W. and Ikeda, Hisako (1961). Effect of amobarbital sodium on the flicker-intensity function for the human fovea. *Psychopharmacologia*, **2**, 258–267.
6. Granger, G. W. and Ikeda, Hisako (1961). Effect of hyperventilation on foveal critical flicker frequency. *Vision Res.*, **1**, 287–300.
7. Ikeda, Hisako (1963). Effects of ethyl alcohol on the evoked potential of the human eye. *Vision Res.*, **3**, 155–169.
8. Ikeda, Hisako and Granger, G. W. (1962). Action of alcohol on visual and retinal responses to intermittent illumination. In *Proc. Third Int. Conf. Alcohol & Road Traffic.* London: British Medical Association.
9. Mahneke, A. (1956). Flicker fusion thresholds: the significance of frequency acceleration. *Acta Ophthal., Kbh.*, **34**, 113–120.
10. Mandelbaum, J. (1941). Dark adaptation: some physiologic and clinical considerations. *Arch. Ophthal., N.Y.* **26**, 203–239.
11. Skoglund, C. R. (1943). On the influence of alcohol on the pupillary light reflex in man. *Acta physiol. scand.*, **6**, 94–96.
12. Stiles, W. S. and Crawford, B. H. (1933). The luminous efficiency of rays entering the eye pupil at different points. *Proc. roy. Soc. B.*, **112**, 428–450.
13. Swets, J. A., Tanner, W. P. and Birdsall, T. G. (1961). Decision processes in perception. *Psychol. Rev.*, **68**, 301–340.

PROPRIOCEPTION, VISION AND DEPRESSANT DRUGS

D. Legge

Department of Psychology, University College London

Central nervous system depressant drugs generally impair performance of skilled tasks. Performance decrements have been described in detail for the effects of alcohol on a skill resembling driving (Drew, Colquhoun and Long, 1959) and the effects of nitrous oxide on handwriting (Legge, Steinberg and Summerfield, 1964) and on a number of other perceptual-motor tasks (Steinberg, 1954). The way in which these drugs produce their effects may be described not only at biochemical and physiological sites of action, but also at what may be called psychological sites of action. Psychological sites of action can only be determined if it is possible to describe in psychological terms the constituent processes underlying the performance which is being measured. However, psychopharmacological experiments sometimes throw light both on the basic psychological processes underlying behaviour and on the mode of action of the drugs (cf. Summerfield, 1964; Kornetsky and Mirsky, 1960; Legge, 1965).

In general, perceptual or input processes may be distinguished from motor or output processes. Perceptual-motor skills depend upon the co-ordinated activity of both processes and when a skill breaks down it is legitimate to enquire whether this breakdown is mainly localized in one or other of these constituent processes. The most important perceptual modalities for perceptual-motor skills are vision and proprioception and in order to perform these skills the information mediated by these two modalities must usually be integrated. The way in which nitrous oxide and alcohol impair skilled performance has been investigated experimentally, particularly by examining their effects on constituent psychological processes. The results show that these depressant drugs affect behaviour systematically, making it more variable. The pattern of the drug effects may be most simply accounted for by a relatively specific effect of the drugs at a perceptual site of action. There is no evidence to support the notion of a generalized depressant effect on all the constituent psychological processes.

Experimental methods

In these experiments the main task was to align a movable stylus to a target line. This task was chosen because it could be performed using various controlled combinations of visual and proprioceptive information. In addition, alignments could be made in two ways. If the subject was allowed to match the movable stylus to the target line, correcting his settings without restriction, any remaining misalignment could be attributed to errors or imprecision of perception. Alternatively the subject could be instructed to align an initially displaced stylus with a target line using a single, smooth, very rapid movement completed in less than half a second. Such movements are called ballistic. The accuracy of alignments made using ballistic movements reflects the combined accuracy of both perceptual and motor processes.

In detail, subjects had to move the point of a vertical stylus, controlled by the right hand, to a position in line with a horizontal target line slightly to the left of and perpendicular to the forward line of sight. The stylus could only be moved in a straight line at right angles to the target. There was a gap between the target line and the stylus, so the subject had to position the stylus on an imaginary extension of the target line rather than upon the line itself. This gap made it possible to prevent the subject from looking at either the target line or the stylus by inserting screens. In this way subjects could be forced to combine visual and proprioceptive information in order to perform the alignment task.

The processes underlying performance of this alignment task may be described in general terms. Three processes are involved in a perceptual matching task where the subject is allowed to correct the position of the stylus: (1) perception of the location and orientation of the target, (2) perception of the location of the stylus, and (3) comparison of these two pieces of information to yield an estimate of the misalignment of the stylus with the target. It is assumed that the subject will terminate the trial when this estimated misalignment is zero. If the alignment response is made using a ballistic movement two further processes are required. First it is necessary to determine quantitatively the change in the position of the stylus that would eliminate the initial misalignment, and then an appropriate motor response has to be organized to effect this change.

In the first experiment (Legge, 1965) the effects of sub-anaesthetic doses of nitrous oxide on this alignment task were investigated. By interposing screens the perceptual conditions were varied. Four perceptual conditions were used:

both target and stylus perceived visually (condition VV),
target perceived visually and stylus proprioceptively (condition VP),
target perceived proprioceptively and stylus visually (condition PV),
both target and stylus perceived proprioceptively (condition PP).

The subjects were instructed to match the stylus to the target, correcting its position until alignment had been attained. The experimental design involved repeated measurements in which each subject acted as his own control. An air control and three doses of nitrous oxide were used, 10%, 20% and 30% nitrous oxide in oxygen.

Results

The results of this experiment were analysed by calculating the logarithm of the variance of the several alignments which subjects made under each experimental treatment. This performance score provides a suitable measure of variable error. The mean variable error scores are shown in Fig. 1. Analysis of vari-

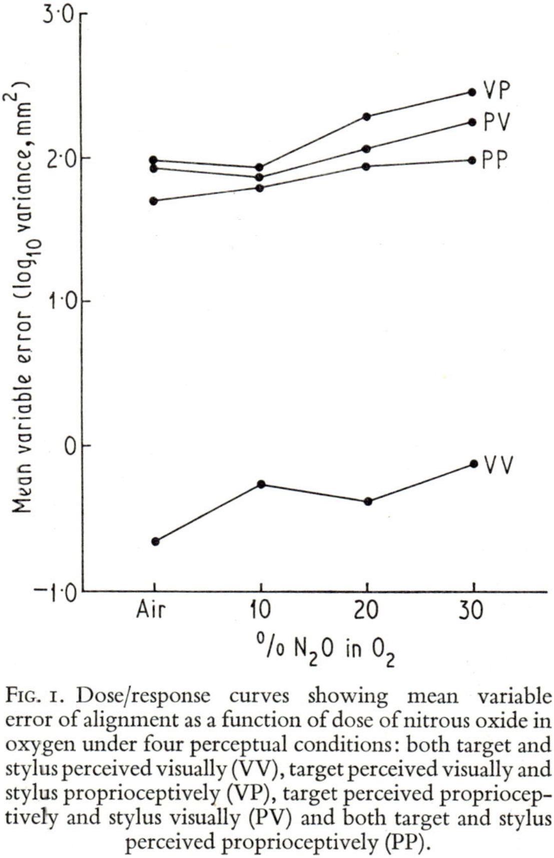

FIG. 1. Dose/response curves showing mean variable error of alignment as a function of dose of nitrous oxide in oxygen under four perceptual conditions: both target and stylus perceived visually (VV), target perceived visually and stylus proprioceptively (VP), target perceived proprioceptively and stylus visually (PV) and both target and stylus perceived proprioceptively (PP).

ance of the data showed that the four dose/response curves in Fig. 1 were best described by four straight lines, each with the same slope. The difference in the general level of the dose/response curves indicates that subjects were more accurate under some perceptual conditions than others. The uniformity of slope of the four curves shows that nitrous oxide affected alignment performance equally, regardless of the perceptual conditions. In other words, nitrous oxide had the same effect on alignment accuracy no matter whether the alignment depended solely on visual information or solely on proprioceptive information or whether both modalities were involved in an inter-modal task.

The uniformity of this effect might suggest that the drug produced a general deterioration of perceptual accuracy. However, closer examination of the data reveals that the effects can be more plausibly explained in terms of a specific action of the drug on a particular perceptual process. This conclusion is suggested by the fact that the two inter-modal dose/response curves (those for conditions VP and PV) lie above those for the two intra-modal perceptual conditions (VV and PP). Since the inter-modal condition is less accurate than the less accurate intra-modal condition, inter-modality performance must depend upon a special process that allows the integration of information from different modalities and is not perfectly accurate in operation. However, it seems that this process is unaffected by the drug because such an effect would have been revealed by a steeper slope to the inter-modal dose/response curves than to the intra-modal curves. Clearly there is no evidence of a generalized depressant effect on all perceptual processes. Different specific effects which could produce the observed results are discussed below.

The hypothesis of a generalized depressant effect also fails to be confirmed by the results of a second experiment, using alcohol. Subjects attempted to align the stylus with the target using either matching or ballistic responses. The target was always perceived visually but screens were used to hide the stylus when it was to be perceived by proprioception alone. The experimental design was similar to that of the previous experiment. Subjects acted as their own controls. A control and three small doses of alcohol were used (0·2, 0·4 and 0·6 g./kg.), calculated to produce blood alcohol levels well below 100 mg./100 ml.

Variable error scores were calculated as before and submitted to an analysis of variance. Alcohol increased variable errors irrespective of how the stylus was perceived or of the kind of

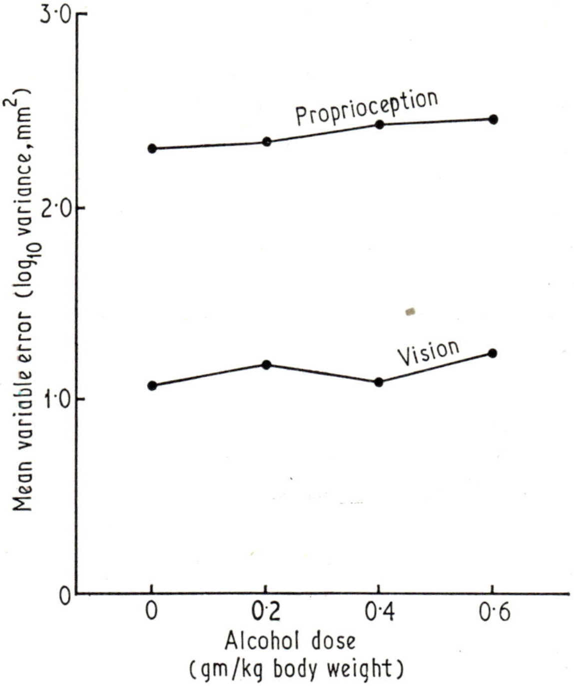

FIG. 2. Dose/response curves showing mean variable error of alignment as a function of dose of alcohol under different perceptual conditions. Subjects aligned a stylus that could be perceived either visually or proprioceptively, with a visually perceived target.

alignment response that was made. The uniform dose/response curves are shown in Fig. 2 and Fig. 3. Figure 2 shows that although variable errors were larger when the stylus was perceived proprioceptively, alcohol had no more effect on them then, than when the stylus could be seen. Similarly Fig. 3 shows that although the variable errors of ballistic responses were generally greater than those of matching responses the two drug effects were the same.

The uniformity in Fig. 2 corresponds to that in Fig. 1 and shows that alcohol affected inter-modal and intra-modal alignments

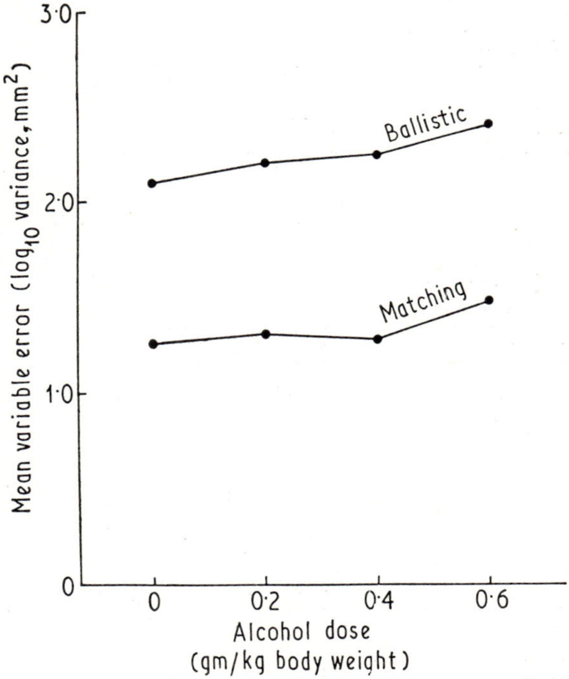

FIG. 3. Dose/response curves showing mean variable error of alignment as a function of dose of alcohol for matching and ballistic responses. Correction was allowed for matching responses but ballistic responses had to be uncorrected and completed in less than half a second.

equally. Figure 3 shows that there was no effect of alcohol on the motor processes; the dose/response curve for ballistic responses was no steeper than that for matching responses. If alcohol was to affect all processes equally it would be expected to make the motor processes less efficient and thus to inflate the variable error of ballistic responses more than that of matching responses.

Discussion

The results of these experiments show that no increased drug effect was found either when an additional perceptual process was introduced (during inter-modal alignments) or when motor processes were introduced (during the making of ballistic responses). The most likely reason for this is that the relatively small doses of drugs given acted preferentially on some perceptual process. There are two likely forms of this preferential effect. Either the drugs affected vision and proprioception equally or they affected some process common to all alignment conditions. The latter is the more plausible hypothesis, especially since Burns, Robson and Welt (1960) have reported some evidence that proprioception is not always affected to the same extent as other modalities such as vision, hearing and touch. The most likely single process to be affected by the drugs and to give rise to these data, would be the process that compares information about the target and the stylus and calculates misalignment. This process is required regardless of the conditions under which the subject works. The observed results would be produced if the drugs acted on such a process and made it function less precisely than normal. This reduction in sensitivity to misalignment would result in some misalignments going undetected and therefore being inadequately corrected. This explanation is attractive since it describes the drug effects economically in terms of a specific effect on a single constituent process.

Although the data imply a specific effect of these drugs, more experiments are needed to determine whether this apparent specificity is simply a dose effect. Some processes might be differentially sensitive to these drugs, so that large enough doses might affect several processes. This pattern of action may be compared with that of complete specificity in which only some processes are affected no matter how big the administered dose. With the low and moderate doses used in these experiments there was no sign of a dose effect: the drug effects may have been completely specific.

This analysis of the effects of nitrous oxide and alcohol provides a basis for describing how these drugs impair driving performance and make subjects' writing larger than usual (Legge, 1965). However, it would be unwise to attribute all these effects to a simple effect on a supra-modality perceptual process. Many perceptual-motor skills demand more than those constituent processes in the alignment task. The dynamic coordination of ballistic responses which characterizes many skills was not studied in these experiments and may be particularly sensitive to depressant drugs. For example, Drew *et al.* (1959) consider that alcohol may impair skills primarily by upsetting the timing of responses. However, with this reservation, it may be said that both the decreased control of a simulated car reported by Drew *et al.* (1959) and the increased size of handwriting caused by both nitrous oxide and alcohol may both be plausibly accounted for in terms of simple drug effects on a supra-modality perceptual process (Legge, 1965). Many of the effects of depressant drugs on skills may be due to effects on perception.

These experiments have been valuable in several ways. By providing an opportunity to analyse psychologically the effects of depressant drugs the old question of a generalized depressant effect has been raised. The evidence here suggests that it may be more useful to treat these effects as relatively specific to some processes. It has also been possible to consider how drugs affect behaviour by postulating a variety of alternative psychological sites of action. One way in which depressants impair skills appears to be by acting on a supra-modality perceptual process and reducing its sensitivity. Perhaps by evaluating the physiological and anatomical aspects of the actions of these drugs it may eventually be possible to point to an anatomical site or a physiological system which could be identified with this supra-modality psychological process.

REFERENCES

Burns, B. D., Robson, J. G. and Welt, P. J. L. (1960). The effects of nitrous oxide upon sensory thresholds. *Can. Anaes. Soc. J.*, **7**, 411–422.

Drew, G. C., Colquhoun, W. P. and Long, H. A. (1959). *Effect of small doses of alcohol on a skill resembling driving*. London: H.M.S.O.

Kornetsky, C. and Mirsky, A. F. (1966). On certain psychopharmacological and physiological differences between schizophrenic and normal persons. *Psychopharmacologia*, **8**, 309–318.

Legge, D. (1965). Analysis of visual and proprioceptive components of motor skill by means of a drug. *Brit. J. Psychol.*, **56**, 243–254.

Legge, D., Steinberg, H. and Summerfield, A. (1964). Simple measures of handwriting as indices of drug effects. *Percept. Motor Skills*, **18**, 549–558.

Steinberg, H. (1954). Selective effects of an anaesthetic drug on cognitive behaviour. *Quart. J. exp. Psychol.*, **6**, 170–180.

Summerfield, A. (1964). Drugs and human behaviour. *Brit. med. Bull.*, **20**, 70–74.

DISCUSSION

Quilliam: Have you studied any drugs other than alcohol? From experience in operating a decompression chamber to show aircrew the effects of oxygen lack, I wondered whether you have had an opportunity of using your techniques on anoxic human beings, for I suspect some of the changes which you report with ethanol may mimic those with anoxia.

Legge: I have used no drugs apart from those I mentioned. However, there seems to be some evidence that reduced oxygen tension may produce similar effects to those of nitrous oxide.

Harper: Could I just clarify one point. Did you plot as your ordinate the amount of error or the variability?

Legge: I plotted the variability. The actual index was the logarithm variance.

Turner: I would like to comment on the potential value of critical flicker fusion (CFF) measurement in three directions: (1) In assessment of drug action on the C.N.S. we have found that amylobarbitone 60 and 120 mg. and chlorpromazine 10 and 25 mg. produce significant depression when compared with a placebo. (2) In studying the interaction of drugs, I have found that while amylobarbitone 100 mg. depresses CFF, a combination of amylobarbitone 100 mg. with dexamphetamine 15 mg. is indistinguishable from a placebo in its effects (Turner, P. *J. Pharm. Pharmacol.*, 1965, **17,** 388). (3) It is a useful tool in demonstrating the differences in drug action produced by physiological changes. For example, I have found that the effect of amphetamine on CFF is both enhanced and prolonged if the urine is alkaline compared with that under acid conditions, which correlates with the changes in urine excretion of amphetamine under these conditions (Smart, J. V. and Turner, P. *Brit. J. Pharmacol.*, 1966, **26,** 468).

Finally, in relation to Dr. Besser's findings (p. 199), we have demonstrated a similar adaptation of CFF to intermittent light of varying frequency, which is not influenced by any drug so far investigated (Turner, P., Patterson, D. S. and Smart, J. V. *Nature* (*Lond.*), **209,** 813).

Herxheimer: Would Dr. Arden like to comment on the visual effects of nalidixic acid (Negram)?

Arden: I have investigated a few people who have suffered from side effects of nalidixic acid. There are a considerable number of reports now of visual disturbances—generally of moving patterns of light. A few people have complained of classical migrainous figures. We have looked to see whether there is an alteration of the peripheral mechanism, using the same techniques that Dr. Siegel mentioned (p. 210) and we haven't found any really clear-cut results—nothing like those we found with furaltadone or troxidone. Colour hallucinations have been reported but I think that in view of the very 'central' nature of the most common disturbances, these too are possibly related to something which is well supra-retinal.

Malcolm: Can I ask the flicker-fusion experts why they persist in using flicker fusion? To a neuro-physiologist this seems odd because a far more accurate measure of the recovery cycles from stimulus 1 to stimulus 2 is obtained when you allow a considerable time interval between tests and simply use a pair of stimuli—one conditioning and one testing, unless what they are really looking for is the prolonged 'hangover' from the repetitive stimulation, which reflects fatigue processes or very much delayed recovery processes.

Arden: One does not use critical fusion frequency to study one particular frequency. In this sort of system, for example, it is very well established that whatever information is obtained by the receptors from the stimulus is centrally filtered selectively for a frequency —and a spatial or temporal frequency may be involved. For convenience we use a shutter, which makes the light go off and on, but it is much better and is far more sensitive to use a light which is sinusoidally modulated to various depths. In this way one can treat the system with engineering techniques: this is the classical approach by Fourier Analysis to the 'black box' problem. When this is done, one finds that the system behaves as though there were an upper limit to the bandpass, and the critical fusion frequency is just one measure of attenuation at a cut-off level. This Fourier analysis is extremely useful because over quite large changes of stimulus parameter the visual system does respond linearly. Dr. Granger and Dr. Ikeda showed that the first electroretinogram was large, then there was electrical silence for a few flashes and then the responses came back to an equilibrium voltage level; what they were doing was measuring the equilibrium amplitudes and with square light pulses. On looking at the Fourier series it is plain that the bandpass hypothesis completely explains not only the response to the first flash, but also the ensuing silence and then the equilibrium response level. The conclusion is that these drugs affect the upper bandpass attenuation characteristics; this could explain why the drugs affect the cone system selectively, because they lower the cut-off frequency of the filter so that the more rapid responses seem to be affected before the slow ones. When one tests the rod system which only responds slowly in its peripheral part, one doesn't notice the effect. There then would be no magic in a drug visibly affecting cones rather than rods, and this is rather nice to know, because of course the information all goes by the same channels up to the brain. Early on in the retina the cones and the rods are joined to the same interneurones, and it would be very surprising indeed if a drug had a highly selective effect on rods and cones beyond this point, but this does not seem to be the case. A drug may merely modify the bandpass characteristics of the channels slightly, so that they limit the more rapid responses, i.e. responses to stimuli which cones alone can follow. This same type of mechanism possibly accounts for the effect of Altafur that Dr. Siegel and I mentioned (p. 218). We were emphasizing its selective effect on colour vision. If this drug had a similar effect on the rod system, we would not necessarily be able to detect it. Our suggestion is that the inhibitory interactions which enable one to see hundreds of hues from three pigments are disrupted by furaltadone. There is however only one rod pigment and therefore no hue discrimination. If similar inhibitory interactions are interrupted for the rod system, the subjective effect will be different—possibly not noticeable. But the removal of inhibition might lead to the most annoying dazzle that, as we emphasized, the patient was really worried about. So perhaps all these drugs, including furaltadone, have a quite simple neurophysiological action, and when we translate this into terms of perception we merely pick up the dramatic effects that occur when particular parts of the frequency responses of our visual system are affected.

Session V

Central Effects

Chairman: J. A. B. Gray

THE ACTION OF DRUGS ON THE SENSORY CORTEX

J. L. Malcolm and Phyllis J. Spear

Department of Physiology, University of Aberdeen

Drugs have long been a useful tool in the elucidation of the anatomical, physiological and chemical processes which are involved in the normal functioning of the nervous system. Previous contributors have discussed the influence of different drugs on both peripheral and central sensory mechanisms, and, in particular, those of the 'special' senses of smell, taste, hearing and vision. The actions of drugs on peripheral sensory processes have yielded valuable information, but of course eventually the sensory cortex itself becomes involved, either indirectly, from the disturbance of afferent volley patterns, or directly, by the actions of substances crossing the blood-brain barrier. An analysis of such central actions is of obvious importance, but is limited by our lack of knowledge of the physiological processes that accompany activity in the sensory cortex, and also by uncertainty about what is the appropriate phenomenon to observe. The choice is wide. For instance, one may examine the spontaneous electrical activity of the brain (the EEG) at many points simultaneously and observe the effects of drugs given by mouth or injected into the circulation. Many such studies have been made, and with a variety of drugs (Toman and Davis, 1949; Bradley and Elkes, 1957; Faulconer and Bickford, 1960; Bradley, 1963; Brazier, 1963, 1964; Grundfest, 1964; Millichap, 1965). However, although the drug-induced changes are clear-cut, the actual site and mode of action of the drug are not. Hence evaluation of the data can only be speculative.

Another line of investigation entails the examination of drug effects upon individual neurones whose spike activity is recorded by extracellular microelectrodes. Several workers favour this method and it is a common practice to stimulate a quiescent or a sporadically-firing cell with an iontophoretic application of certain excitatory aminoacids, such as L-glutamate or DL-homocysteic acid, to enable a greater number of neurones to be studied (Curtis and Andersen, 1962; Curtis and Davis, 1962; Krnjević and Phillis, 1963a, 1963b, 1963c; Crawford, Curtis, Voorhoeve and Wilson, 1963; Crawford and Curtis, 1964; Andersen and Curtis, 1964; Krnjević, Randić and Straughan, 1964; Randić, Siminoff and Straughan, 1964; Biscoe and Straughan, 1965; Curtis, 1965; Krnjević, 1965; Bloom, Costa and Salmoiraghi, 1965). This method is excellent for single-cell studies, but, in an organ as complex as the brain, it may be misleading to study the action of drugs on the spike activity of individual nerve cells and to ignore the slow wave activities which are so characteristic of groups of neurones, whether composed of few or of many cells. These slow waves—allegedly postsynaptic, and probably involving the activity of the dendrites rather than of the soma and axons (Eccles, 1951; Li and Jasper, 1953; Li, Cullen and Jasper, 1956; Mountcastle, Davies and Berman, 1957; Grundfest, 1957; Purpura, 1959; Chang, 1959; Amassian, Waller and Macy, 1964)—are very sensitive to many drugs and often show a different pattern of pharmacological reactions from that of the spike activity.

That the two phenomena *sometimes* correspond is well known. However, such correlations are not always apparent and drug effects on single-cell spike activity should therefore be interpreted cautiously, taking into account the drug-induced changes seen in slow waves. Further research involving the study of drug actions on both phenomena would be profitable.

For those who employ drugs as tools of brain research, there arises the important problem of where and how to apply the drug. Each of the four main routes that has been used has advantages and disadvantages.

The drug may be given via the systemic circulation, as already mentioned. This method immediately involves the neurone in direct and indirect drug effects, obtained from central and peripheral actions, and it also encounters the variations in permeability to drugs of the blood-brain barrier. This may differ in various parts of the cerebral vascular bed as a result of a change in membrane selectivity from site to site. Often, however, impermeability is relative, and may be overcome by raising the drug concentration in the circulation. The drawbacks of this method are that the exact quantity of drug reaching any neurone cannot be estimated; that one cannot readily discover whether high doses of drug—needed to overcome the impermeability of the blood-brain barrier—produce any effects which mask the neuronal drug-induced changes; and that, as already mentioned, the precise site of action of the drug cannot be pin-pointed.

On the other hand, the introduction of drugs via the cerebral ventricles—a technique developed and used especially by Feldberg and his colleagues (see reviews by Feldberg, 1963; Feldberg and Fleischhauer, 1965)—overcomes the problems imposed by the blood-brain barrier, and by this method a single injection may exert its effects locally by acting directly upon the cortex. Abnormal neuronal discharges other than those caused directly by drugs may however arise from pressure changes or from the interruption of cerebrospinal fluid flow, both of which may result from either injection or perfusion of drugs into or through the cerebral ventricles. Such procedures may cause powerful indirect excitation or inhibition of the cortex (Feldberg, Malcolm and Darian Smith, 1957).

Thirdly, drugs can be applied to single neurones by iontophoresis. This method, originally used by Nastuk (1951, 1953) and del Castillo and Katz (1955, 1957) to study the pharmacological properties of muscle end-plates, was later adapted by Curtis and

Eccles (1958) for the study of spinal neurones. Since then, the technique has been widely used to investigate drug effects on many parts of the nervous system (see reviews by Salmoiraghi, Costa and Bloom, 1965; Curtis, 1965; Krnjević, 1965; Bradley and Wolstencroft, 1965; Phillis, 1965). It involves the active ejection of ions by the passage of a small electric current, from the tip of a micro-electrode placed at a desired depth in brain tissue. Small quantities of drugs may thus be applied to individual nerve cells in a very localized area. Such a technique has obvious advantages (Curtis, 1965) which no doubt account for its extensive use. However, it also has disadvantages (Curtis, 1965), including the uncertainty of the exact extent of the site of action of the drug, the relatively high drug concentrations needed to achieve an effect, and the unknown effects of the accompanying ionic movements which, though apparently innocuous in themselves, may condition the cell's response or lack of response to applied drugs. In addition there may be significant changes in pH during iontophoresis, and the introduction of the broad-tipped multi-barrelled pipettes into the brain substance itself must be assumed to cause pressure changes, vascular disturbances, rupture of nerve and glial cells and possible oedema in the area surrounding the neurone under study.

Fourthly, drugs can be applied locally to the pia. This method has often involved the use of drug-soaked pledgets of filter paper placed topically on a desired cortical area. Such methods calling for frequent placement and replacement of material are very prone to produce spreading depression of the underlying cortex (Leão, 1944; Leão and Morison, 1945; van Harreveld, Stamm and Christenson, 1956; Marshall, 1959; Grafstein, 1961) as a result of the mechanical manipulations, sudden pressure changes or drying of the pial surface. In addition, such manoeuvres are liable to disturb recording conditions. Most experimenters with this technique have applied excessively high concentrations of drugs, sometimes dissolved in distilled water—itself likely to injure cells (e.g. Chatfield and Purpura, 1954; Chatfield and Lord, 1955). The local application of drugs to the pia has several disadvantages. Diffusion, or in some cases active transport, has to be relied upon as the mechanism by which drugs reach neurones at any depth, despite the fact that the pia itself is a barrier, though it is less selective than the blood-brain barrier. Moreover, one cannot know exactly which neurones are affected by the drug applied, nor estimate with precision the final concentration of drug that reaches them.

The drawbacks and uncertainties which immediately confront the experimenter who wants to apply drugs to the brain appear to present a gloomy and confused picture of the chances of accurately assessing drug-induced changes. But even if present methods seem so inadequate we must increase our knowledge of the normal physiology of the brain before we can talk intelligently about the action of drugs on the cortex. In this context we shall summarize briefly some data from our laboratory, obtained from experiments on rats under allobarbital-urethane anaesthesia.

We have observed the slow-wave response evoked in the primary sensory area by electrical stimulation of the skin of the rat's forepaw. The spontaneous activity (the EEG) has not passed unnoticed or unrecorded. In the cat Marshall, Woolsey and Bard (1941) demonstrated that the area of sensory cortex involved in the reception of evoked responses varies with the magnitude of the peripheral stimulus, and in fact showed that there are three main receiving areas. This phenomenon is less apparent in the rat and there seems to be only one particular region of the sensory cortex from where an 'optimum' evoked response may be recorded either from the cortical surface or from a desired depth. A surface recording of a response evoked by a shock of 20 V lasting for 0·1 msec. and delivered once every 2 seconds, consists of a positive-negative slow-wave sequence. The positive wave is divided into two peaks, which arise 7 and 10 msec. respectively from the time of stimulation. The amplitude of the negative wave is more variable than that of each positive wave, but its peak normally occurs 17–20 msec. after the stimulus. The response recorded from the deeper layers is, as is well known, essentially a reversal of a surface record, and consists of a large negative wave which may be followed by a positive one, depending on the depth of the recording point within the cortex. One can usually discern a small positive deflection on the upstroke of the negative wave, which corresponds with the peak of the first positive wave seen on the surface recording. Similarly the peak of the deep negative wave corresponds with that of the second surface-positive peak.

We have applied drugs topically to the pial surface, avoiding the complication of inconstant recording conditions and the possibility of spreading depression by injecting drugs into a small perspex ring (volume 0·025 ml.) which is placed on the appropriate area of the somatosensory cortex and whose edges are sealed with soft paraffin. This ensures a leak-proof pool of fluid over the area under study and also minimizes pulsations caused by respiration. The drugs, made up in an artificial c.s.f. solution, buffered to pH 7·4 (Merlis, 1940), are delivered into the ring from hypodermic syringes by means of fine polythene tubes. Two recording electrodes are used to monitor the evoked response: one is an insulated silver wire electrode which records from the surface of the cortex, and the other is a KCl-filled microelectrode, of tip diameter 1–2 μ and resistance 15–20 megohms, which records from a depth of 400–600 μ.

The evoked responses are recorded either on a Mingograf ink-jet recorder (which, having a top frequency response of 700 c.p.s., faithfully records the full amplitude of the slow waves), or on a Southern Instruments pen recorder with shortened pens so that only slight attenuation of the response could occur.

In an attempt to elucidate the role of the well known peripheral transmitter substances in the sensory cortex, and to learn something of the physiology of chemical transmission, we have looked particularly at the actions and interactions of noradrenaline and acetylcholine on the evoked response and on the EEG.

Noradrenaline when applied in a 1 mM concentration for 15 seconds to the pial surface typically inhibits the evoked response for a period of 3–6 minutes. This inhibitory effect, particularly apparent upon the surface and the deep negative waves, can be blocked by a previous application of the adrenergic α-blocker phenoxybenzamine, in a 3 mM concentration. Other α-blockers (ergotamine tartrate, 0·76 mM, dihydroergotamine, 1·47 mM, and tolazoline, 5·1 mM) have similar effects, although not to the same extent as does phenoxybenzamine. The β-blocker propranolol, 3·40 mM, does not block the noradrenaline-induced inhibition.

A 30-second application of a 2 mM solution of acetylcholine, in the presence of the anticholinesterase physostigmine (0·7 mM), shows an exactly similar inhibition. In addition there is a later-developing marked stimulation of the background activity, producing fast, spike-like waves which vary in amplitude according to the length of time that the drug is in contact with the cortex. These two cholinergic effects are shared by two cholinomimetic substances—carbamylcholine (2·75 mM) and acetyl-β-methylcholine bromide (2·1 mM). Atropine (0·3 mM) blocks both the inhibitory effect of cholinergic compounds upon the evoked slow waves and stimulant effect on the background activity.

If one crosses these experiments and applies acetylcholine in the presence of phenoxybenzamine, the inhibitory action is again blocked. This seems not to be an atropine-like action of phenoxybenzamine, for the acetylcholine-induced repetitive EEG activity still appears. On the other hand, the typical inhibition by noradrenaline of the evoked responses occurs as usual in the presence of atropine.

It is possible to explain these findings in a variety of ways, but we suggest the following simple, but by no means proven, organization. We propose the existence of adrenergic inhibitory cells within the primary somatosensory cortex of the rat, which can suppress to some extent all cortical activity, including the incoming primary evoked responses. Further we suggest that these inhibitory cells are excited by cholinergic synapses which either arise directly from neurones occurring in the main sensory pathway, or else from interneurones which the latter excite. Such an arrangement would explain the double action of cholinomimetic substances, i.e. the inhibition of the primary cortical response, and the excitation of the EEG, both of which are blocked by atropine. It would account for the block by phenoxybenzamine of the acetylcholine-induced inhibition, and not of the cholinergic EEG excitation. Finally it would explain why the noradrenaline-induced inhibition is blocked by adrenergic blockers but not by atropine.

There are, of course, big gaps in the evidence for this hypothesis. We badly need to know how rapidly substances penetrate from the pia into the cortical substance. We have followed the penetration rates of a number of substances, but the most striking demonstration of speed is the detection by the Falck fluoroscopic technique (Falck and Owman, 1965) of noradrenaline applied only briefly to the pia. This method shows that within 1 minute of application, a 1 mM solution of noradrenaline can penetrate over 100 μ into the superficial layers of the cortex where it has its initial and main effect. The action would seem therefore to be direct.

Another important question is: what evidence is there for the presence of cholinergic and adrenergic cells and synapses within the cortex? Thanks to the beautiful study of Krnjević and Silver (1965), the histological evidence for a cholinergic mechanism in the cat cortex is good. The depth at which they found cholinesterase-staining endings corresponds approximately to that in the rat at which we found the excitatory effects of cholinomimetic substances to be most marked, and this provides supporting evidence for the existence of cholinergic mechanisms. As regards adrenergic mechanisms, it has been shown by Csillik and Erulkar (1964), Fuxe (1965) and by our colleague Mr. G. Arbuthnott, using

Falck's fluorescent technique, that there are many fibres staining for noradrenaline in the superficial layers of the cortex. Arbuthnott has also shown that many cells in deeper layers take up the applied catecholamine and fluoresce vividly.

We think therefore that there is good evidence for both cholinergic and adrenergic mechanisms in the sensory cortex of the rat, and that our method of local application of drugs gives an indication of how they may be interrelated.

REFERENCES

Amassian, V. E., Waller, H. J. and Macy, J., Jr. (1964). *Ann. N.Y. Acad. Sci.*, **112**, 5.
Andersen, P. and Curtis, D. R. (1964). *Acta physiol. scand.*, **61**, 85.
Biscoe, T. J. and Straughan, D. W. (1965). *J. Pharm. Pharmacol.*, **17**, 60.
Bloom, F. E., Costa, E. and Salmoiraghi, G. C. (1965). *J. Pharmacol. exp. Therap.*, **150**, 244.
Bradley, P. B. (1963). *In* Physiological Pharmacology (ed. Root, W. S. and Hofmann, W. G.), **1**, 17. New York: Academic Press.
Bradley, P. B. and Elkes, J. (1957). *Brain*, **80**, 77.
Bradley, P. B. and Wolstencroft, J. H. (1965). *Brit. med. Bull.*, **21**, 15.
Brazier, M. A. B. (1963). *In* Physiological Pharmacology, **1**, 219 (ed. Root, W. S. and Hofmann, W. G.). New York: Academic Press.
Brazier, M. A. B. (1964). *Clin. Pharmac. Therap.*, **5**, 102.
Chang, H.-T. (1959). *In* Handbook of Physiology, Section 1, Neurophysiology, vol. 1, 299 (ed. Field, J., Magoun, H. W. and Hall, V. E.) Washington: American Physiological Society.
Chatfield, P. O. and Lord, J. T. (1955). *EEG clin. Neurophysiol.*, **7**, 553.
Chatfield, P. O. and Purpura, D. P. (1954). *EEG clin. Neurophysiol.*, **6**, 287.
Crawford, J. M. and Curtis, D. R. (1964). *Brit. J. Pharmacol.*, **23**, 313.
Crawford, J. M., Curtis, D. R., Voorhoeve, P. E. and Wilson, V. J. (1963). *Nature, Lond.*, **200**, 579.
Csillik, B. and Erulkar, S. D. (1964). *J. Pharmacol. exp. Therap.*, **146**, 186.
Curtis, D. R. (1965). *Brit. med. Bull.*, **21**, 5.
Curtis, D. R. and Andersen, P. (1962). *Nature, Lond.*, **195**, 1105.
Curtis, D. R. and Davis, R. (1962). *Brit. J. Pharmacol.*, **18**, 217.
Curtis, D. R. and Eccles, R. M. (1958). *J. Physiol.*, **141**, 435.
Del Castillo, J. and Katz, B. (1955). *J. Physiol.*, **128**, 157.
Del Castillo, J. and Katz, B. (1957). *Proc. R. Soc. B*, **146**, 339.
Eccles, J. C. (1951). *EEG clin. Neurophysiol.*, **3**, 449.
Falck, B. and Owman, C. (1965). *Acta Univ. lund.* **2**, 6.

Faulconer, A., Jr. and Bickford, R. G. (1960). Electroencephalography in Anaesthesiology. Springfield: C. C Thomas.
Feldberg, W. (1963). A Pharmacological Approach to the Brain from its Inner and Outer Surface. Evarts Graham Memorial Lectures, 1961. London: Edward Arnold.
Feldberg, W. and Fleischhauer, K. (1965). *Brit. med. Bull.*, **21**, 36.
Feldberg, W., Malcolm, J. L. and Darian Smith, I. (1957). *J. Physiol.*, **138**, 178.
Fuxe, K. (1965). *Acta physiol. scand.*, **64**, Suppl. 247, 39.
Grafstein, B. (1961). *Brain Function*, **1**, U.C.L.A. Forum in Med. Sci., No. 1, ed. Brazier, M. A. B., p. 87. Los Angeles: University of California Press.
Grundfest, H. (1957). *Physiol. Rev.*, **37**, 337.
Grundfest, H. (1964). *Ann. Rev. Pharmacol.*, **4**, 341.
Krnjević, K. (1965). *Brit. med. Bull.*, **21**, 10.
Krnjević, K. and Phillis, J. W. (1963a). *J. Physiol.*, **165**, 274.
Krnjević, K. and Phillis, J. W. (1963b). *J. Physiol.*, **166**, 296.
Krnjević, K. and Phillis, J. W. (1963c). *Brit. J. Pharmacol.*, **20**, 471.
Krnjević, K. Randić, M. and Straughan, D. W. (1964). *J. Physiol.*, **175**, 21P.
Krnjević, K. and Silver, A. (1965). *J. Anat.*, **99**, 711.
Leão, A. A. P. (1944). *J. Neurophysiol.*, **7**, 359.
Leão, A. A. P. and Morison, R. S. (1945). *J. Neurophysiol.*, **8**, 33.
Li, C.-L., Cullen, C. and Jasper, H. H. (1956). *J. Neurophysiol.*, **19**, 111.
Li, C.-L. and Jasper, H. H. (1953). *J. Physiol.*, **121**, 117.
Marshall, W. H. (1959). *Physiol. Rev.*, **39**, 239.
Marshall, W. H., Woolsey, C. N. and Bard, P. (1941). *J. Neurophysiol.*, **4**, 1.
Merlis, J. K. (1940). *Amer. J. Physiol.*, **131**, 67.
Millichap, J. G. (1965). *Post-grad. med. J.*, **37**, 22.
Mountcastle, V. B., Davies, P. W. and Berman, A. L. (1957). *J. Neurophysiol.*, **20**, 374.
Nastuk, W. L. (1951). *Fed. Proc.*, **10**, 96.
Nastuk, W. L. (1953). *Fed. Proc.*, **12**, 102.
Phillis, J. W. (1965). *Brit. med. Bull.*, **21**, 26.
Purpura, D. P. (1959). *Int. Rev. Neurobiol.*, **1**, 47.
Randić, M., Siminoff, R. and Straughan, D. W. (1964). *Expl. Neurol.*, **9**, 236.
Salmoiraghi, G. C., Costa, E. and Bloom, F. E. (1965). *Ann. Rev. Pharmacol.*, **5**, 213.
Toman, J. E. P. and Davis, J. P. (1949). *Pharmacol. Rev.*, **1**, 425.
Van Harreveld, A., Stamm, J. S. and Christenson, E. (1956). *Amer. J. Physiol.*, **184**, 312.

DISCUSSION

Herxheimer: What happens in different parts of the sensory cortex that normally receive inputs from all kinds of different modalities? Are they similar as far as you can tell, or do you find any differences?

Malcolm: No, I think they are quite different and I really limit what I have said specifically to the S.1 area. If you examine the visual area, for example, the catechol amines have no effect whatsoever. There must be a different mechanism, or the patterns of pharmacological types of neurones are quite different. If we were investigating nalidixic acid we would look at the visual cortex rather than the sensory cortex.

Salmoiraghi: Could Professor Malcolm remind us of the evidence that the effects are not due to vascular actions of the agents or to metabolic effects such as those reported by the Hokins?

Malcolm: I can't rule out 'metabolic actions'—no, but I don't think these substances arrive in the cells in the concentration that the Hokins required for the interference with phospholipid turnover and so on. As for vascular effects, noradrenaline in this situation actually dilates the vessels. After the application the area under the ring is quite obviously a brighter red than the surrounding.

Salmoiraghi: What does the increased oxygen tension do to the activity?

Malcolm: It has no comparable effect on the evoked responses but I couldn't increase the oxygen tension significantly, as the animal was in very good condition.

Salmoiraghi: Can you explain your data in the light of the findings by Krnjević, that none of the major cortical pathways is cholinergic? This evidence, of course, does not exclude the possibility that some other pathway may be cholinergic.

Malcolm: Krnjević and Silver's own paper shows very nicely cholinergic synapses—the synapses with cholinesterase-staining material around them and at about the appropriate level. How many of these are local transcortical neurones, and how many are conveying incoming volleys from further afield, I cannot say.

Salmoiraghi; I had the impression from Krnjević's evidence that the reticular formation may be cholinergic.

Malcolm: The inhibitory pathway is not excited first by the incoming volley; it is more frequently associated with the second arrival which is possibly via the reticular formation or some other sensory pathway. It could even be via some neighbouring cortical pathway and therefore I would be looking at the end of a short transcortical neurone and exciting that with my acetycholine. This could still be the neurone that Krnjević excited with his acetycholine and the one which he shows contains cholinesterase-staining material in the cat. I think this is compatible.

Salmoiraghi: How do you reconcile your findings of fluorescence with those of the Swedish workers?

Malcolm: I think the difference is that we are using the rat, and also the neurones that you saw were the result of loading the tissue with pial application of noradrenaline. There may be not very much basic fluorescent material in the neurone, although we find neurones that do show fluorescence which we have accentuated by allowing those neurones to take up more than their normal amount of noradrenaline. It seems to be necessary to do this to be able to see them with this technique. The fibres, though, are normal rat fibres; they are not 'loaded'.

Whitfield: Have you looked at any individual neurone responses? We have found that when we put our manipulator on, unless we are extremely careful, the preparation can be depressed for two hours, and perhaps 40% of neurones don't respond, and I wonder what the effect of the ring was.

Malcolm: I think the ring actually stabilizes the cortex—it helps to damp pulsations so that the cortex remains in a very steady position. The ring is supported quite rigidly by a holder at the side; it doesn't float on the cortex, which is wide open. The freer the cerebrospinal fluid is to flow, the less pulsation there is. When the cortex in the rat is half open one gets pulsation, oedema and general distortion of the cortex.

DRUG-INDUCED HALLUCINATIONS IN PRIMATES

LEONARD A. COHEN

Department of Physiology, Albert Einstein Medical Center, Philadelphia

IN most investigations involving sensory function, experiments on humans have the advantage that the subject can describe his sensations and mental images to the investigator. At first sight this appears to be particularly true of research on hallucinogenic drugs, since the best method for obtaining information about hallucinations that have been experienced would seem to be to ask a human subject to describe verbally what he felt and saw. In truth, however, this method is very unreliable. In general, verbal descriptions of subjective sensations are very poor substitutes for objective quantitative data. Furthermore, a hallucination is by definition an erroneous perception of actual physical reality, and consequently, a hallucinating brain is a very poor tool indeed for logically analyzing its own hallucination. Finally, when a patient must wait until he has recovered from his hallucinations before he can coherently report them to the investigator, the complex factor of recall enters in and even further compromises the scientific validity of the subject's verbal descriptions. It is therefore essential to develop and use quantitative objective tests of hallucinogenic activity.

Previous techniques to obtain objective quantitative information about hallucinations can be grouped into five categories:

1. electrical recording and stimulation of brain activity;
2. surgical ablation;

3. recording related physiological phenomena;
4. comparison of drug effects;
5. direct measurement of hallucinations.

1. Recording of deep brain potentials in monkeys given lysergide (9) has revealed only highly specific alterations in potentials, but it has not been possible to correlate these with behavioural features, and certainly not with the behavioural features described by humans who have experienced lysergide hallucinations. Furthermore, even the more generalized electroencephalograms, which represent electrical activity of larger brain areas than do depth electrodes, have not yielded any specific wave forms that can be correlated with specific features of hallucinatory behaviour. Indeed, even the relatively distinct EEG sleep-arousal response has not provided the correlations between specific electrical response and specific aspects of hallucinations which we so urgently need (3, 4). For example, when a 'drowsy' pattern appears in the EEG during hallucinatory activity, does this mean that the subject's sensory cortical areas have been *excited* in such a way as to mimic the feeling of quiescence, or does it mean the subject's cortical sensory areas have been *inhibited* with the result that the brain is really in a quiescent state? These are opposite conditions, yet with present techniques for recording electrical activity of the brain, we cannot distinguish between them. Another fundamental question here is whether the EEG is an infallible indicator of behaviour. For example, dogs given atropine display a sleep-pattern EEG simultaneously with excited behaviour (15). Electrical stimulation of specific brain areas is equally uncertain as a technique for objectively analyzing hallucinatory activity. For example, stimulation of the ventral hypothalamus to activate the 'emotion centre' yielded behavioural activity which only superficially resembled true emotional states (12).

2. Surgical ablation experiments in primates have been similarly unsuccessful. Although, at first sight, it might seem that

removal of specific parts of the brain could identify the structures for drug-induced hallucinations, in practice this has not been so: 'Indeed, our seemingly most "exact" neurosurgical studies in animals confirmed yet another clinical maxim; that the effects of a cerebral lesion depend perhaps less on its site or extent than on the previous "personality" and current treatment of the patient, i.e.: his significant pretraumatic or preoperative experiences and the physical and psychiatric care given him during crucial periods of physical recovery, retraining and rehabilitation.' (12). This is true for monkeys as well as for man. The personality differences between normal monkeys are vast and changeable. Furthermore, monkeys subjected to neurosurgery commonly show a change in personality and behaviour in tests which may appear for the first time many months following surgery. Fortunately, as a result of an unusually long and unexpected delay, we discovered these cases before giving any hallucinogenic drugs postoperatively. Furthermore, monkeys routinely tested for response to hallucinogens will occasionally change their response even after many months of stable, objective, quantitative test responses. The handling which is part of normal animal care practices has been shown to influence the responses to drugs in rats, for example (14). Thus, behavioural changes can occur (a) spontaneously at any time (b) as a result of surgery, even many months postoperatively, and (c) as a result of continuous hallucinogenic experimentation. This makes the interpretation of postoperative responses to hallucinogens highly unreliable.

3. Attempts to obtain objective measurements of hallucinations by recording such functional indicators of nervous activity as blood pressure and respiration are neither better nor worse than the techniques mentioned earlier, for the functions recorded only indirectly indicate hallucinogenic activity and are compared with the observer's impression of the monkey's hallucinated behaviour.

4. Drug comparisons are familiar in psychopharmacology, and some investigators who have previously worked with the more

specific techniques described above, have subsequently used this approach (3, 4, 12, 13). This approach, again, does not give us objective quantitative measures of hallucinogenic activity which we need.

5. Direct measurement of hallucinations has been relatively neglected, though it appears to be a very promising approach. The rest of this paper therefore deals with it in some detail. The studies were conducted on macaque nemestrina monkeys, but the general problems of objective testing are of course the same for humans as for these animals.

One of the most prominent features of hallucinations is the spatial disorientation of the subject, and this aspect has been selected for analysis below. A hallucinating subject can no longer accurately judge the physical relationship existing between his body and his immediate environment. Indeed, a subject often has a false impression of his bodily posture, and of the position of his individual limbs. Furthermore, he may be completely unaware of his immediate physical surroundings, or may have an erroneous perception of the spatial relationship existing between surrounding objects and his body (1, 2, 10, 11, 13). Thus, he may reach for objects which do not exist in his environment, or he may reach in the wrong place for objects which do exist in his environment. A hallucinated organism can be defined as being out of accurate physical contact with its environment, that is, disoriented in space and time. By this definition, any individual in a 'state of hallucination' would have to display spatial disorientation in any valid test for spatial disorientation. However, the presence of spatial disorientation in an organism does not *necessarily* indicate a state of hallucination.

Very little real progress has been made over the years in developing objective quantitative tests which measure the accuracy of spatial orientation. Subjects are still tested by finger-to-finger and finger-to-nose tests with eyes closed, by a body sway test, standing with eyes closed, and by looking for nystagmus. These tests are very imperfectly controlled and are generally non-quantitative. Total body balance has been studied quantitatively in humans by a new test which requires patients to walk along rails of various widths (7). The most noteworthy advance has been in the development of electronystagmography, which automatically records eye movements. Typically, a recording electrode is placed on each external canthus and voltage output is amplified and recorded (Fig. 1A). However, although nystagmus can be objectively

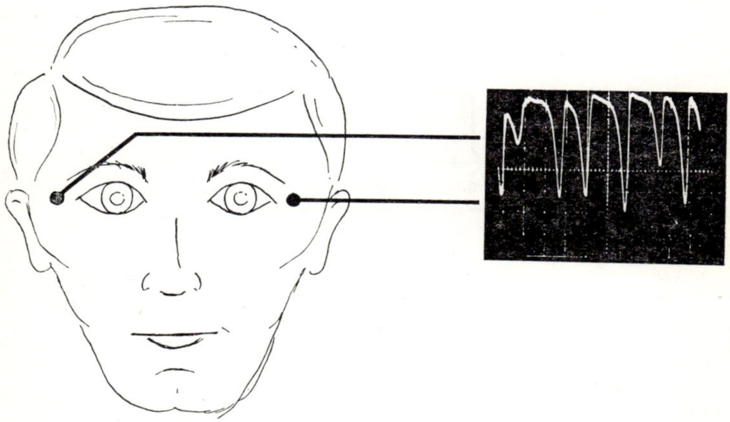

FIG. 1A. Drawing of location of horizontal nystagmus electrodes and of assc-ciated left and right electronystagmograms.

and quantitatively studied, it is a poor indicator of body spatial orientation because normally it only occurs in response to atypical physiological stimuli, and its physiological significance is unknown. Nonetheless, for our purposes, nystagmography should be very useful for obtaining records of all eye movements occurring during hallucinatory activity. Eye movements must surely be important correlates of the visual images which are such a prominent feature of hallucinations. This approach should be exploited. For this purpose, the recording arrangement shown in Fig. 1B is suggested, since it will record all directions and amounts of eye movements.

Total spatial orientation has been recorded in primates (5–7), by measuring the ease and accuracy with which the subjects could perform certain specialized motor activities which depend on accurate spatial placement of limbs. The principal motor acts tested involved climbing up and down a special ladder and a pegboard. The pegboard represented a greater challenge since the monkeys had to place their limbs exactly on the pegs or an obvious miss, and a delay in climbing time, were recorded; whereas

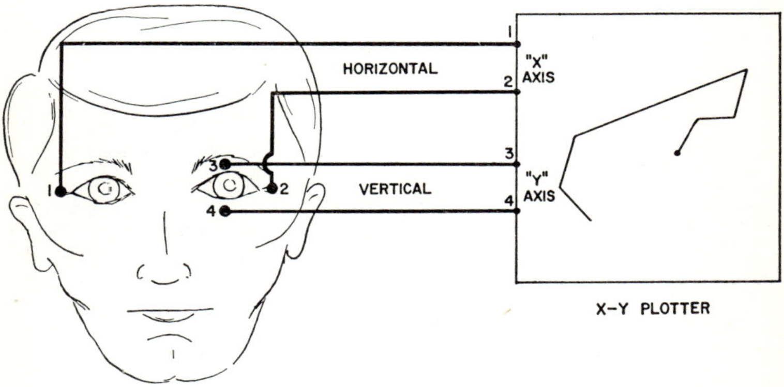

FIG. 1B. Suggested placement of electrodes for recording all eye movements.

the animals could use sweeping movements of the arms in order to grasp a rung of the ladder, and lateral errors of several centimetres made little difference. Animals were always tested under the same food motivation, and other experimental conditions were also kept constant.

Repeated testing over a period up to 6 months was necessary before standard normal performance times were obtained for each experimental animal being subjected to drugs. The spatial disorientation associated with lysergide (LSD 0·05 mg./kg.), phencyclidine (Sernyl 0·2 mg./kg.) and Ditran (4·0 mg./kg.) were recorded and compared with the normal state. These doses produced definite spatial disorientation without incapacitating the animals (7). The performances at such doses were clearly below normal (Fig. 2). High doses so incapacitated the animals that they would usually stay in one place as if in a stupor, and make occasional arm movements as if reaching for imaginary objects. In such a state the animals sometimes walked into objects, or otherwise indicated complete unawareness of their immediate

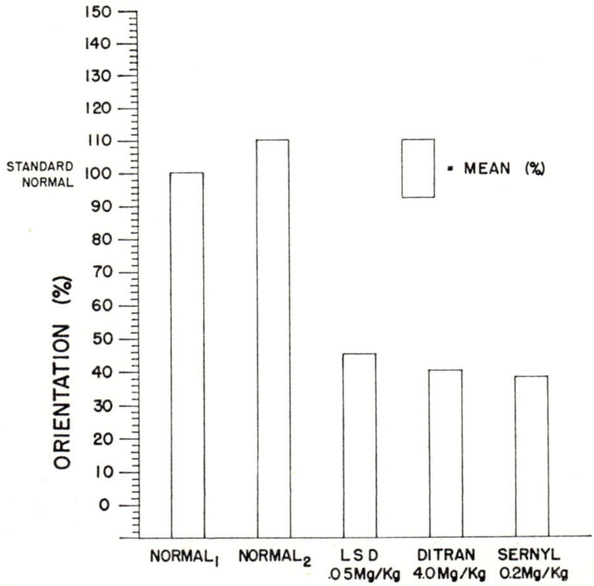

FIG. 2. Mean orientation ability for the population of animals. Normal-1 was selected as the standard normal representing 100% orientation ability.

surroundings. Such animals did not perform in the spatial orientation tests, because they seemed unaware of the food cues and thus would not use the testing equipment, even if they had been fasted as long as 2 days. Obviously, for such deep levels of hallucination new tests must be devised which do not depend on the animal's awareness of environmental stimuli, if objective quantitative data are to be obtained. This will be discussed later.

This method reveals some significant subtleties of information which would be lost if subjective non-quantitative information were used. Thus, Fig. 3 shows that the development of disorientation in an animal following administration of a hallucinogen follows the same time course at all doses except the one just below

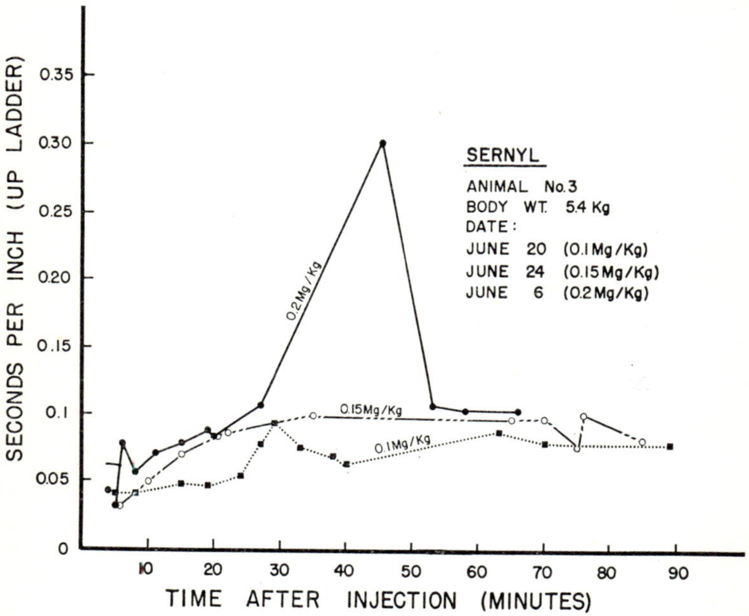

FIG. 3. Onset and course of disorientation in a single animal after three different doses of the same drug. Disorientation is plotted on the *y* axis as climbing rate, represented by seconds per inch so that slower rates will give increasing values and thus depict increasing disorientation.

the incapacitating dose. At this dose, a sharp high peak of disorientation typically emerges from the 'broad hump', which suggests involvement of a different orientation mechanism than that which underlies the broad hump (7).

Studies of hallucinations in primates have also been combined with other spatial disorienting procedures to study the mechanism of hallucinogenic disorientation. The spatial orientation tests for primates were originally used to measure the contribution of neck proprioceptors to spatial orientation of the body (5). Elimination of cervical sensation by bilateral block of C 1, 2, 3 dorsal roots in the monkey was shown to cause severe spatial disorientation of a severity matching that produced by labyrinthectomy. In our studies monkeys were first tested for normal orientation. The cervical component of orientation was then interrupted surgically and orientation measured again. Operated animals were given lysergide and spatial orientation was again tested. Operated monkeys showed severe orientational defects which were greatly intensified by subsequent administration of lysergide. Indeed, the animals were 'sensitized' to the drug since 0·0125 mg./kg., one fourth the normal dose, now caused a 50% decrease in normal orientation. This implies that hallucinogens affect the central physiological mechanism for orientation, since hallucinogenic disorientation summates with cervical disorientation.

Generally, lysergide, even in doses as low as 0·0125 mg./kg. inhibited the animals so that they did not climb the special apparatus, although they walked around on the floor and thus could not be said to be incapacitated. The objective quantitative test had therefore to be changed to a subjective pseudoquantitative test where the observer evaluated orientation on a 4-point scale to obtain data from operated animals that had received a hallucinogen. Further objective quantitative tests for measuring spatial orientation were thus needed to measure more severe disorientation.

Most urgently needed are tests for orientation which automatically stimulate the subject for the desired response to be measured, without requiring the conscious participation of the subject. Any test which requires the subject to participate consciously, such as to become aware of presented food and to respond to it, will fail since the severely disoriented animal is unaware of his surroundings and will not respond. This is just as important for studying human reactions to hallucinogens.

Tests are now being planned for measuring spatial orientation objectively and quantitatively even in a deep hallucinatory state. The new equipment includes a tilt platform which will measure the amount of tilt necessary before the primate staggers, and apparatus for measuring dynamic body balance. The flexor reflex will be recorded in response to cutaneously applied electrical stimuli, and will be recorded by electronystagmography.

These new tests will conform to an important principle that has been previously neglected, namely, the development and use of objective quantitative tests for animals which can also be used in man. It then becomes possible to compare objective data between animals and man regardless of the underlying mechanism. If we can make sure that our human and animal data are obtained by identical experimental procedures we will have made a major advance.

REFERENCES

1. Abood, L. G. and Meduna, L. J. (1958). Some effects of a new psychotogen in depressive states. *J. nerv. ment. Dis.*, **127**, 546–550.
2. Abood, L. G., Ostfeld, A. and Biel, J. H. (1959). Structure-activity relationships of 3-piperidyl benzilates with psychotogenic properties. *Arch. internat. Pharmacodyn.*, **120**, 186–200.
3. Bradley, P. B. (1959). Methods and analysis of drug-induced behaviour in animals. *In* Neuro-psychopharmacology, p. 11, ed. Bradley, P. B., Deniker, P. and Radouco-Thomas, C. Amsterdam: Elsevier.
4. Bradley, P. B. (1964). EEG correlates of drug effects. *In* Animal Behaviour and Drug Action (ed. Steinberg, H., de Reuck, A. V. S. and Knight J.), p. 119. Ciba Foundation Symp. London: Churchill.
5. Cohen, L. A. (1961). The role of eye and neck proprioceptor mechanisms in body orientation and motor coordination. *J. Neurophysiol.*, **24**, 1–11.
6. Cohen, L. A. (1964). Analysis of induced disorientation in primates. *Aerospace Med.*, **35**, 16–20.
7. Cohen, L. A. (1965). Hallucinogenic spatial disorientation. *Internat. J. Neuropsych.*, **1**, 347–351.
8. Graybiel, A. and Fregly, A. R. (1965). A new quantitative ataxia test battery. *NASA Joint Report*. NSAM–919. March, 1965.
9. Heath, R. G. and Leach, B. E. (1956). Changing Concepts of Psychoanalytic Medicine. New York: Grune and Stratton.

10. Hoch, P. H., Cattell, J. P. and Pennes, H. H. (1951). Effects of mescaline and lysergic acid (d-LSD-25). *Amer. J. Psych.*, **108,** 579–584.
11. Luby, E. D., Cohen, B. D., Rosenbaum, G., Gottlieb, J. S. and Kelly, R. (1959). Study of a new schizophrenomimetic drug—Sernyl. *A.M.A. Arch. Neurol. Psych.*, **81,** 363–369.
12. Masserman, J. H. (1959). Behavioral pharmacology in animals. *In* Neuro-psychopharmacology (ed. Bradley, P. B., Deniker, P. and Radouco-Thomas, C.), p. 97. Amsterdam: Elsevier.
13. Melander, P. and Martens, S. (1959). A pharmacological test-system for demonstration of psychotomimetic activity in animals. *In* Neuro-psychopharmacology (ed. Bradley, P. B., Deniker, P. and Radouco-Thomas, C.), p. 374. Amsterdam: Elsevier.
14. Rushton, Ruth and Steinberg, Hannah (1964). Modification of behavioural effects of drugs by past experience. *In* Animal Behaviour and Drug Action (ed. Steinberg, H., de Reuck, A. V. S. and Knight, J.), p. 207, Ciba Foundation Symp. London: Churchill.
15. Wikler, A. (1952). Pharmacologic dissociation of behavior and EEG 'sleep patterns' in dogs: morphine, N-allyl-normorphine and atropine. *Proc. Soc. exp. Biol. Med. N.Y.*, **79,** 261–265.

DISCUSSION

Summerfield: If one is talking about hallucinations, one is talking psychology or behaviour, one is not talking physiology. At the very best, therefore, physiological methods only give indirect evidence on the subject of hallucinations.

Cohen: Pavlov thought his greatest contribution was that he claimed for physiology the entire organism, the mind as well as the physical body. We usually think of Pavlov as a psychologist, but apparently he thought of himself as a physiologist. So perhaps this is a semantic problem.

Bradley: I wonder if Dr. Cohen has tested the effects of bromolysergide (BOL 148) on his monkeys, because it seems to me he is hardly justified in relating these beautiful objective studies of behavioural effects to hallucinations in these animals unless he can show that they are produced specifically by drugs which produce hallucinations.

Cohen: I did not test bromolysergide, and I agree it would be worth testing.

Salmoiraghi: Unless in your tests you have used drugs known not to produce hallucinations in man, an essential control is missing. Have you used drugs in your experiments which produce positive results in your terms which can't produce them in man?

Cohen: Well, we have used phencyclidine and Ditran. Phencyclidine certainly was not as good as lysergide in producing hallucinations. Ditran was much worse, and we have stopped using it. Here was a drug reported to produce hallucinations in man and yet we couldn't get consistent data to confirm it in our monkeys, so this may be an even more critical test inasmuch as it was a weakly 'hallucinating' drug in man but we couldn't demonstrate such an effect with our monkeys.

Grossman: Dr. Cohen's idea of getting objective measures of hallucinations is fascinating, but I share Dr. Bradley's misgivings. It seems to me that to some extent you are assuming that which you presume to measure. Could you, on the basis of the time it takes the monkey to go up the wall to the reinforcement or his skill in doing so, differentiate the effect of lysergide from the effect of a variety of other drugs which might be selected so as to impair the animal's sensory or motor ability, or his interest in the reward? I believe that it would be possible to compile a list of drugs which would come very close to duplicating your objective lysergide results, without inducing lysergide-like hallucinations.

Cohen: I should like to make two points in reply to that. First, on controls, one must recognize that there is a threshold for a statistically significant state of disorientation which represents a deviation, from a 'norm' that had been established over a long period of time. This is true for lysergide as well as for phencyclidine and Ditran, so that there were many experiments where we were using too low a dose to get anything significant. Second, this method was used originally to measure the effect of neck proprioceptors on total body balance and orientation. These studies were done some years ago at Oxford (Cohen, L. A. *J. Neurophysiol.*, 1961, **24**, 1) and I have repeated them again in Philadelphia. Normal orientation scores were obtained, the first three dorsocervical roots were cut, and the animals were retested with the same method. Here we were removing one important information input for the total ability of the animal to orientate itself. These animals that were deprived of neck sensation went on for weeks with severe spatial disorientation. This is similar to a typical neurophysiological ablation experiment for studying a physiological defect, in which all variables are controlled except the one under study. Some of these animals have now been used to study drug effects, and it takes one-fourth the dose of lysergide to produce a significant disorientation, so there is summation of a known physiological spatial orientation component and the effect we are measuring with lysergide.

THE QUANTIFICATION OF RAPID-EYE-MOVEMENT SLEEP

STUART A. LEWIS

Department of Psychiatry, University of Edinburgh

SINCE Aserinsky and Kleitman (1955) demonstrated the presence of rapid synchronous jerky eye movements during the stage of sleep when the electroencephalograph is of low voltage and is desynchronized, it has become well known that there are two different types of sleep. (See Oswald (1965) for a discussion of this.) Their characteristics are illustrated in Fig. 1. The upper record, of orthodox sleep, shows high-voltage slow wave activity and, if it were possible to subtract the electrical activity originating in the brain from that coming from the eyes, the eyes would be found to be motionless, or at most, executing very slow rolling movements. The lower record, of rapid-eye-movement sleep (also variously known as 'periodical', 'rhombencephalic' or 'dream' sleep), shows a low-voltage desynchronized EEG and is not dissimilar to that found in the waking subject. The jerky synchronous movements of the eyes give this type of sleep its name.

In the Edinburgh Sleep Laboratory we have tried to find a pharmacological explanation for these two types of sleep, REM and orthodox. To this end subjects have been given a variety of drugs. Our measurements have all related to the effects these drugs have on the proportion of the night spent in REM sleep. Since drugs such as amphetamine tend to shorten the total time spent asleep it is pointless to consider merely the absolute time spent in this type of sleep, for one night could not then be compared with another, nor indeed one drug with another. Hence, in line with other sleep laboratories, we have used the percentage

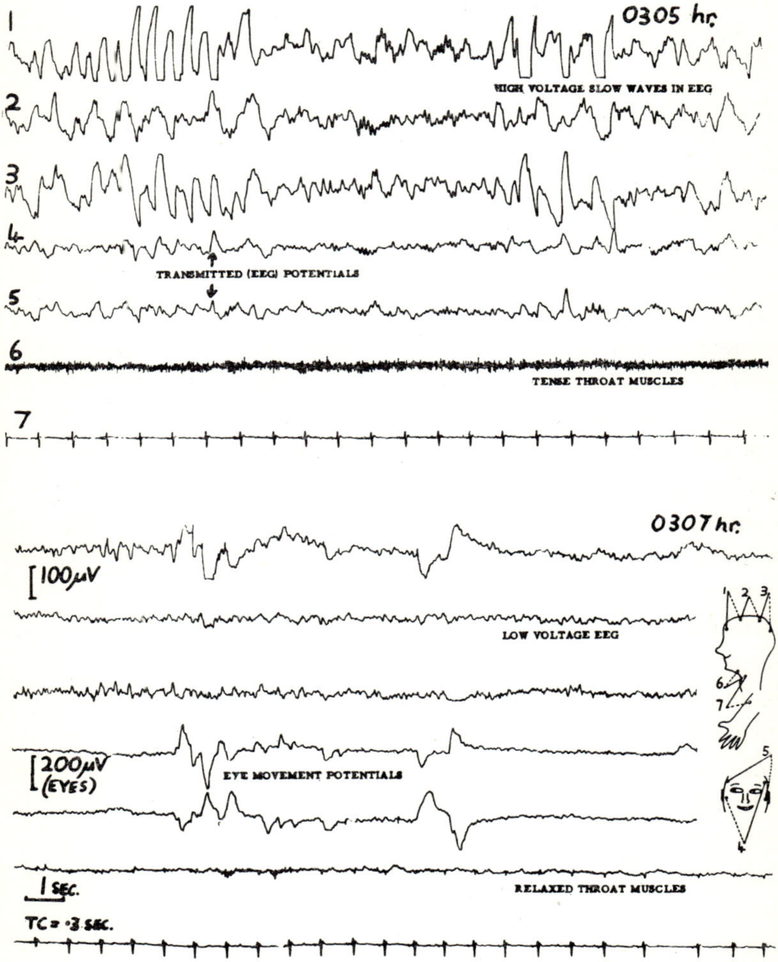

FIG. 1. Two kinds of sleep (see text). Reproduced with the permission of Dr. I. Oswald.

of the night spent in REM sleep. This method unfortunately makes it impossible to awaken the subject to obtain dream reports.

Longitudinal study of the effects of drugs on the sleep cycle in man, has brought to light the so-called 'rebound' phenomenon (Oswald and Priest, 1965; Lewis, 1965), which can only be observed if the study is extended beyond the cessation of drug administration. On the first few nights after the subject has stopped taking the drug, the proportion of the total sleep time which is spent in REM sleep increases dramatically. During this period the experimenters have many times been told by the subject when he was finally awakened in the morning that he had experienced a 'nightmare'. It is worth emphasizing here that the classification of night mentation into nightmares and non-nightmares is entirely subjective. The experimenter cannot legitimately call a dream a nightmare; what he can do is classify the dream experience according to the reported activity which took place. These reports were obtained quite incidentally to the studies, and written reports are not available. It would have been impossible to compare the EEG and other records against the reports obtained in the mornings, because the REM phase appears several times throughout the night. However, it was noticed that in scoring the records to obtain the REM percentage for the night, the REMs were very much easier to distinguish during the first few records after medication had ceased.

If the eye movements do change, it may be possible to obtain an electrophysiological measure of 'activity'—thereby adding a second dimension to the study of rapid-eye-movement sleep. (This electrophysiological 'activity' is not to be equated with the activity in dream reports though later study may well enable them to be considered as homologous.) Dr. J. I. Evans (personal communication, 1966) has repeated the amylobarbitone experiment mentioned earlier but used a lower dose, 200 mg. instead of 600 mg. Although he obtained results analogous to those

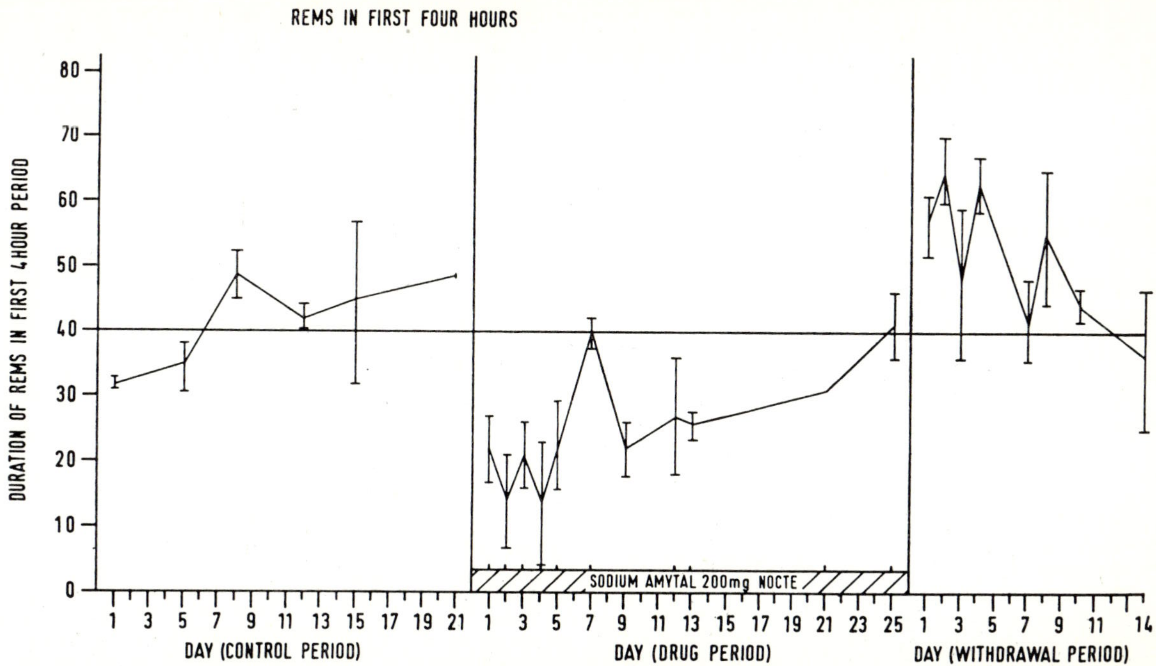

FIG. 2. Analysis of first 4 hours of sleep before, during and after a period of night sedation. Reproduced with the permission of Dr. J. I. Evans.

of Oswald and Priest, but with a shorter time course, his analysis of the percentage of REM sleep in the first 4 hours demonstrated that this was still well above the control values even though the percentage for the whole night had returned to the control value (Fig. 2). This indicates that a more sensitive measure of REM sleep is needed than that previously used in our laboratory.

The eye movements occurring during the paradoxical phase of sleep have several characteristic features (see Fig. 3). For our purposes one of the most important features is that the 'take-off' is always very sudden, between 80° and 90°. We therefore wondered whether in a physiologically very active REM phase or a phenomenologically very active dream there might be an increase in the number of eye movements. Before describing the results of our efforts to count the number of eye movements one or two features of earlier results must be recalled.

One of the effects of amylobarbitone sodium, and of amphetamine, is to delay the onset of the first REM phase. Furthermore, this first REM phase tends to last only about 5 minutes, and has no readily defined starting point or stopping point. We therefore decided to limit the quantifications for this preliminary study to the first REM phase to occur after 4 a.m. (0400 hours). This period tends—whether before, during or after drug administration—to last for about 15 to 45 minutes. A further reason for taking only REM phases after 0400 is that the bursts of eye movements increase in amplitude as the period progresses. Thus at this time maximum REMs were most likely to occur.

Having now outlined our reasons for considering the 'dream periods' described, let us return to the problem of counting the 'take-offs'. As with most electrophysiological records there are slow shifts in the base-line potential. An artificial base-line was therefore drawn parallel to the edge of the paper to facilitate recognition of the eye movements. A cursor with a series of 80° angles marked on it was then moved along this base-line and any pen deflections greater than 80° were marked. A cumulative

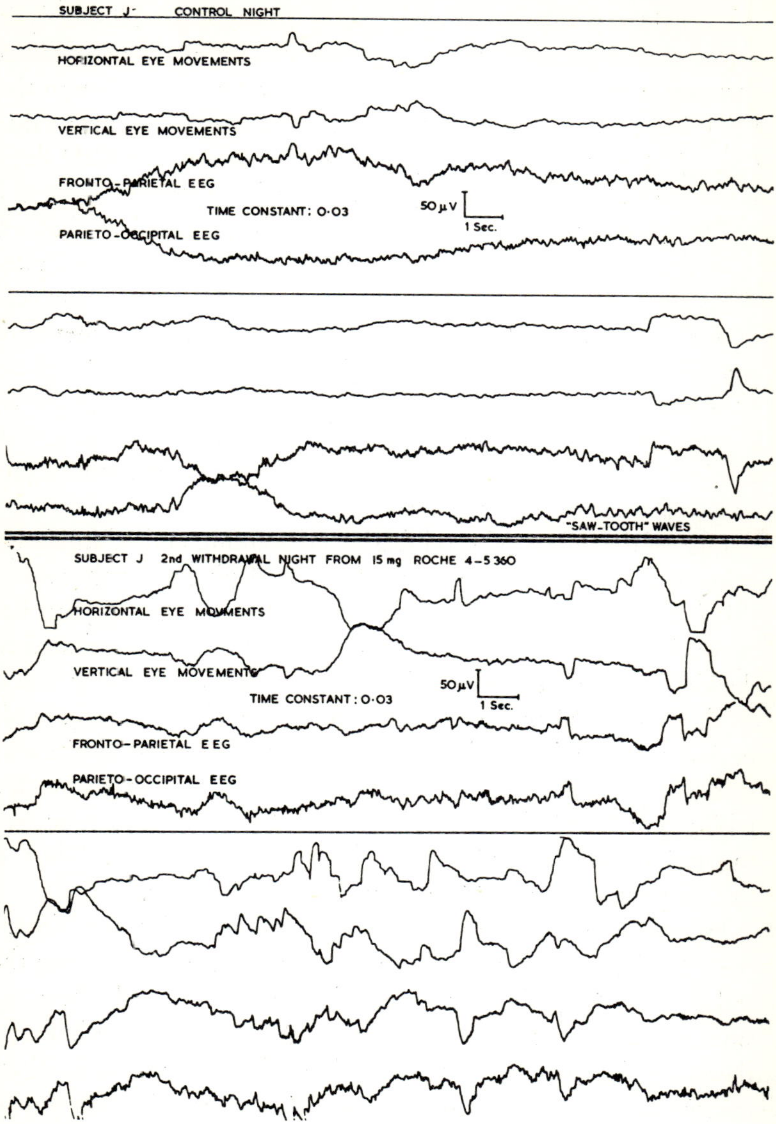

FIG. 3. Two varieties of rapid eye-movements. *Upper record:* short bursts of low amplitude eye potentials. *Lower record:* continuous high amplitude eye potentials after withdrawal of medication with nitrazepam (Mogadon).

count of the number of eye movements is shown in Fig. 4. The rapid eye movements occur in bursts, and plateaux represent time intervals with very few eye movements.

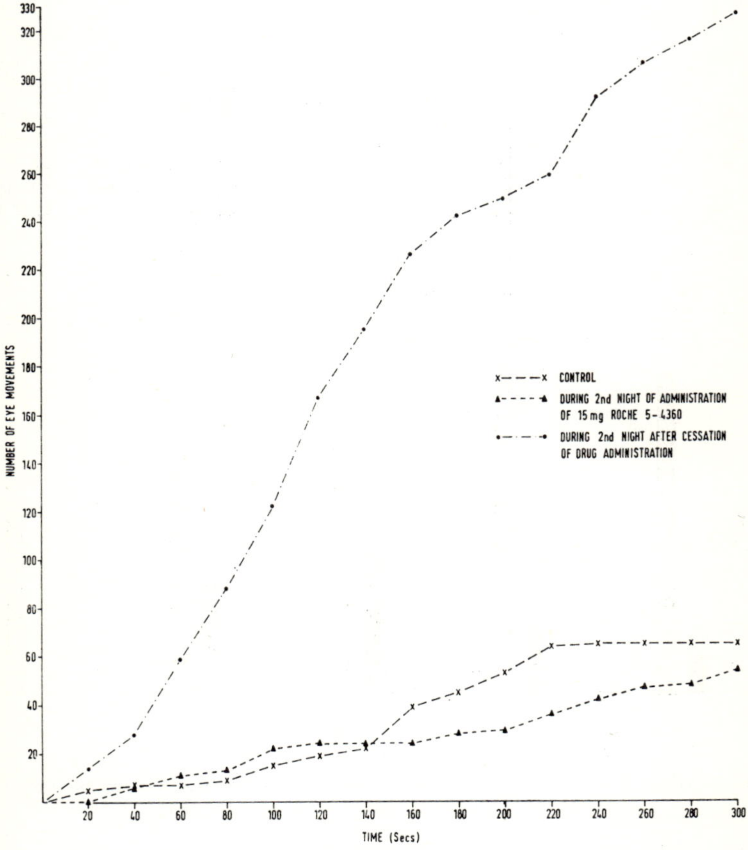

FIG. 4. Cumulative record of eye movement counts for a 5-minute period during a rapid-eye-movement phase of sleep.

More detail can be seen in a histogram of the mean number of eye movements during successive time intervals throughout the REM phase (Fig. 5).

Statistical analysis by Wilcoxon's (1964) variation of Kruskal-Wallis' method of a 5-minute sample of the REM appropriate to the conditions outlined above, was used to compare the number of eye movements occurring in successive 20-second periods.

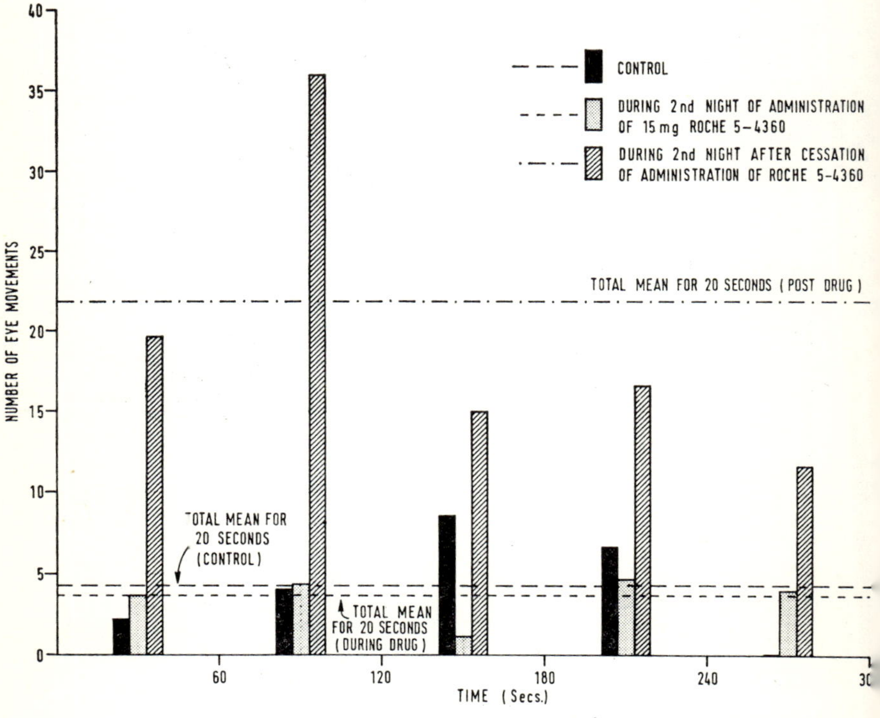

FIG. 5. Mean number of eye movements during successive 20-second periods of 5 minutes of a rapid eye-movement phase of sleep.

Table 1 gives the results of this two-tail ranking method for the comparison of several treatments. The post-drug REM sample is significantly different from both the pre-drug and during-drug samples, but it is surprising that the during-drug sample does not differ significantly from the pre-drug one. Although less of the

Table 1

Analysis of REM count for 20-second intervals of a 5-minute sample from the 1st REM period after 0400 hours

	Sum of ranks	Pre-drug 254·0	During-drug 307·0	Post-drug 556·0
Pre-drug	254·0			
During-drug	307·0	53·0		
Post-drug	556·0	302·0*	249·0*	

* p ⩽ 0·01

night was spent in REM sleep, it does not appear that the periods were any less 'active' on this electrophysiological measure.

A possible explanation for the difference found between the post-drug sample and the other two would be that there was a greater variance in the score per unit of time, i.e. that eye movements come spasmodically and that each burst is more active. Table 2 demonstrates that this hypothesis can be rejected. This means that any increase in the spread of the scores cannot account for the significant increase in the scores for the time unit used. It is, however, still possible that the differences could have arisen from the shortness of the time interval used, 20 seconds. The same statistical test was applied to the data grouped into 1-minute intervals (Table 3); the same statistically significant differences were found. Oswald *et al.* (1963) have described not dissimilar results.

A legitimate criticism of this preliminary attempt at quantification of rapid-eye-movement sleep would be that it takes a 5-minute sample from a REM period ranging in total duration from 34

Table 2

F ratios for standard deviations

	Standard deviation	*df*	*Variance*	*F*	*p*
Pre-drug	1·58	14	0·1343		
During drug	1·6	14	0·1143	1·174	>0·05
Post-drug	3·23	14	0·2307	1·718	>0·05

Table 3

Analysis of REM count for 1-minute intervals of a 5-minute sample from the 1st REM period after 0400 hours

		Pre-drug	During drug	Post-drug
	Sum of ranks	29·5	25·5	65
Pre-drug	29·5			
During drug	25·5	4		
Post-drug	65	35·5*	39·5*	

* $p \leqslant 0.01$

minutes for the post-drug period to 15 minutes for the control period. However, this attempt is only a preliminary to the design of an automatic counter. Manual scoring is tedious and several important variables may well not have been included. For example, when scoring the all-night records for the proportion of the night spent in REM sleep, all the Edinburgh workers have commented that the general voltage level of the eye movements appears to be greater during the first few nights after the subject stops taking the drug. Thus, apart from there being more eye movements at this time, the lateral deviations of the eyes might also be increased. Another difference that has been noticed is that the individual eye movements during drug withdrawal appear to last longer than during control night REM phases, i.e. when the eyes move out of the mid-line they tend to remain out of it for longer during the post-drug phases. As yet these possible variables have merely been remarked upon; no attempt has been made to quantify them.

The manual analysis that I have outlined shows that real differences in the nature of the eye movements can be measured. But manual methods do not attract much enthusiasm and so, with the help of Mr John Foster of the Dept. of Electrical Engineering, Napier Technical College, Edinburgh, we have made a start on automation of the process.

Accepting the same criteria as for the manual analysis, an

analogue computer has been modified to count the eye movements. The machine has a discriminative function built into it. This is necessary since many potentials of cerebral origin are recorded on the eye channel. Thus it would be all too easy to obtain a spuriously large score. The discriminant function operates in such a way that any eye channel potential which occurs in phase with a potential in the parieto-occipital channel is not recorded. A problem which arises with this is that true eye movements of large potential tend to be recorded (as a much lower potential) as far posterior as the parieto-occipital region. This latter recording of the eye movement may be of neural origin or it may be myoclonic as Bickford (e.g. 1964) has suggested in the case of auditory evoked potentials. But whatever its origin, it presents a problem. As yet, the machine is in a very rudimentary stage and has not been tested in the 'real' situation. However, it has been tested using a wave-form generator and will discriminate in-phase and out-of-phase waves. It may be that if the subject wakes during the night the REM counter will register eye blinks that occur since they are of the same order of rise time and of large enough voltage. If this does happen, the experimenter will probably have to count these manually and adjust the total count. His task will, however, be considerably lightened since eye blinks are well defined and not very frequent.

In summary, then, it is gradually becoming possible to show that drugs have effects on rapid-eye-movement sleep. What has in the past seemed to be a state of confusion due to the diversity of the drugs having an apparently similar effect on the proportion of the night spent in REM sleep, may become less chaotic as more detailed analysis of this stage of sleep advances.

Acknowledgements

The work reported was carried out while the author held a Medical Research Council Grant for Training in Research Methods (G 65/1176). The author thanks Professor G. M. Carstairs for making facilities available, and Dr. J. I. Evans for his help and advice in the preparation of the paper.

REFERENCES

Aserinsky, E. and Kleitman, N. (1955). *J. appl. Physiol.*, **8**, 1.

Cody, D. T. R., Jacobson, J. L., Walker, J. C. and Bickford, R. G. (1964). *Ann. Otol. (St. Louis)*, **73**, 164–177.

Lewis, S. A. (1965). Paper read to British Psychological Society (*Bull. Brit. Psychol. Soc.* 1966, **19**, 7A).

Oswald, I. (1964). *In* The Scientific Basis of Medicine Annual Reviews (ed. Paterson Ross, J.). London: Athlone Press.

Oswald, I., Berger, R. J., Jaramillot, R. A., Keddie, K. M. G., Olley, P. C. and Plunkett, G. B. (1963). *Brit. J. Psychiat.*, **109**, 66–78.

Oswald, I. and Priest, R. G. (1965). *Brit. med. J.*, **ii**, 1093–1099.

Wilcoxon, F. and Wilcoxon, R. A. (1964). Some rapid approximate statistical procedures. Lederle Laboratories, American Cyanamid Company, Pearl River, N.Y.

THE INFLUENCE OF DRUGS ON DREAMS*

MILTON KRAMER, ROY M. WHITMAN,
BILL BALDRIDGE, and PAUL H. ORNSTEIN,

Department of Psychiatry, University of Cincinnati, Ohio

Introduction

THE discovery in 1953 by Aserinsky and Kleitman (4–6) that dreaming was accompanied by conjugate rapid eye movements, which Trumbull Ladd had suggested 60 years before (95), has led to the elaboration of the sleep-dream cycle (18, 20, 22, 26–29, 87, 88, 113, 164, 165). It has been repeatedly confirmed that in the adult a dream episode occurs about every 90 minutes (26, 29, 42, 135) during sleep. The dream is the psychological manifestation (6, 18, 27, 43, 48, 123, 134, 137, 164, 165) of a state of total activation (8, 88) which includes conjugate rapid eye movements, autonomic irregularities (3, 5, 21, 80, 137, 140, 141) in the respiratory and cardiovascular system, a decrease in postural muscle tone (12, 21, 74), and an emergent Stage I EEG which is characterized by a low-voltage fast activity free of spindling (4–6).

The first dream of the night comes on about 1–2 hours after sleep onset (39, 58) and the dream periods vary from 15–60 minutes in length (39). The cycles get longer as the night progresses (26, 27). An adult spends about 20–25% of his time asleep in the dream state (2, 125, 144). When subjects are awakened from these rapid-eye-movement (REM) periods, the recall of dreaming is

* This paper has appeared under the title of 'The Pharmacology of Dreaming' in *Enzymes in Mental Health*, edited by Gustav J. Martin, Sc.D., and Bruno Kisch, M.D., published by J. B. Lippincott Co., 1966.

six to eight times greater than if they are awakened during non-rapid-eye-movement—periods (6, 18, 27, 43, 48, 123, 134, 137, 164, 165).

Because of its unique qualities along so many parameters, Snyder has characterized this state of the organism as the third organismic state (39, 74, 114, 135, 138). This designation of a part of sleep as a third state underlines its difference from both the waking state and non-dreaming sleep. In this third state, the organism's responsiveness to external stimuli is different from what it is either during waking or during the non-dreaming portion of sleep (11, 26, 61, 115, 162, 163).

The notion that there is a third organismic state is supported both by phylogenetic (1, 22, 26, 69, 72, 86, 105, 127, 133, 136, 138, 149, 151) and ontogenetic studies (2, 117, 125, 126, 144). So far all mammals that have been studied, and these include the rat (105, 149), mouse (149), sheep (68), goat (127), cat (22), dog (133), rabbit (86, 130, 149), monkey (151), chimpanzee (1) and opossum (138), have demonstrated the existence of this third state. A homologous pattern has been observed in birds (72, 142) but not in reptiles (72, 136). In newborn animals the percentage of sleep spent in this state is high (39, 58, 135); with maturity it decreases (125). It is estimated that at about 24–30 weeks gestational age in the human foetus, 100% of sleep is in this third state; in the 1-day-old neonate, 50% (117, 126).

How is the striking periodicity of the dream-sleep cycle regulated? In a series of experiments utilizing transection at various brain levels and direct electrical stimulation, Jouvet (70, 73, 74, 77) has shown that a centre in the ventral pons (nucleus pontis caudalis) initiates the activated state of which the dream is the psychological accompaniment. This centre is near the ascending reticular activating system of the pons, but lies ventral to it and has separate cerebral connections. This pontine centre fires anteriorly along a ponto-limbic pathway (Nauta) and posteriorly along a ponto-bulbar path. These ponto-bulbar connections account for the concomitant autonomic and muscular manifestations of the REM state.

The delineation of the anatomical centre and pathways which govern the initiation of the third organismic state does not tell us what mechanisms might serve to stimulate or act as a trigger to this pontine centre. Jouvet and Mounier (78), noting a lag between stimulation of the pontine centre and initiation of the REM state, as well as a refractory period of 10–15 minutes before another period could be initiated, suggested that some neurohumoral mechanism was involved in initiating the action of the REM state centre.

Speculations about the possible neurohumoral mechanisms involved in REM state initiation have been contradictory and confusing. Effects found in one species have not been found in other species. However, experimental work has shown that both cholinergic and adrenergic mechanisms are involved. The REM state can be initiated or sustained by cholinergic drugs (47, 55, 63, 76, 78), blocked or reduced by anti-cholinergic drugs (78, 150), and stimulated by noradrenaline (102a) or its precursor DOPA (103).

Two other substances (58, 148) have been implicated as possible neuromodulators in the triggering of the REM state if not as actual neurotransmitters. These are γ-aminobutyric acid (GABA) and 5-hydroxytryptamine (5-HT).

The REM state can be initiated by sodium butyrate and related short-chain fatty acids (75, 104). Naturally occurring rises and falls have been found in serum free fatty acids (FFA) in man associated with REM state (131). These rises and falls in FFA correlate with the anxiety expressed in the dream reports from the REM periods as measured by a verbal anxiety scale (50).

The work on 5-HT is perhaps the most confusing of all. Hartmann (58) has noted an increase in REM time and Azima (7) observed increased dream reporting in subjects given reserpine, a substance which reduces brain 5-HT. Mandell *et al.* (101) have noted an increase in REM time in man given 5-hydroxytryptophan (5-HTP), a precursor of 5-HT. In contrast, Spooner and Winters (142) gave 5-HTP to chicks and stimulated only slow-wave sleep. Jouvet and Matsumato (103) by giving cats reserpine reduced slow-wave sleep and abolished REM sleep. They then gave 5-HTP to these reserpine-treated cats and induced only slow-wave sleep.

A neurohumoral mechanism is undoubtedly involved in the stimulation of the REM state. Possible roles have been suggested for acetylcholine, noradrenaline, GABA, and 5-HT in REM state regulation. The function of these substances in the natural ocurrence of the REM state remains uncertain.

Besides the exploration of substances which may be neurohumours in affecting the REM state, the role of hormones in the initiation and cessation of the REM state has been investigated. Secretions of the pituitary, for example, do have effects on the third organismic state. Anterior pituitary products such as the gonadotrophins (129, 130) can initiate and corticotrophin (84) can block the appearance of REM state in the rabbit. However, both Weitzman (152) and the Mandells (102) report changes in 17-OH corticoids which would be consistent with corticotrophin secretion in the REM state. Before the REM era of dream research, Finley (38) had pointed out changes in dream content associated with giving a patient pituitary and adrenal extract, and Kant (81) had suggested using changes in dream content to monitor the effects of hormone therapy in psychiatric patients. Antidiuretic hormone (ADH), a posterior pituitary secretion, has been shown to initiate the REM state in animals (34) and ADH effects have been demonstrated in man (102) at the start of a REM period.

The role of gonadal hormones in the REM state has also been investigated. Sawyer and his co-workers (129, 130) report the stimulation of REM state in the rabbit with luteinizing hormone. Hartmann (58) was able to show a cyclic variation in REM time associated with the menstrual cycle; it was longest in the late progestational phase. Benedek and Rubenstein (10) had earlier demonstrated a cyclic variation in dream content associated with various hormonal phases of the menstrual cycle.

The recognition of the existence of the third organismic state has led to inquiries concerning its possible function in the adaptive economy of the organism. The most striking approach in this field has been made in experimentally depriving subjects of this dreaming portion of sleep. Dement and Fisher (19, 23–25, 40–42) found that trying to reduce a subject's dreaming required more frequent awakenings on successive nights (from 7 on the first night to 30 on the fifth night) because of earlier and earlier dream onset. They noted that after several nights (4 to 7), of such efforts at dream deprivation, the subject's behaviour showed increased anxiety and startle reaction, increased irritability and hostility, increased difficulty in memory, concentration and motor coordination, and increased appetite. Using photic stimulation on dream-deprived subjects, they were able to show a heightened tendency to the development of hallucinations. None of these effects were obtained from control groups in which subjects were awakened a similar number of times during non-dreaming sleep.

Findings of behavioural change were not noted in all subjects in whom dream deprivation was attempted (139). The individual's response to dream deprivation is probably related to his specific vulnerability to dream deprivation and to the difficulty, if not impossibility, of achieving total deprivation. The impact on behaviour of sleep deprivation in man (153) and total REM deprivation in animals (71) sheds some further light on the possible adaptive function of the REM state.

Total sleep deprivation results, after about 100–120 hours, in psychotic phenomena, including hallucinations and delusions. As in the dream deprivation studies, hunger and increased appetite are stimulated. But most importantly, it was observed in totally sleep-deprived subjects that, especially at night, these psychotic phenomena occurred every 90–120 minutes, the length of the usual dream cycle. One possible implication might be that the psychotic phenomena in sleep deprivation are a break-through of the dream hallucination into waking life because of the deprivation of REM state that accompanies total sleep loss.

Jouvet achieved total REM-state deprivation in cats by destroying the pontine triggering centre. Many of these cats showed 'hallucinatory-like' behaviour and ate ravenously. One such animal, with a complete lesion of his pontine centre, lived for 30 days without paradoxical sleep, finally became insomniac and overactive, with increased heart rate and decreased body temperature, and died in a 'manic state'.

The intriguing, if ancient, hypothesis (33) is again suggested to us that the hallucination is the break-through of dreaming into waking life. The invitation to study the dream, to learn about hallucinations, to solve the problem of psychosis is again offered by the new work on the sleep-dream cycle. Unfortunately, the work of Rechtschaffen (122), comparing the state of the waking schizophrenic to that of the dreamer, yielded negative results. Consistent changes in REM time in depressed (32, 53, 60, 114) and schizophrenic patients (36, 37, 56, 90) could not be found. Nevertheless, 70% of psychiatric patients have sleep disturbances (31), and Hartmann (58) has suggested that this insomnia, with its concurrent REM-state deprivation, may account for some of the behavioural changes and hallucinations which accompany acute psychotic episodes.

Drug studies

Realizing that suppression of the REM state leads to disturbed behaviour, one becomes intrigued to explore the possible effects of drugs on the dream-sleep cycle. Particularly one wonders about the effects on the dream state of drugs, such as the tranquillizers, which are known to modify anxiety, hallucinations and delusions. The anatomical proximity of the supposed locus of action of the tranquillizers to that of the dream-initiating centre stirs curiosity all the more about the possible effects of these drugs on dreaming.

Clinical reports of the effect of tranquillizers on dreams (7, 16, 96) suggested a stimulation of dream recall early in the treatment process, with such major tranquillizers as chlorpromazine and reserpine, followed by a gradual suppression of the ability to recall dreams as drug treatment continued. With a minor tranquillizer such as meprobamate, most (132) but not all (119) studies report a decrease in dream recall. However, these reports were of morning dream recall, without waking the patient to report his dreams or monitoring the time spent in dreaming. Our own work on dream recall (157) indicates that this process of reporting dreams is so influenced by intra- and interpersonal factors that an adequate estimate of dream time cannot be based on morning dream-recall frequency. Nevertheless, clues about patterns of effects are available from reports of morning dream-recall (i.e. the increase and decrease of dream recall by major tranquillizers described in morning reports of remembered dreams was later confirmed with REM time studies.) In reviews (65, 82, 91, 112, 158) over the last 5 years of the English-language literature on tranquillizing drugs, by ourselves and our departmental colleagues, the effect of tranquillizing drugs on dream recall is strikingly absent.

A. *REM time studies*

1. *Psychotropic drugs*

Phenothiazine tranquillizers such as chlorpromazine (36, 62) and trifluoperazine (42) tend to have similar effects on REM time which are related to dose and duration of administration. In large doses and over short periods, namely one to two nights, these drugs tend to stimulate an increase in REM time because of an atypical Stage I EEG period at the onset of sleep; chronically administered, and perhaps in more modest doses, these drugs tend to decrease REM time about 15% and even more markedly to reduce the frequency of eye movements.

The work on reserpine is contradictory. In man, Hartmann (59) has reported an increase in REM time; while in cats, Jouvet (103) has described a total suppression of REM state.

Meprobamate is the only minor tranquillizer reported on so far with which the eye movement technique has been used. Meprobamate seems to reduce the amount of time spent dreaming (44) as well as the frequency of dream episodes (159).

Thus both major tranquillizers (chlorpromazine, trifluoperazine, and perhaps reserpine) and minor ones (meprobamate) tend to suppress dream time. This would lend support to a hypothesis that sees the action of a tranquillizer on psychotic symptoms as a function of the suppressant effect of those drugs on some subcortical centres which may control the production of the hallucination, of the dream, and of psychosis. We have suggested this suppressant action as the mechanism of action for both the tranquillizers and the antidepressants (158).

Some studies on an antidepressant, imipramine (147, 161) have noted a decrease in dream frequency and dream time which supports the proposed suppressant function of the psychotropic drugs. Other work on imipramine noted no effect on REM time (128). A study in cats of a hydrazine monoamine oxidase (MAO) inhibitor noted only a decrease in slow-wave (non-REM) sleep (103).

2. *Psychotogens*

The initial studies of the effects of drugs on the third organismic state were at least partially determined by speculations which related the dream to psychotic phenomena, particularly hallucinations. Similarly, with the psychotogens, the interest in their effect on the REM state was invited by the presumed similarity between the hallucinations induced by them and those which occurred in the dream. Investigators wondered if the mechanism underlying the hallucination in the two states—psychedelic and dreaming—were perhaps similar. This view of similarity was held despite the descriptive differences in hallucinations in the two states pointed out by Bliss and Clark (13) and the striking discrepancy in the colourful description given by Weir Mitchell (107) of his visual experiences with mescal and Peter Knapp's (89) characterization of the typical dream as like a silent, black and white movie.

The psychotogens are hallucinogenic substances and might be expected to produce an increase of REM state if the underlying mechanism of dreams and hallucinations are the same. The suppressant effect of the tranquillizers on psychotogenically induced hallucinations and on REM state would tend to encourage a view that the mechanism of formation of the hallucination in both are similar.

Lysergide (LSD) has been the psychotogen studied for its effect on REM state, and the results are contradictory. Muzio (109) and Green (51) both noted that the drug was capable of selectively lengthening one of the REM periods to a significant degree. Muzio noted a slight increase in total REM time, while Green, in a single case report, noted a marked increase in REM time. Interestingly, Green observed a rebound increase on the night after the drug was given, which would be associated with REM suppression rather than stimulation. Hobson (64) noted no increase in REM time in cats given lysergide, though the dosage he gave may have been excessive and arousal effects may have then predominated. Lysergide seems to stimulate both arousal and REM state, i.e. both the ascending reticular system and the ponto-limbic system.

Evarts' (33) reminder that not all hallucinatory phenomena need be a function of the same neurophysiological mechanism may well be in order, not only in these, but in all studies in this general area.

3. *Alcohol*

Continuing to pursue the possible relationship between psychotic-like states with hallucinations and dreaming, investigators have become interested in the effects of alcohol on REM state because hallucinations commonly occur in delirium tremens.

Interestingly, the Iroquois Indians have used alcohol to stimulate dreaming as part of their 'Vision Quest' (15). These Indians saw the intoxicated state as indistinguishable from the dream state.

Gresham *et al.* (54) have demonstrated that alcohol depresses REM time in normal subjects. Greenberg and Pearlman (52) noted a 40% REM time in patients with delirium tremens which persisted for up to a week after alcohol withdrawal. They were not sure whether they were getting a rebound phenomenon from prior alcohol suppression of dream time alone or whether dream deprivation was compounded with sleep deprivation.

The hallucinated state in delirium tremens could be a breakthrough of the dream state into the waking state. The resultant picture then becomes a mixture of the two usually separate states of the organism (58).

4. *Stimulants and depressants*

Given the anatomical proximity of the dream centre to the ascending reticular activating system and the similarity of the emergent Stage I EEG to the EEG in arousal, studies have been performed which reasoned that stimulants should increase REM time and that depressants should reduce it. (The previously discussed work on lysergide is an example of the effect of a stimulant, and alcohol of a depressant, on the REM state.)

Many studies on various barbiturates (23, 36, 62, 114) have noted a reduction in dream time and eye movement frequency in patients taking these drugs. It is of clinical interest that in psychiatric patients Detre *et al.* (31) noted that those who had been taking barbiturates made more suicide attempts than those who had not. Were their suicide attempts related to a disturbance enhanced by their barbiturate-induced dream deprivation?

Studies on stimulants have included an examination of the effects on REM time of caffeine (54) and amphetamine (116, 121). Caffeine given to normal volunteers had no effect on REM time, but the dosage may have been insufficient.

Amphetamine on the other hand reduced dream time abruptly in normal volunteers (121). In chronic users of amphetamine the REM time was normal (116). However, in such chronic users, when the amphetamine was withdrawn, there was a rebound increase of up to 48% REM time. The overall effect of amphetamine is to suppress dream time. The psychosis seen in amphetamine addicts may come on as a result of chronic amphetamine suppression of dream time, analogous to the situation in extended sleep deprivation. An alternative view is that the amphetamine psychosis results from the rebound increase in dream time during the withdrawal period with the break-through of the dream into the waking state, analogous to what has been reported in delirium tremens.

The vivid reports of dreams from literary figures such as DeQuincey (30) and Coleridge (17), both of whom were addicted to opiates, raise questions about the possible dream-stimulating qualities of opium and its derivatives. There is a suggestion in the literature that the vividness of a dream may be a function of dream time (2, 97).

In a heroin addict Kaufman *et al.* (83) noted a high dream time during addiction, which fell during withdrawal. The authors suggest that the narcotic may be a stimulant of REM state. Roffwarg (124), however, reports no change in REM time in an addict withdrawn on methadone rather than morphine.

The vividness of dreams induced by opiates remains unexplained (67). The reports on the influence of opium and its derivatives on the REM state are too anecdotal to permit conclusions.

Stimulation of dreams by various anaesthetic gases has been reported (35, 66, 98–100, 108), but no study of REM time during such gas-induced states is available. There is a distinct possibility that REM state may be obliterated during prolonged deep anaesthesia (14).

B. *Dream content studies*

Much less attention has been paid to the impact of drugs on the psychological content of dreams than to the effect of drugs on the physiology of the REM state. Rechtschaffen (120) has aptly observed: 'If we don't keep our attention on the psychology of the dream, we might find out a lot of biology without knowing very well what it is the biology of.'

Before the REM state was discovered, observations had been made on the effect of tranquillizers on dream frequency and dream content (7, 16, 96, 119, 132). Of course, these were all morning recall studies. Lesse (96) gives a detailed report of the effect of chlorpromazine and promazine on dreams. He noted an initial stimulation of dream recall in anxious patients given phenothiazine tranquillizers. This increased recall or awareness of dreams was associated with the period of initial anxiety reduction in the patient. Reduction in a patient's anxiety was often preceded by a decrease of excessive motor activity in his dreams.

Lesse further observed, in patients taking the phenothiazine tranquillizers, that the emotional impact of the dream was altered before the dream content was affected. After anxiety had been reduced to a certain level, specific for the individual patient, the dream content began to change. As the anxiety of the patient was reduced to pre-morbid levels, the dream recall also returned to what was usual for the patient.

Cohen (16) confirmed that chlorpromazine can stimulate dream recall. A similar increase in dream recall was observed by Azima (7) with reserpine and by Prigot *et al.* (119) in patients receiving meprobamate. Selling (132) found that meprobamate suppressed dream recall when disturbing dreams were the source of the patient's complaint.

Cohen, Azima and Prigot have all remarked that patients on drugs report their dreams as more vivid than usual. Azima studied the content of dreams produced by patients while on reserpine and on a placebo. He could not detect any difference in dream content between the drug and placebo states. Cohen pointed out that the anxiety in the dreams of patients on chlorpromazine was disproportionately small. Similarly, Prigot observed that the dreams reported by patients receiving meprobamate were seldom frightening.

Workers with psychotogens have not reported the content of their subjects' dreams, but they have reported the content of their subjects' hallucinatory experiences. Bliss and Clark (13) have excellently summarized the descriptive differences in the hallucination of the dreamer, of the schizophrenic, of the sleep-deprived, and of the subject given lysergide. The difference has already been noted between Weir Mitchell's (107) description of his mescal-induced visions and Knapp's (89) characterization of the dream.

The dreams of patients with delirium tremens have not been specifically investigated, though their hallucinations of snakes, bugs, and elephants are common knowledge. We could not find reports of the effects of caffeine, the barbiturates or amphetamine on dream content. Detre (31) has reported a decrease of dream recall in patients taking barbiturates.

Finley (38) reported the effects on dream recall and dream content of pituitary and adrenal extract. While receiving pituitary extract, the patient recalled dreams more frequently and more vividly. The dreams were generally delightful, colourful and filled with hope. When the patient then received adrenal extract the dreams were less vivid, less easily recalled, and totally colourless. They were all unpleasant and filled with anger and fear.

Benedek (10) obtained dreams and vaginal smears from patients in psychoanalysis. She could predict the hormonal phase of the menstrual cycle from the content of the patients' dreams.

Opium and its derivatives have been reported to increase the vividness and colourfulness of dreams (17, 30, 67). DeQuincey has given a highly literary description of the effect of opium on dreams in "Confessions of an English Opium Eater" (30). He summarized the effects of opium on his dreams as being four-fold: (1) it greatly increased the splendour of the dream; (2) it enhanced the anxious, melancholic feeling in the dream; (3) it greatly expanded space and time in the dream; and (4) it led to the recall of childhood incidents in the dream which would never have been recaptured by him while awake. Coleridge in his "Literary Reminiscences" suggests that the inspiration for his poem "Kubla Khan" came to him in an opium-stimulated dream (17).

Interestingly, the problem-solving function of the dream was noted by Mittelman (108) in the dreams of one patient who dealt repetitively, in several dreams induced by anaesthesia, with his reaction to being put to sleep, The problem-solving function and sequential relationship in dreams had been dealt with by Freud (46), Jung (79), Stekel (143), French (45), and Hall (57) in the pre-REM era; and by Trosman (146), Offenkrantz (111), Rechtschaffen (120) and our group in Cincinnati (94) using the REM technique.

The essentially anecdotal reports of dreams recalled after gas-induced states concern themselves mainly with the cosmic nature of the experience (35, 66, 98, 108). Oliver Wendell Holmes (66) described one such gas-induced dream, in which 'the veil of eternity was lifted, the one great truth that underlies all human experience flashed upon him in a sudden revelation'. He noted that children may smile, but that wise men will ponder. Describing his dream of revelation he notes: 'A strong smell of turpentine prevails throughout.'

Tart (145) has observed that research on the effect of drugs on dream content is 'still very exploratory and no definite conclusions can be drawn'. Nevertheless, we would like to report the studies of our research group at the University of Cincinnati on the effects of drugs on dream content (92, 93, 154, 155, 159–161). Keeping Dr. Holmes' insight firmly in mind, our dream research group has primarily focused on the study of the *content of dreams* rather than on the *physiological process of dreaming* Certainly our therapeutic orientation has considerably influenced and guided our work in this direction. We feel that as poetry will never be completely understood in electrophysiological terms, dreams cannot be explained solely from a description of eye movements and activated Stage I EEG's. Even 'granting the physiological and biological primacy of REM sleep, we are still left with the problem of the function of the concomitant psychic activity of dreaming, which cannot simply be reduced to the underlying somatic and physico-chemical processes. What Seymour Kety (85) said about memory, that we may sometimes have a biochemistry of memory but never of memo*ries*, holds true for dreaming and dreams' (39) as well.

Initially we have tried to use the dream, now that the vagaries of dream recall could be substantially bypassed, to examine the psychological shifts which accompany the taking of tranquillizing drugs. As clinicians, we view the dream as representing the most significant, condensed, psychological product of the organism (154). Our intent was to *psychoassay* the newer drugs by examining their effects on dream content. To this end we have studied the influence on dream content of various types of psychoactive drugs: prochlorperazine (161), a phenothiazine tranquillizer; imipramine (92, 93, 161), an antidepressant; meprobamate (159), a minor tranquillizer; and phenobarbitone, a sedative (161).

After recording baseline nights of dreaming, we start the subject on medication, and finally obtain additional dreams from the subject after he has taken the drug for at least several days. The subjects sleep in our laboratory at either the General Hospital or the V.A. Hospital in Cincinnati. Dreaming is determined by eye-movement indicators (9). Subjects are awakened to report dreams after 5 minutes of dreaming to keep the dream reports somewhat comparable (49). The subject reports his dream into a tape-recorder from which typed scripts are prepared. These typed dream reports are then rated along seven dimensions using rating scales we have devised (161). The dimensions along which the dreams are rated include hostility, dependency, heterosexuality, homosexuality, anxiety, intimacy and motility.

The psychoassay of tranquillizing drugs has yielded some interesting results. The most striking finding is the tendency of imipramine to stimulate the expression of hostility in dreams (161). We speculated that this increase of hostility discharge in dreams could result in a reduction of aggressive instinctual pressure. If this were so, then the discharge of hostility in the fantasy of the dream might be linked with the antidepressant effects of imipramine. Our idea is that the blocked self-directed aggression, so common in the depressed, was finding some release in the hostility expressed in dreams. Our work on enuresis (118), in which enuretic episodes were found to substitute for dream periods, supports this notion that the dream has a discharge function.

The major specific effect on dream content that we found for meprobamate (159) could also be seen as an example of the discharge function of the dream. Scores on the motility scale were significantly raised above the baseline in a subject taking meprobamate. This change may perhaps reflect a compensatory discharge of motility in the dream resulting from the alleged muscle-relaxant properties of meprobamate blocking motor discharge via peripheral motor channels.

Both imipramine and meprobamate led to a decrease in the number of dreams reported per night. This may relate to the suppression of REM time described for most tranquillizing medication (36, 42, 62, 103).

Phenobarbitone and prochlorperazine tended to increase the scores on the sexual scales, the former on the homosexual scale and the latter on the heterosexual scale (161), but these trends did not reach statistical significance. Nevertheless, we wondered if phenobarbitone, because of its relaxant qualities, might have fostered a passive state which was reflected in expressions of homosexuality in the dream. This does not fit our thesis of the discharge quality of the dream which we have described above. The tendency for prochlorperazine to elevate heterosexual scores remains unexplained.

A series of identical changes occurred in several of the other scales with all the drugs studied (159, 161). These changes were probably related less to the pharmacological effect of the medication and more to the experimental setting and the doctor-patient relationship engendered by the giving of drugs. With all the drugs a rise occurred in scores on the anxiety and dependency scales and a decrease on the intimacy scale. The experimental setting tends to provoke anxiety and stimulates many concerns which are inevitably reflected in the dreams of the subjects (160). The distancing implied by a decrease in intimacy scores could well be seen as the defensive manoeuvre of an anxious patient (93, 156). That being given a tablet would foster an increase in dependency is to be expected, as it often raises hopes of further care from the giver. The introduction of medication into the doctor-patient relationship could tend to decrease the intimacy of the relationship.

We feel encouraged that by utilizing the dream, the most central intrapsychic product of the organism, we can, by quantifying the psychological forces in the dream along traditional psychological vectors, begin to evaluate the psychological effects of the tranquillizing drugs in a meaningful way.

The striking effect of imipramine on the dreams of normal

subjects led us to study its effect on the dreams of the depressed (92, 93). We obtained two nights of dreaming from ten depressed patients while they were on an imipramine placebo. They were then switched to the active medication and had their dreams collected one night a week for three additional weeks. At the end of the fourth week when the last dreams were collected, all the patients had improved.

We could not demonstrate any shift concurrent with clinical improvement in the frequency of dream recall or in any of the dream theme parameters we examined. These parameters included themes of hopelessness, helplessness, low self-regard, deprivation, self-criticism and self-blame, overwhelming problems and duties, self-commands and injunctions, and escape and suicide. We have not yet examined these dreams to explore for possible shifts in hostility expression concomitant with clinical improvement.

It is clear from our observations of the dreams of depressed patients, as reflected in dream-recall percentages and various dream themes, that their dreams do not mirror their waking clinical state. Apparently the dream lags qualitatively behind the clinical state in indicating change. If the intrapsychic indicators do ultimately change, one might consider that the lag reflects the still precarious adaptation of the depressed patient. If this is so, decisions about recovery and readiness for discharge from the hospital should take this fact into account.

As has been indicated, the primary interest of our group in Cincinnati is in the dream more than in dreaming. We cannot accept Nelson's comment made in 1888 (110), which seems echoed today in the flurry of studies on dream time with little or no interest in dream content, that it's not what you dream that matters but only how much.

A piece of verse by a graduate student (106) may explain our romantic commitment to the richness of dream content rather than to the sterility of dream time:

One mystery alone remains
Of my beloved's sleep:
We've solved the movement of her eyes
And why they do repeat,
We know what brings her breath in sighs,
We've tracked her EEG;
The haunting doubt that still remains
Is does she dream of me?

What better reason could one have?

REFERENCES

APSS is the abbreviation for the Association for the Psychophysiological Study of Sleep.

*These publications are excellent review works on the current research in sleep and dreams.

1. Adey, W. R., Kado, R. and Rhodes, J. (1963). Sleep: Cortical and subcortical recordings in the chimpanzee. *Science*, **141**, 932–933.
2. Antrobus, J. S., Dement, W. and Fisher, C. (1964). Patterns of dreaming recall: An EEG study. *J. abnorm. soc. Psychol.*, **69**, 341–344.
3. Aserinsky, E. (1965). Periodic respiratory pattern occurring in conjunction with eye movements during sleep. *Science*, **150**, 763–766.
4. Aserinsky, E. and Kleitman, N. (1955). A motility cycle in sleeping infants as manifested by ocular and gross bodily activity. *J. appl. Physiol.*, **8**, 11.
5. Aserinsky, E. and Kleitman, N. (1953). Regularly occurring periods of eye motility and concomitant phenomena during sleep. *Science*, **118**, 273.
6. Aserinsky, E. and Kleitman, N. (1955). Two types of ocular motility occurring in sleep. *J. appl. Physiol.*, **8**, 1.
7. Azima, H. (1958). The possible dream inducing capacity of the whole root of *Rauwolfia Serpentina*. *Canad. psychiat. Assoc. J.*, **3**, 47–51.
8. Baldridge, B. J., Whitman, R. M. and Kramer, M. (1965). The concurrence of fine muscle activity and rapid eye movements during sleep. *Psychom. Med.*, **27**, 19–26.
9. Baldridge, B. J., Whitman, R. M. and Kramer, M. (1963). A simplified method for detecting eye movements during dreaming. *Psychosom. Med.*, **25**, 78–82.

10. Benedek, T. and Rubenstein, B. B. (1952). Psychosexual Functions in Women. New York: Ronald Press Co.
11. Berger, R. J. (1963). Experimental modification of dream content by meaningful verbal stimuli. *Brit. J. Psychiat.*, **109,** 722–740.
12. Berger, R. J. (1961). Tonus of extrinsic laryngeal muscles during sleep and dreaming. *Science*, **134,** 840.
13. Bliss, E. L. and Clark, L. D. (1959). Visual Hallucinations. *In* Hallucinations (ed. West, L. J.) New York: Grune and Stratton.
14. Brazier, M. B. (1964). The effect of drugs on the electroencephalogram of man. *Clin. Pharmacol. Ther.*, **5,** 102–116.
15. Carpenter, E. S. (1959). Alcohol in the Iroquois dream quest. *Amer. J. Psychiat.*, **116,** 148–151.
16. Cohen, I. M. (1956). Complications of chlorpromazine therapy. *Amer. J. Psychiat.*, **113,** 1115–1121.
17. Coleridge, S. T. (1947). How a dream inspired the poem 'Kubla Khan'. *In* The World of Dreams (ed. Woods, R. L.), pp. 859–862. New York: Random House.
18. Dement, W. (1955). Dream recall and eye movements during sleep in schizophrenics and normals. *J. nerv. ment. Dis.*, **122,** 263.
19. Dement, W. (1960). The effect of dream deprivation. *Science*, **131,** 1705.
20. *Dement, W. C. (1964). Experimental Dream Studies. *In* Science and Psychoanalysis (ed. Masserman, J.), vol. 7, pp. 129–184. New York: Grune and Stratton.
21. Dement, W. C. (1964). Eye movements during sleep. *In* The Oculomotor System (ed. Bender, M.). New York: Harper and Row.
22. Dement, W. (1958). The occurrence of low voltage, fast electroencephalogram patterns during behavioral sleep in the cat. *Electroenceph. clin. Neurophysiol.*, **10,** 291–296.
23. Dement, W. and Fisher, C. (1963). Experimental interference with the sleep cycle. *Canad. psychiat. Assoc. J.*, **8,** 395–400.
24. Dement, W. and Fisher, C. (1960). Studies in dream deprivation and satiation. *Psychoanal. Quart.*, **29,** 671.
25. Dement, W. and Fisher, C. (1960). Studies in dream deprivation and satiation. An experimental demonstration of the necessity for dreaming. *Bull. Phila. Assoc. Psychoanal.*, **10,** 30.
26. Dement, W. and Kleitman, N. (1957). Cyclic variations in EEG during sleep and their relation to eye movements, body motility, and dreaming. *Electroenceph. clin. Neurophysiol.*, **1,** 673–690.
27. Dement, W. and Kleitman, N. (1957). The relation of eye movements during sleep to dream activity: an objective method for the study of dreaming. *J. exp. Psychol.*, **53,** 339–346.
28. Dement, W. and Wolpert, E. A. (1958). The relation of eye movements, body motility and external stimuli to dream content. *J. exp. Psychol.*, **55,** 543–553.

29. Dement, W. and Wolpert, E. A. (1958). Relationships in the manifest content of dreams occurring on the same night. *J. nerv. ment. Dis.*, **126,** 568–578,

30. DeQuincey, T. (1947). The Dreams of the English Opium Eater. *In* The World of Dreams (ed. Woods, R. L.), pp. 863–870. New York: Random House.

31. Detre, T., Davis, J. and Spaulding, P. (1965). Sleep disturbance in mental patients. APSS, Washington, D.C.

32. Diaz-Guerro, R., Gottlieb, J. S. and Knott, J. R. (1946). The sleep of patients with manic-depressive psychosis, depressive type. *Psychosom. Med.*, **8,** 399–404.

33. Evarts, E. V. (1962). A neurophysiologic theory of hallucinations. *In* Hallucinations (ed. West, L.). New York: Grune and Stratton.

34. Faure, J. (1962). La phase 'paradoxale' du sommeil chez le lapin (ses relations neurohormonales). *Rev. neurol.*, **106,** 190–196.

35. Federn, P. (1944). A dream under general anesthesia: studies in egocathexis. *Psychiat. Quart.*, **18,** 422–438.

36. Feinberg, I., Koresko, R., Gottlieb, F. and Wender, P. H. (1964). Sleep electroencephalographic and eye movement patterns in schizophrenic patients. *Comprehens. Psychiat.*, **5,** 44–53.

37. Feinberg, I., Koresko, R., Heller, N. and Steinberg, H.R. (1965). Case report: Unusually high dream time in an hallucinating patient. *Amer. J. Psychiat.*, **121,** 1018–1020.

38. Finley, C. S. (1921). Endocrine stimulation as affecting dream content. *Arch. Neurol. Psychiat. (Chic.)*, **5,** 177–181.

39. *Fisher, C. (1965). Psychoanalytic implications of recent research on sleep and dreaming. *J. Amer. psychoanal. Assoc.*, **8,** 197–303.

40. Fisher, C. and Dement, W. (1961). Experimental manipulation of the dream-sleep cycle. Paper read at 3rd World Congr. Psychiat.

41. Fisher, C. and Dement, W. (1962). Manipulation experimentale du cycle rêve-sommeil par rapport aux états psychopathologiques. *Rev. Méd. psychosom.*, **4,** 5.

42. Fisher, C. and Dement, W. C. (1963). Studies on the psychopathology of sleep and dreams. *Amer. J. Psychiat.*, **119,** 1160–1168.

43. Foulkes, W. D. (1962). Dream reports from different stages of sleep. *J. abnorm. soc. Psychol.*, **65,** 14–25.

44. Freeman, F., Agnew, H., Jr. and William, R. (1965). An electroencephalographic study of the effects of meprobamate on human sleep. *Clin. Pharmacol. Ther.*, **6,** 172–176.

45. French, T. M. (3 volumes, 1952, 1953, and 1958). Integration of Behavior. Chicago: University of Chicago Press.

46. Freud, S. (1958). Interpretation of Dreams. New York: Basic Books.

47. George, R., Haslett, W. O. and Jenden, D. J. (1964). A cholinergic mechanism in the brain stem reticular formation: Induction of paradoxical sleep. *Int. J. Neuropharmacol.*, **3,** 541–552.
48. Goodenough, D. R., Shapiro, H. and Steinschriber, L. (1959). A comparison of 'dreamers' and 'non-dreamers': eye movements, electroencephalograms, and the recall of dreams. *J. abnorm. soc. Psychol.*, **59,** 295–302.
49. Gottschalk, L. A., Gleser, G. C., Springer, K. J., Kaplan, S. M., Shanon, J. and Ross, W. D. (1960). Effects of perphenazine on verbal behavior patterns. *Arch. gen. Psychiat.*, **2,** 632–639.
50. Gottschalk, L. A., Stone, W. N., Gleser, G. C. and Iacono, J. M. (1966). Relationship of changes in plasma free fatty acids to anxiety levels in the dreams of sleeping subjects. *Science*, **153,** 654.
51. Green, W. J. (1965). The effect of LSD on the sleep-dream cycle. *J. nerv. ment. Dis.*, **140,** 417–426.
52. Greenberg, R. and Pearlman, C. (1964). Delirium tremens and dream deprivation. APSS, 1964.
53. Gresham, S. C., Agnew, H., Jr. and Williams, R. L. (1965). The sleep of depressed patients. *Arch. gen. Psychiat.*, **13,** 503–507.
54. Gresham, S. C., Webb, W. B. and Williams, R. L. (1963). Alcohol and caffeine: effect on inferred visual dreaming. *Science*, **140,** 1226–1227.
55. Grob, D., Lilienthal, J., Harvey, A. and Jones, B. (1947). Administration of DFP to man. *Bull. Johns Hopk. Hosp.*, **81,** 217–244.
56. Gulevich, G. and Dement, W. (1964). All-night sleep recordings on a group of schizophrenic patients in remission. APSS.
57. Hall, C. G. (1953). A cognitive theory of dreams. *J. gen. Psychol.*, **49,** 273–282,
58. *Hartmann, E. L. (1965). The D-State: A review and discussion of studies on the physiologic state concomitant with dreaming. *New Engl. J. Med.*, **273,** 30–35, 87–92.
59. Hartmann, E. L. (1965). Serotonin and dreaming sleep. APSS.
60. Hartmann, E., Verdone, P. and Snyder, F. (1964). A longitudinal study of sleep and dream patterns in psychiatric patients. APSS.
61. Hawkins, D. R., Puryear, H. B., Wallace, C. D., Deal, W. B. and Thomas, E. S. (1962). Basal skin resistance during sleep and 'dreaming'. *Science*, **136,** 321–322.
62. Hendley, C. D. (1963). Effects of drugs on sharp waves from the lateral geniculate nucleus and eye movements during low-voltage sleep in the cat. APSS.
63. Hernández-Peón, R., Chavez-Ibarra, G., Morgane, P. J. and Timo-Iaria, C. (1963). Limbic cholinergic pathways involved in sleep and emotional behavior. *Exp. Neurol.*, **8,** 93–111.
64. Hobson, J. (1964). Effect of LSD on sleep cycle in cat. *Electroenceph. clin. Neurophysiol.*, **17,** 52–56.

65 Hofling, C., Winslow, W. W. and Stone, W. N. (1966). Drug therapy. *In* Progress in Neurology and Psychiatry (ed. Spiegel E. A.). New York: Grune and Stratton.

66. Jastrow, J. (1947). Anesthesia dreams. *In* The World of Dreams (ed. Woods, R. L.), pp. 531–535. New York: Random House.

67. Jelliffe, S. E. (1944). Two morphine color dreams with note on etiology of opium habit. *Psychoanal. Rev.*, **31,** 128–132,

68. Jouvet, D. and Valatx, J. L. (1962). Étude polygraphique du sommeil chez l'agneau. *C.R. Soc. Biol.* **156,** 1411–1414.

69. Jouvet, M. (1962). Ontogenetic and phylogenetic studies of sleep. APSS.

70. Jouvet, M. (1962). Recherches sur les structures nerveuses et les mécanismes responsables des differentes phases du sommeil physiologique. *Arch. ital. Biol.*, **100,** 125.

71. Jouvet, M. (1961). Research on the neurophysiological mechanisms of sleep and attention. Technical Final Report, Air Force Office of Scientific Research of the Air Research and Development Command, U.S. Air Force, European Office, Contract Af 61 (052) 109.

72. Jouvet, M. (1964). Studies on rhombencephalic sleep. APSS.

73. Jouvet, M. (1962). Sur l'existence d'un système hypnique ponto-limbique et ses rapports avec l'activité onirique. Physiologie de L'Hippocampe. *Colloq. int. Cent. nat. Rech. sci.*, No. 107, 297.

74. *Jouvet, M. (1960). Telencephalic and rhombencephalic sleep in the cat. *In* The Nature of Sleep (ed. Wolstenholme, G. E. W. and O'Connor, M.). London: Churchill.

75. Jouvet, M., Cier, A., Mounier, D. and Valatx, J. L. (1961). Effets du 4-butyrolactone et du 4-hydroxybutyrate de sodium sur l'E.E.G. et le comportement du chat. *C.R. Soc. Biol.* **155,** 1313–1316.

76. Jouvet, M. and Michel F. (1960). Nouvelles recherches sur les structures responsables de la 'phase paradoxale' du sommeil. *J. Physiol.* (*Paris*), **52,** 130–131.

77. Jouvet, M. and Michel, F. (1956). Recherches sur l'activité électrique cerebrale au cours du sommeil. *C. R. Soc. Biol.*, **152,** 1167.

78. Jouvet, M. and Mounier, J. (1962). Neurophysiological mechanisms of dreaming. *Electroenceph clin. Neurophysiol.*, **14,** 424.

79. Jung, C. G., quoted by Mackenzie, N. (1965). Dreams and Dreaming, p. 221. New York: The Vanguard Press, Inc.

80. Kamiya, J. (1961). Behavioral, subjective, and physiological aspects of drowsiness and sleep. *In* Functions of Varied Experience (ed. Fiske, D. and Maddi, S. R.), pp. 145–174. Illinois: The Dorsey Press.

81. Kant, O. (1942). Dreams of schizophrenic patients. *J. nerv. ment. Dis.*, **95,** 335–347.

82. Kapp, F. T. and Gottschalk, L. M. (1962). Drug therapy. *In* Progress in Neurology and Psychiatry (ed. Spiegel, E. A.), Chapter 32. pp. 536–558. New York: Grune and Stratton.

83. Kaufman, E., Roffwarg, H. and Muzio, J. (1964). Alterations in the sleep EEG configuration during narcotic addiction, withdrawal and post-withdrawal states. APSS.

84. Kawakami, M., Negro, H. and Terawara, E. (1965). Influence of immobilization stress upon the paradoxical sleep (EEG) afterreaction in the rabbit. *Jap. J. Physiol.*, **15**, 1–16.

85. Kety, S. S. (1960). A biologist examines the mind and behavior. *Science*, **132**, 1861.

86. Khazan, N. and Sawyer, C. H. (1963). 'Rebound' recovery from deprivation of paradoxical sleep in the rabbit. *Proc. Soc. exp. Biol. (N.Y.)*, **114**, 536–539.

87. *Kleitman, N. (1960). The nature of dreaming. *In* The Nature of Sleep (ed. Wolstenholme, G. E. W. and O'Connor, M.). London: Churchill.

88. *Kleitman, N. (1963). Sleep and Wakefulness. 2nd Edition, Chicago: University of Chicago Press.

89. Knapp, P. H. (1956). Sensory impressions in dreams. *Psychoanal. Quart.*, **25**, 325–347.

90. Koresko, R. L., Snyder, F. and Feinberg, I. (1963). 'Dream time' in hallucinating and non-hallucinating schizophrenic patients. *Nature, Lond.*, **199**, 1118–1119.

91. Kramer, M., Ornstein, P. H. and Whitman, R. M. (1965). Drug therapy, *In* Progress in Neurology and Psychiatry (ed. Spiegel, E. H.), Chapter 33, pp. 723–753. New York: Grune and Stratton.

92. Kramer, M. Whitman, R. M., Baldridge, B. J. and Lansky, L. M. (1965). Depression: Dreams and defenses. *Amer. J. Psychiat.*, **122**, 411–419.

93. Kramer, M., Whitman, R. M., Baldridge, B. J. and Lansky, L. M. (1966). Dreaming in the depressed. *Canad. psychiat. Assoc. J.*, **11** (Suppl.), 178–192.

94. Kramer, M., Whitman, R. M., Baldridge, B. J. and Lansky, L. M. (1964). Patterns of Dreaming: The interrelationship of the dreams of a night. *J. nerv. ment. Dis.*, **139**, 426–439.

95. Ladd, G. T. (1892). Contribution to the psychology of visual dreams. *Mind*, **1**, 299.

96. Lesse, S. (1959). Experimental studies on the relationship between anxiety, dreams and dream-like states. *Amer. J. Psychother.*, **13**, 440–455.

97. Lewis, H. B. (1963). Individual differences among nonreporters in failure to recall dreams. APSS.

98. Lind, J. E. (1914). Partial analysis of an ether anesthesia dream. *Alienist and Neurologist*, **35**, 310–317.

99. Lindsay, J. S. B. (1953). Abreaction and dreams. *Brit. J. med. Psychol.*, **26**, 36–48.

100. Lovett Doust, J. W. (1951). Studies of the physiology of awareness: The incidence and content of dream patterns and their relationship to anoxia. *J. ment. Sci.*, **97**, 801–811.

101. Mandell, M. P. *et al.* (1964). Biochemical and neurophysiological studies of paradoxical sleep. *Recent Advances Biol. Psychiat.*, **7,** 115–122.
102. *Mandell, A. J. and Mandell, M. P. (1965). Biochemical aspects of rapid eye movement sleep. *Am. J. Psychiat.*, **122,** 391–401.
102a. Marczynski, T., Yamaguchi, N. and Ling, C. (1963). Effects of bufotenine and melatonin applied in crystalline form to the preoptic region or nucleus centralis medialis in unrestrained cats. *Pharmacologist*, **5,** 175.
103. Matsumato, J. and Jouvet, M. (1964). Effets de reserpine, dopa et 5-HTP sur les deux états de sommeil. *C.R. Soc. Biol.* **158,** 2137–2140.
104. Matsuzaki, M., Takagi, H. and Tokizane, T. (1964). Paradoxical phase of sleep: its artificial induction in the cat by sodium butyrate. *Science*, **146,** 1328–1329.
105. Michel, F., Klein, M., Jouvet, D. and Valatx, J. (1961). Étude polygraphique du sommeil chez le rat. *C.R. Soc. Biol.* **155,** 2289–2290.
106. Miller, M. (1965). On building bridges. *In* Psychoanalysis and Current Biological Thought, Chapter 1 (ed. Greenfield, N. S. and Lewis, W. D.), Madison: University of Wisconsin Press.
107. Mitchell, S. W. (1947). The visions induced by mescal. *In* The World of Dreams (ed. Woods, R. L.), pp. 421–425. New York: Random House.
108. Mittelman, B. (1945). Psychoanalytic observations on dreams and psychosomatic reactions in response to hypnotics and anesthetics. *Psychoanal. Quart.*, **14,** 498–510.
109. Muzio, J., Roffwarg, H. and Kaufman, E. (1964). Alteration in the young adult human sleep EEG configuration resulting from d-LSD-25. APSS.
110. Nelson, J., quoted by Mackenzie, N. (1965). Dreams and Dreaming, Chapter 10. New York: The Vanguard Press.
111. Offenkrantz, W. and Rechtschaffen, A. (1963). Clinical studies of sequential dreams. *Arch. gen. Psychiat.*, **8,** 497–505.
112. Ornstein, P. H. and Whitman, R. M. (1963). Drug therapy. *In* Progress in Neurology and Psychiatry (ed. Spiegel, E. A.), Chapter 34, pp. 631–658. New York: Grune and Stratton.
113. *Oswald, I. (1962). Sleeping and Waking. New York: Elsevier.
114. Oswald, I., Berger, R. J., Jaramillo, R. A., Keddie, K. M., Olley, P. C. and Plunkett, G. B. (1963). Melancholia and barbiturates: A controlled EEG, body and eye movement study of sleep. *Brit. J. Psychiat.*, **109,** 66–78.
115. Oswald, I., Taylor, A. M. and Treisman, M. (1960). Discriminative responses to stimulation during human sleep. *Brain*, **83,** 440.
116. Oswald, I. and Thacore, U. R. (1963). Amphetamine and phenmetrazine addiction: Physiological abnormalities in the syndrome. *Brit. med. J.*, **ii,** 427–431.

117. Parmelee, A. H., Akiyama, Y., Wenner, W. H. and Flescher, J. (1964). Activated sleep in premature infants. APSS.
118. Pierce, C. M., Whitman, R. M., Mass, J. W. and Gay, M. (1961). Enuresis and dreaming: Experimental studies. *Arch. gen. Psychiat.*, **4,** 166–170.
119. Prigot, A., Barnes, A. L. and Barnard, R. D. (1957). Meprobamate therapy. *Harlem Hosp. Bull.*, **10,** 63–77.
120. Rechtschaffen, A. (1964). A Discussion of: Dement, W., Part III Research Studies: Dreams and Communication. *In* Science and Psychoanalysis, **7.** New York: Grune and Stratton.
121. Rechtschaffen, A. and Maron, L. (1964). The effect of amphetamine on the sleep cycle. *Electroenceph. clin. Neurophysiol.*, **16,** 438–445.
122. Rechtschaffen, A., Mednick, S. A. and Schulsinger, F. (1964). Schizophrenia and physiological indices of dreaming. *Arch. gen. Psychiat.*, **10,** 89–93.
123. Rechtschaffen, A., Verdone, P. and Wheaton, J. (1963). Reports of mental activity during sleep. *Canad. psychiat. Assoc. J.*, **8,** 409–414.
124. Roffwarg, H., quoted in Fisher, C. (1965). Psychoanalytic implications of recent research on sleep and dreams. *J. Amer. psychoanal. Assoc.*, **8,** 197–303.
125. Roffwarg, H., Dement, W. and Fisher, C. (1964). Preliminary observations of the sleep-dream pattern in neonates, infants, children and adults. *In* Mono. on Child Psychiatry No. 2, (ed. Harms, E.), pp. 60–72. New York: Pergamon Press.
126. Roffwarg, H., Muzio, J., and Dement, W. C. (1963). A sleep EEG-rapid eye movement cycle in newborn infants associated with specific physiological variations. APSS.
127. Ruckebusch, Y. and Bost, J. (1962). Activité corticale au cours de la somnolence et de la rumination chez la chèvre. *J. Physiol. (Paris)*, **54,** 409–410.
128. Ryba, P. (1965). Physiological and psychological changes during several months of observation of a depressed patient: Sleep, dream reporting and waking behavior. APSS.
129. Sawyer, C. H. (1963). Some effects of sex hormones on brain functions. *Proc. 3rd World Cong. Psychiat.*, pp. 118–120.
130. Sawyer, C. H. and Kawakami, M. (1959). Characteristics of behavioral and electroencephalographic after-reactions to copulation and vaginal stimulation in the female rabbit. *Endocrinology*, **65,** 622–630.
131. Scott, J. (1964, 1965). Fatty acids and sleep. APSS.
132. Selling, L. (1955). Clinical study of a new tranquilizing drug. *J. Amer. med. Ass.*, **157,** 1594–1596.
133. Shimazono, Y., Horie, T., Yanagisawa, Y., Hori, H., Chikazawa, S. and Shozuka, K. (1960). The correlation of the rhythmic waves of the hippocampus with the behavior of dogs. *Neurol. Med. Chir.*, **2,** 82–88.

134. Snyder, F. (1960). Dream recall, respiratory variability and depth of sleep. Paper delivered at Roundtable on Dreams Research, Annual Meeting of the American Psychiatric Association.
135. *Snyder, F. (1963). The new biology of dreaming. *Arch. gen. Psychiat.*, **8,** 381–391.
136. Snyder, F. (1964). Observations concerning REM-state in a 'living fossil'. APSS.
137. *Snyder, F. (1965). The organismic state associated with dreaming. *In* Psychoanalysis and Current Biological Thought (ed. Greenfield, N. S. and Lewis, W. C.), pp. 275–315.
138. *Snyder, F. (1965). Progress in the new biology of dreaming. *Amer. J. Psychiat.*, **122,** 377–391.
139. Snyder, F. (1962). Theoretical comment on the significance of the 'dream deprivation' findings. APSS.
140. Snyder, F., Hobson, J. A. and Goldfrank, F. (1963). Blood pressure changes during human sleep. *Science*, **142,** 1313.
141. Snyder, F., Hobson, J., Morrison, D. and Goldfrank, F. (1964). Changes in respiration, heart rate, and systolic blood pressure in human sleep. *J. appl. Physiol.*, **19,** 417.
142. Spooner, C. E. and Winters, W. D. (1965). Evidence for the direct action of monoamines on the chick central nervous system. *Experientia* **21,** 256–258.
143. Stekel, W. H. (1943). Interpretation of Dreams. New York: Liveright.
144. Strauch, I. H. (1963). Sleep-dream cycle in female subjects between the ages of 33 and 45. APSS.
145. *Tart, C. T. (1965). Toward the experimental control of dreaming. *Psychol. Bull.*, **64,** 81–91.
146. Trosman, H., Rechtschaffen, A. and Offenkrantz, W. (1960). Studies in psychophysiology of dreams. *Arch. gen. Psychiat.*, **3,** 602–607.
147. Toyoda, J. (1964). The effects of chlorpromazine and imipramine in the human nocturnal sleep EEG. *Psychiat. Neurol. jap.*, **18,** 198–221 (as quoted in Snyder, F. (1965). *Amer. J. Psychiat.*, **122,** 377–391).
148. *U.S.P.H.S. (1965). Current Research on Sleep and Dreams, Publication #1389.
149. Weiss, T. (1964). Sleep cycles in rodents. APSS.
150. Weiss, T., Bohdanecky, A., Fifkova, E. and Roldan, E. (1964). Influence of atropine on sleep cycle in rats. *Psychopharmacologia* (*Berlin*), **5,** 126–135.
151. Weitzman, E. (1960). A note on EEG and eye movement during behavioral sleep in monkeys. *Electroenceph. clin. Neurophysiol.*, **13,** 113–120.
152. Weitzman, E. *et al.* (1965). Plasma 17-hydroxycorticosteroid levels during sleep in man. APSS.
153. West, L. J., Janszen, H. H., Lester, B. K. and Cornelisoon, F. S., Jr. (1962). The psychosis of sleep deprivation. *Ann. N.Y. Acad. Sci.*, **96,** 1.

154. Whitman, R. W. (1963). Drugs, dreams, and the experimental subject. *Canad. psychiat. Assoc. J.*, **8,** 395–399.
155. Whitman, R. M. (1963). Remembering and forgetting in psychoanalysis. *J. Amer. psychoanal. Assoc.*, **11,** 752–774.
156. Whitman, R. M., Kramer, M. and Baldridge, B. J. (1963). Experimental study of supervision of psychotherapy. *Arch. gen. Psychiat.*, **9,** 529–535.
157. Whitman, R. M., Kramer, M. and Baldridge, B. J. (1963). Which dream does the patient tell? *Arch. gen. Psychiat.*, **8,** 277–282.
158. Whitman, R. M., Ornstein, P. H. and Kramer, M. (1964). Drug therapy. *In* Progress in Neurology and Psychiatry (ed. Spiegel, E. A.), Chapter 32, pp. 606–630. New York: Grune and Stratton.
159. Whitman, R. M., Pierce, C. M. and Maas, J. W. (1960). Drugs and dreams, *In* Drugs and Behavior (ed. Uhr, L. and Miller, J.), pp. 591–595. New York: Wiley.
160. Whitman, R. W., Pierce, C. M., Maas, J. W. and Baldridge, B. J. (1962). The dreams of the experimental subject. *J. nerv. ment. Dis.*, **134,** 431–439.
161. Whitman, R. W., Pierce, C. M., Maas, J. W. and Baldridge, B. J. (1961). Drugs and dreams II: imipramine and prochlorperazine. *Comprehens. Psychiat.*, **2,** 219–226.
162. Williams, H. L., Hammack, J. T., Daly, R. L., Dement, W. C. and Lubin, A. (1964). Responses to auditory stimulation, sleep loss and the EEG stages of sleep. *Electroenceph. clin. Neurophysiol.*, **16,** 269.
163. Williams, H. L., Tepas, D. I. and Morlock, H. C., Jr. (1962). Evoked responses to clicks and EEG stages of sleep in man. *Science*, **138,** 685.
164. Wolpert, E. A. (1960). Studies in psychophysiology of dreams. II. An electromyographic study of dreaming. *Arch. gen. Psychiat.*, **2,** 231–241.
165. Wolpert, E. A. and Trosman, H. (1958). Studies in psycho-physiology of dreams: I. Experimental evocation of sequential dream episodes. *Arch. Neurol. Psychiat. (Chic.)*, **79,** 603–606.

DISCUSSION

Robertson: I think there is a lot of confusion about dreams, particularly because we tend to interest ourselves in more dramatic dreams and for this reason alone the psychoanalytic Freudian hypothesis has on the whole predominated. But what I feel Dement showed is that dreaming of the most ordinary and banal kind is important and that when people are deprived of it they have a mental breakdown (Dement, W. *Science*, 1960, **131,** 1705). This, together with much that Dr. Kramer mentioned goes to support a new hypothesis of dreaming which Evans and Newman published quite recently (Evans, C. R. and Newman, E. A. Dreaming: analogy from computers *New Sci.*, 1964, **24**, 577; Newman, E. A. and Evans, C. R. Human dream processes as analogous to computer programme clearance *Nature* (*Lond.*) 1965, **206**, 534). It turns out that if you develop a very large computer which controls on line some complicated process—indeed this is really a definition of a man—if you develop a computer of this sort full of adaptive programmes and with a very large store of information, some of which is being added to the whole time, then the machine has to be off line for quite a large proportion of its working life in order to reorganize itself, otherwise it becomes hopelessly cluttered with trivia, or useless data which it collects. We do this during the day, and it should not be difficult for us to understand why we spend a third of our life sleeping. It is becoming clearer, I think, that we dream not only during REM sleep, when we have on the whole dreams associated with vision, but during quite a lot of the rest of sleep, when we have proprioceptive dreams, hearing dreams and so forth. One of the examples that Dr. Kramer mentioned was somebody given progressive anaesthesia who naturally enough kept dreaming about being put to sleep. I think this is the sort of thing that turns up; it is not surprising that people under amphetamine whose dreaming is suppressed become more and more psychotic. They can't get rid of the mass of data cluttering up their computer which wishes to get on with the main business.

Kramer: Your analogy is very apt for our times. Robert writing in the late 19th century, not being burdened with computers, used alimentary analogies to describe the process of the relieving oneself of clutter. I think that if you listen to patients' dreams even in the consulting room, the dramatic dream proves the exception rather than the rule. I believe this is one of the descriptive problems one gets into in trying to relate the dream to the hallucination, in the usual clinical sense. The descriptions do not match closely enough; one becomes concerned that at the surface level one is dealing with disparate phenomena. Some of the too easy transitions from the dream to the hallucination are very difficult to follow.

The effects of deprivation studies are not universal. For example, dream-deprived subjects, who are not sleep-deprived, will not show invariably behavioural change. One could choose to ignore the people who are not disturbed, but I believe one must explain what happens and what fails to happen. That is, why doesn't the 17-year-old man develop the psychotic symptoms that are supposed to occur in sleep-deprived subjects? (Gulevich, G., Dement, W. and Johnson, L. Psychiatric and EEG observations on a case of prolonged (264 hours) wakefulness. *Arch. gen. Psychiat.*, 1966, **15**, 29).

The rather primitive data we have now are openly contradictory and one has a smorgasbord of information; one can select whatever one likes.

Robertson: I think that with all due respect, that this isn't so! If you deprive human beings you undoubtedly get disturbed states.

Kramer: This to my knowledge has not been substantiated. Snyder who repeated Dement's dream deprivation study did not find behavioural changes (Snyder, F. Theoretical Comment on the Significance of the 'Dream Deprivation' Findings. APSS, 1962). Dement himself points out that severe behavioural change was not universal in all his dream-deprived subjects (Dement, W. 'Studies on the function of rapid eye movement (paradoxical) sleep in human subjects', *in* Jouvet, M., ed.: Aspects Anatomo-Fonctionnels de la Physiologie du Sommeil, p. 571 Paris: Centre de la Recherche Scientifique, 1965). He reported particular incidents that illustrated a point, not a universal phenomenon. It is no criticism of Dement's speculation that perhaps there is only a trend in this. We must explain not only why subjects develop behavioural change with dream deprivation but also why some do not.

Epstein: Would you speculate further perhaps, that the periodicity with which psychotic symptoms were observed in certain sleep-deprived subjects is actually a manifestation of an inherent biological or metabolic rhythm which is independent of personality? A pertinent example in neurohumoral systems is found in Quay's finding of a 9-fold variation in the serotonin content of pineal glands of rats, associated with a circadian rhythm (Quay, W. B., in *Progress in Brain Research*, **8**, 1964, Elsevier).

Kramer: Yes, I agree that the periodicity is biologically determined and the psychological changes are concomitant. Dr. Kleitman has suggested that this is analogous to speech being superimposed on respiration (Kleitman, N. The nature of dreaming, *in* Wolstenholme, G. E. W.

and O'Connor, M., eds. The Nature of Sleep, p. 347, Churchill, London, 1960). The basic biological rhythm underlies the visual dream that the subject reports, and I think this is what West found in his 'disc jockey' in New York (West, L. J., Janzen, H. H., Lester, B. K. and Cornelisoon, F. S., The psychosis of sleep deprivation. *Ann. N. Y. Acad. Sci.*, 1962, **96,** 1).

INDEX OF SUBJECTS

Printed by Spottiswoode, Ballantyne & Co. Ltd., London and Colchester